Food and the Gut

Food and the Gut

Edited by

J. O. Hunter MA, MD, FRCP
Consultant Physician
Addenbrooke's Hospital
Cambridge

and

V. Alun Jones BA, MB BChir
Clinical Research Fellow
Department of Gastroenterology
Addenbrooke's Hospital
Cambridge

Baillière Tindall   London Philadelphia Toronto
Mexico City Rio de Janeiro Sydney Tokyo Hong Kong

Baillière Tindall 1 St Anne's Road
W. B. Saunders   Eastbourne, East Sussex BN21 3UN, England

West Washington Square
Philadelphia, PA 19105, USA

1 Goldthorne Avenue
Toronto, Ontario M8Z 5T9, Canada

Apartado 26370—Cedro 512
Mexico 4, DF Mexico

Rua Evaristo da Veiga 55,20° andar
Rio de Janeiro—RJ, Brazil

ABP Australia Ltd, 44–50 Waterloo Road
North Ryde, NSW 2113, Australia

Ichibancho Central Building, 22–1 Ichibancho
Chiyoda-ku, Tokyo 102, Japan

10/fl, Inter-Continental Plaza, 94 Granville Road
Tsim Sha Tsui East, Kowloon, Hong Kong

First published 1985

Typeset by Photo·Graphics, Honiton, Devon
Printed and bound in Great Britain by Biddles Ltd of Guildford.

British Library Cataloguing in Publication Data

Food and the gut.
 1. Intestines——Diseases   2. Diet
 I. Hunter, J.O.   II. Alun Jones, V.
 616.3′4   RC860

 ISBN 0–7020–1090–1

Contents

Contributors

T. E. Adrian PhD, MRCPath, Senior Research Fellow, Royal Postgraduate Medical School, Hammersmith Hospital, Ducane Road, London.

V. Alun Jones BA, MB BChir, Clinical Research Fellow, Department of Gastroenterology, Addenbrooke's Hospital, Cambridge.

I. Bjarnason MSc, MD, Research Clinician, MRC Clinical Research Centre, Harrow; Honorary Senior Registrar, Northwick Park Hospital, Harrow, Middlesex.

S. R. Bloom MD, DSc, FRCP, Professor of Endocrinology, Royal Postgraduate Medical School; Consultant Physician, Hammersmith Hospital, Ducane Road, London.

Jonathan Brostoff MA, DM, FRCP, FRCPath, Reader in Clinical Immunology and Honorary Consultant Physician, Middlesex Hospital Medical School, London.

Alice Bullen MD, MRCP, Clinical Teacher in the Faculty of Medicine, University of Leicester; Consultant Physician, George Eliot Hospital, Nuneaton, Warwickshire.

John H. Cummings MA, MSc, FRCP, Member of the Scientific Staff, MRC Dunn Clinical Nutrition Centre, Cambridge; Honorary Consultant Physician, Addenbrooke's Hospital, Cambridge.

Michael L. G. Gardner BSc, PhD, DSc, Research Fellow, Department of Biochemistry, University of Edinburgh Medical School, Edinburgh. *Present address*: School of Biomedical Sciences, University of Bradford, Bradford, West Yorkshire.

Kenneth W. Heaton MA, MD, FRCP, Reader in Medicine, University of Bristol, Bristol; Honorary Consultant Physician, Bristol and Weston Health Authority.

Michael J. Hill PhD, Director, Bacterial Metabolism Research Laboratory, PHLS Centre for Applied Microbiology and Research, Porton Down, Salisbury, Wiltshire; Honorary Consultant Research Bacteriologist, St Mark's Hospital, City Road, London.

J. O. Hunter MA, MD, FRCP, Consultant Physician, Addenbrooke's Hospital, Cambridge.

J. D. Maxwell MD, BSc, FRCP, Senior Lecturer in Medicine, St George's Hospital Medical School; Consultant Physician, St George's Hospital, London.

P. J. Milla MSc, MB BS, MRCP, Senior Lecturer in Child Health, Institute of Child Health; Honorary Consultant Paediatric Gastroenterologist, Hospital for Sick Children, Great Ormond Street, London.

Graham Neale MA, BSc, MB ChB, FRCP, Associate Lecturer in Medicine, University of Cambridge; Consultant Physician, Addenbrooke's Hospital; Member of the Clinical Scientific Staff, MRC Dunn Clinical Nutrition Unit, Cambridge.

T. J. Peters MSc, PhD, FRCP, FRCPE, FRCPath, Head of Division of Clinical Cell Biology, Clinical Research Centre, Harrow; Visiting Professor, University of London; Consultant Physician, Northwick Park Hospital, Harrow, Middlesex.

N. W. Read MD, Reader in Physiology, University of Sheffield; Honorary Consultant Gastroenterologist, Royal Hallamshire Hospital, Sheffield.

P. I. Reed MB, FRCP, Honorary Senior Lecturer in Medicine, Royal Postgraduate Medical School, London; Consultant Physician, Hammersmith Hospital, London and East Berkshire Health District.

Glenis K. Scadding MA, MD, MRCP, Senior Registrar in Clinical Immunology and Allergy, Middlesex Hospital, London.

Denis R. Stanworth DSc, FRCPath, Reader, Department of Immunology, and Head, Rheumatology and Allergy Research Unit, University of Birmingham, Birmingham.

Alison M. Stephen PhD, Research Assistant, Department of Environmental and Preventive Medicine, The Medical College of St Bartholomew's Hospital, Charterhouse Square, London.

John A. Walker-Smith MD(Sydney), FRCP(Ed), FRCP(Lond), FRACP, Professor of Paediatric Gastroenterology, Medical College of St Bartholomew's Hospital, London; Honorary Consultant Paediatrician, St Bartholomew's Hospital and Queen Elizabeth Hospital for Children, Hackney Road, London.

C. L. Walters PhD, Section Manager, Biochemistry/Mycotoxin Section, Leatherhead Food Research Association, Leatherhead, Surrey.

I. McL. Welch BSc(Hons), Research Assistant, Clinical Research Unit, Royal Hallamshire Hospital, Sheffield.

Preface

In recent years there has been increasing interest amongst both members of the medical profession and their patients in the possibility that food may be a cause of hitherto unexplained diseases. Unfortunately this interest has produced more excitement and controversy than scientific research, and although evidence is now accumulating to support a role for diet in the management of conditions as diverse as migraine, eczema and Crohn's disease, the mechanisms of the relationship between food and disease remain poorly understood.

The purpose of this book is to clarify the present state of our knowledge in relation to gastro-intestinal physiology and pathology. The gut is daily exposed to a vast number of foreign substances, both foods and chemicals, whose subsequent digestion, metabolism and absorption may have effects which might be not only immunological but also hormonal or pharmacological. It seems feasible that abnormalities in these processes might lead to disease. In this book we have therefore attempted to draw together recent insights into the pathophysiology of the gut, from such diverse areas as intestinal permeability, gastro-intestinal hormones and changes in the microflora. We have concentrated on the potential effects, both local and systemic, of chemicals such as opioids and nitrosamines produced in the gut, and have examined the evidence for the existence of food intolerance and the therapeutic role of diet in a number of gastro-intestinal disorders.

In view of the numerous articles on alcohol and fibre that have appeared in recent years, we felt justified in avoiding specific consideration of these topics (although they are referred to in several chapters), and we were unfortunately unable to include a chapter on effects of diet on the pancreas. Notwithstanding the omissions, the potential importance of food in the pathogenesis of gastro-intestinal disease will be seen to be profound, and we hope that this book will suggest further avenues of research in this extremely important field.

We wish to express our thanks to Glaxo Ltd through whose generous support it was possible for most of the contributors to meet to discuss the project. We also wish to thank Alison Wilson for her most valuable administrative and secretarial help.

J. O. Hunter
V. Alun Jones

Chapter 1
Effect of Feeding on the Development of the Gut

P. J. Milla

The development of the gastro-intestinal tract in all mammals is characterised by the integrated maturation of its many functions. Differentiation of the various tissues of the gastro-intestinal tract follows an inherent species-dependent pattern, upon which extrinsic influences have a facilitating effect. These aspects have been extensively reviewed (Grand et al 1976; Tanner and Stocks 1983) and hence this chapter will be concerned with the development of intestinal transport and motor activity and the effects that luminal nutrition might have upon them.

The fetus in utero makes little demand on the gastro-intestinal tract, its nutritional needs being supplied intravenously via the placenta. At birth, however, the tract is required to sustain rapid body growth, and survival of the newborn infant is dependent on its ability to adapt successfully to extra-uterine life. With the vast improvement in the care of preterm infants with respiratory disease, nutrition has become the critical factor for survival, and this is dependent on the state of development of the gastro-intestinal tract. Thus a sound understanding of the prenatal and perinatal development of the gastro-intestinal tract, and of both adverse and beneficial extrinsic influences upon it, is essential if the clinician is to ensure a successful transition to established extra-uterine life.

DEVELOPMENT OF GASTRO-INTESTINAL FUNCTION

Intestinal motor activity

The intraluminal contents are moved from one specialised region of the gut to another by the co-ordinated contraction of its smooth muscle layers. The pattern of motility is integrated with, and related to, the function of particular regions. The oesophagus acts as a propulsive conduit for the delivery of food into the stomach which is a mixing and storage organ. Gastric secretion reduces the tonicity of chyme and this is discharged intermittently into the small intestine where further digestion and absorption take place. Clear-cut patterns of motor activity have been described in the small intestine, related to its absorptive function. Similarly, colonic movement is related to its role as an organ which conserves water and electrolytes and processes waste material.

1

Swallowing

Fetal swallowing of amniotic fluid has been observed during the second trimester of pregnancy (Pritchard 1966) and would appear to be an important mechanism in the regulation of amniotic fluid volume. It is well established that hydramnios commonly occurs in pregnancies in which the fetus has oesophageal or high small intestinal obstructive lesions (Lloyd and Clatworthy 1958).

Gastric emptying

Amniographic studies (McLain 1963) suggest that the development of gastric emptying is integrated with, and follows, a similar time course to small intestinal motor activity. The few studies that have been performed on infants suggest that modulation of emptying is an effect of food in the small intestine and that energy concentration is important (Husband and Husband 1969). However, delay in gastric emptying occurs in pathological situations such as respiratory distress syndrome and congenital heart disease (Yu 1975; Cavell 1981), presumably due to disturbance of gastroduodenal motility.

Small intestinal motor activity

McLain (1963), using amniography, demonstrated that intestinal transit of contrast medium occurred after 30 weeks gestation and increased as pregnancy progressed. More recently, techniques have been developed which have enabled the fetal and neonatal development of small intestinal motor activity to be studied in the dog and sheep, (Bueno and Ruchebusch 1979) and in the preterm human infant, (Wozniak et al 1983). In all species studied, three patterns characteristic of three stages of development are seen: disorganised; repetitive groups of contraction (fetal complex); and a well organised migrating motor complex pattern. In man these occur at 26–29 weeks, 30–33 weeks, and 34–36 weeks respectively. The first of these patterns is not associated with transit, but transit increases during the later stages. In animals birth is not accompanied by acute changes of the motor profile; indeed, there is a species-dependent timetable for the development of functional processes. The fetal pattern persists for some 10–15 days after birth in dogs but migrating motor complexes (MMC's) start 5–10 days before birth in sheep and some four weeks before term in man.

It is of interest that in man, the regular MMC pattern coincides with the acquisition of the ability to suck and a clear neurological rest/activity cycle, suggesting that neurological development is of the utmost importance. The effects of luminal nutrition are as yet unknown but clearly may also be of major importance.

Digestion and absorption

The stomach

Gastric secretions may be found early in the second trimester but they contain little hydrochloric acid and even at term the pH of the stomach is relatively high. However, in the first 24 hours after birth, the pH falls dramatically (Ahn and Kim 1963). Studies in experimental animals would suggest that this is due to mechanisms for the active secretion of protons and chloride becoming functional. Peptic activity is reduced in the preterm infant but increases in the third trimester (Werner 1948). There is no information concerning the effects of food on the development of gastric proteolytic activity.

Small and large intestine

Brush border enzymes The brush border of the intestine possesses an integrated system for the final digestion and absorption of nutrients. The development of brush border digestive enzymes has been extensively studied and reviewed recently (Lebenthal et al 1983).

The disaccharidases develop according to a species-specific timetable and in man, unlike animals such as the pig (Stoddart and Widdowson 1976), there is no evidence that the provision of luminal substrates enhances enzyme activity. In man, development occurs in a craniocaudal direction with maximal activity in the upper part of the small intestine. Hydrolytic enzymes are present in the colon in the second trimester but disappear during the third trimester. The role of these enzymes is unknown. The glucosidases (maltase, sucrase-isomaltase) develop early in the small intestine, beginning at 12 weeks gestation, and by 32 weeks of gestation they have reached approximately three-quarters of full term levels of activity. In comparison, galactosidase (lactase) is present only in trace amounts until 30 weeks of gestation and then increases rapidly to reach a maximum just prior to birth. The subsequent pattern of postnatal development is genetically determined and is not substrate inducible. Symptoms of lactose intolerance follow a decline in lactase activity to those races in which the habit of drinking milk after infancy is a late acquisition.

This development pattern has obvious implications for feeding practices in preterm infants, especially in the design of milk formulae. At 36 weeks the infant gut can hydrolyse 35g of sucrose per day but only 6g of lactose, and at term, 72g of sucrose and 60g of lactose. In some milk formulae for premature infants glucose polymers have been used in place of lactose, as they have the advantage of increased energy content without a significant increase in tonicity. In view of the known absence of pancreatic amylase at birth, it might be expected that digestion of glucose polymers would be impaired. This is not the case, probably because of the presence of the glycosidase, glyco-amylase (Lebenthal and Lee 1980).

Pancreatic enzymes

Pancreatic proteases can be detected in the intestinal lumen from about 26 weeks of gestation, when they are capable of hydrolysing protein to a mixture of small peptides and free amino acids. Secretion of pancreatic enzymes can be affected by diet. Zoppi et al (1972) showed that a high protein diet resulted in an increase in trypsin and chymotrypsin. A high starch diet also increased luminal amylase tenfold, but this produced no significant improvement in digestive activity as the initial level was very low. The small peptides released by pancreatic proteases are further hydrolysed by brush border peptidases. These peptidases are present in near adult levels of activity from as early as the twelfth week of gestation (Lindberg 1966) and do not limit protein digestion.

Absorption and transport processes

Each day the intestine handles large quantitites of water and solutes. There is no quantitative data available for infancy but the pattern is almost certainly the same as in adult life (Phillips and Giller 1973), with by far the greatest volume of fluid being reabsorbed in the small intestine.

The functional unit of transport is composed of epithelial cells forming a sheet in which the cells are joined peripherally, near their apices, by a tight junction or junctional complex. The cells are polarised so that the apical brush border faces the lumen and the basal border the lamina propria, with a potential space between them, the lateral intercellular space. Our current understanding of water and electrolyte transport suggests that this epithelial sheet acts as a semi-permeable membrane, with the pores at the site of the intercellular junctions. The movement of water is entirely passive, most of it passing paracellularly in response to osmotic gradients created by the transcellular absorption of solutes, sodium playing a key role (Sackin and Boulpaep 1975; Gupta et al 1978). For transcellular absorption of aqueous solutes to occur, specialised transport mechanisms in the lipid-rich brush border membrane of the enterocyte are required; the absorption of hydrophobic lipid compounds does not require specialised mechanisms. In the small intestine, the jejunum is the most permeable area and the sodium-coupled co-transport of organic solutes, such as glucose, galactose, amino acids and di- and tri-peptides, is of prime importance. The ileum is less permeable and here electroneutral coupled sodium chloride transport is probably more important than sodium coupled to organic solutes. The colon is even less permeable and sodium absorption occurs by an active electrogenic mechanism. The baso-lateral border enzyme Na^+-K^+–ATPase is crucial to the functioning of these systems, generating a Na^+ gradient directed into the cell across the apical border.

The development of intestinal transport processes

The development of transport function is closely integrated with the morphogenesis and differentiation of the fetal intestine. The appearance of specialised transport systems in the brush border membrane and the key transport enzymes Na^+-K^+–ATPase (Rosenberg 1966) and adenylate cyclase (Grand et al 1973) closely follows the acquisition of junctional complexes, secondary lumina and microvilli (Moxey and Trier 1978). Thus development proceeds in an integrated fashion up to 10–11 weeks gestation, and by 12 weeks well defined crypts and villi are present and transport function can be demonstrated.

Koldovsky et al (1965), using everted sacs constructed from human fetal jejunum and ileum, showed the presence of active sodium-dependent co-transport of glucose and alanine. At 10 weeks active transport clearly occurred, which had increased threefold by 18 weeks gestation. These studies show the development of specific transport mechanisms that exhibit stereo-specificity and sodium dependence, obey saturation kinetics, are electrogenic, and allow accumulation of a substrate against a concentration gradient.

Elegant potential difference (PD) studies on everted human fetal sacs show the presence of a small endogenous PD of about 1 mV, the mucosa being negative relative to the serosa, from 10 weeks gestation onwards (Levin et al 1968). Marked sodium dependency suggests that this is due to elec-trogenic sodium transfer, while reversal of polarity on lowering the mucosal sodium concentration further suggests that sodium movement was through a negatively charged pore, but whether this was transcellular or paracellular is unknown. With increasing gestational age the endogenous PD increases, suggesting greater transfer of sodium.

Little is known, however, of the effects that changes in fetal nutrition might have on the development of these transport processes. It is clear from recent studies of electrogenic glucose absorption in premature and full term neonates (McNeish et al 1979), that both the state of nutrition and gestational age influence absorption. Full term, appropriate weight-for-dates infants had a greater capacity for glucose absorption than preterm, semi-starved light-for-dates infants. However, whether this was due to a greater number of enterocytes, or to an increase in the number of transport sites on each cell, is not clear. The changes in apparent affinity for glucose are difficult to interpret from in vivo studies, but might indicate a greater avidity of uptake of glucose in starvation. Alternatively, they might merely reflect changes in the unstirred water layer, caused by differences in mucosal thickness. More recently, Mayne et al (1982) have shown that a dramatic surge in glucose transport occurs in the first three weeks of life. The switch to enteral nutrition must be associated with this in some way, and possible mechanisms will be reviewed later. The capacity for glucose absorption continues to increase throughout infancy and childhood into adult life, concomitantly with an increasing capacity for absorbed sodium to promote water absorption. Perfusion studies show that 56 mM glucose will cause twice as much water absorption in the adult as in the young child (Milla 1983).

Little is known of mechanisms for the absorption of other electrolytes but the occurrence of intra-uterine fetal diarrhoea and maternal hydramnios in the second and third trimesters in cases of congenital chloride-losing di-arrhoea (Holmberg et al 1977) and a newly described defect of sodium/hydrogen exchange (Milla et al 1983) suggest that these must exist.

Colonic transport has been studied even less and the only fetal studies are in experimental animals. In the human, rectal dialysis studies at birth have shown that electrogenic sodium absorption and anion exchange are poorly developed, but these improve rapidly over the first few months of life (Heath and Milla 1983). Studies of two infants with pseudohypo-aldosteronism demonstrate the importance of aldosterone in modulating colonic sodium absorption (Savage et al 1982).

ADAPTATION TO EXTRA-UTERINE NUTRITION:
THE EFFECTS OF FEEDING

It is clear from the above discussion that the development of intestinal function follows a defined programme which varies between species and that many developmental steps are scheduled by a 'biological clock'. However, the observation that preterm infants make a satisfactory transition from intra-uterine intravenous nutrition to extra-uterine oral feeding many weeks early, suggests that gut development is also susceptible to external influences. That enteral feeding itself may be an important factor is suggested by many animal studies of structural changes and growth following birth and the onset of oral feeding (Stoddart and Widdowson 1976; Lichtenberger and Johnson 1977), which are supported by some evidence from man (Ducker et al 1980).

The possible mechanisms whereby enteral feeding may induce changes in gut development include the effects of intraluminal nutrients themselves (and other factors in breast milk), the effects of endogenous secretions such as bile and pancreatic juice, and the effects of endocrine secretions from the gut and its related organs.

Intraluminal nutrients

There are many pieces of indirect evidence, largely derived from experimental animals, that the presence of luminal nutrients is associated with improvement in intestinal digestive and absorptive function. As a consequence of jejunal resection and jejunal bypass, the ileum receives nutrients which normally would have been absorbed, resulting in marked mucosal hyperplasia. Other effects include mural thickening, dilatation and elongation of the bowel (Williamson 1982). In addition to morphological changes, Schmitz et al (1980) showed increased jejunal absorption of glucose and increased luminal hydrolysis of sucrose in children, following recovery from small bowel resection. The specific activity of sucrase-isomaltase had not changed, however, suggesting that although there was an increase in function in relation to length of bowel, there was no change in function in relation to the individual cell.

By contrast, starvation causes the intestinal mucosa to become hypoplastic, with diminished segmental absorptive function. However, whether this was due to exclusion of luminal nutrients, or to malnutrition, has only recently become clear. Total parenteral nutrition (TPN) has helped to clarify this point. Experiments in rats (Hughes and Dowling 1980) and in man (Ducker et al 1980) have shown that when oral feeding is stopped, but nutrition is maintained by parenteral feeding, the function of the intestinal mucosa is impaired and it becomes hypoplastic. Figure 1.1 shows galactose absorption in rats fed orally or by TPN. In those fed solely by TPN there is a reduction in both V_{max} and apparent K_m, suggesting that there are fewer transport sites per unit length but that these have a greater affinity for galactose. Alternatively, the reduced apparent K_m could be an effect of unstirred water layers adjacent to the gut wall. Ducker et al (1980) studied infants who were light-for-dates and had suffered intra-uterine starvation and those who were exclusively fed intravenously from birth. The results are

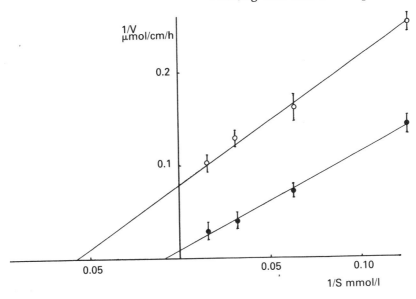

Figure 1.1. Galactose absorption in the jejunum of rats fed orally (closed circles) and fed intravenously for 10 days (open circles). Data as mean ± SEM. Redrawn from Hughes and Dowling (1980).

shown in Figure 1.2. Absorptive function was assessed indirectly by the 1–hour D–xylose absorption test. D–xylose absorption was lower in the light-for-dates babies, compared with the normally nourished, but both groups showed a postnatal improvement suggesting that intra-uterine growth retardation did not permanently affect the light-for-dates babies. In the group which was fed intravenously and was not malnourished, D-xylose absorption at a corresponding postnatal age was markedly reduced.

Additional support for the role of luminal nutrients is provided by animal experiments in which mucosal hypoplasia was induced by TPN (Hughes and Ducker 1982). Forty-eight hours after oral feeding was restarted, mucosal mass had almost returned to the original levels. In a similar study Morin et al (1982) showed that oral fat, in the form of long chain triglyceride, partly prevented TPN-induced mucosal hypoplasia, whereas protein and carbohydrates were ineffective. These data might be explained in several ways. Protein and carbohydrates might be completely absorbed in the upper gut, leaving none to reach the ileum or colon. Alternatively, fat might promote the release of a trophic hormone, perhaps related to pancreatico-biliary secretions.

A variety of hormones are secreted in breast milk, some of which are actively secreted against a concentration gradient; they are listed in Table 1.1. Whether or not these factors might play a role in postnatal gut adaptation is unknown, but epidermal growth factor has been shown to produce mucosal hyperplasia (Dembinski et al 1982), corticosteroids are known to influence

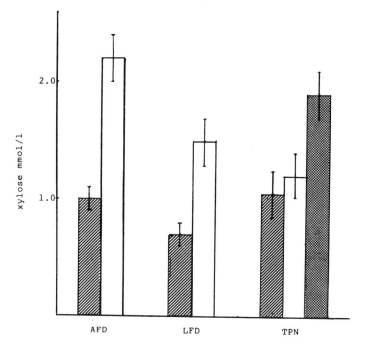

Figure 1.2. Xylose absorption in appropriately grown gestational age neonates (AFD), light for gestational age (LFD), and appropriately grown infants who were fed exclusively by total parenteral nutrition (TPN) from birth. Data are shown as histograms of the mean ± SEM. Histograms show age in weeks after birth:

▨ 1 week   ☐ 3 weeks   ▨ 5 weeks*

*i.e. 3 weeks after the introduction of TPN. Redrawn from Ducker et al 1980.

Table 1.1. Hormones present in breast milk.

Epidermal growth factor	ACTH (adrenocorticotrophic hormone)
Prostaglandins	TRH (thyrotrophin-releasing hormone)
Calcitonin	TSH (thyroid-stimulating hormone)
Melatonin	LHRH (luteinising hormone-releasing hormone)
Prolactin	Gonadotrophins
Erythropoietin	Steroids
	Thyroxine

enterocyte sodium permeability (Field 1980), and it seems likely that breast milk is an important factor in neonatal gut development.

Pancreatico-biliary secretion

TPN also leads to pancreatic hypoplasia and it seems likely that digestive secretions released during oral feeding are trophic. Experiments in animals in which pancreatico-biliary secretions are diverted into the ileum cause an increase in the size of the villi (Altman 1971). In dogs fed by TPN cholecystokinin and secretin given to stimulate pancreatico-biliary secretion completely prevent mucosal hypoplasia, but previously collected pancreatic secretions also remain trophic even after boiling (Hughes et al 1979, 1982). The trophic effects of pancreatico-biliary secretions can therefore be attributed to their nutrient or hormonal peptide content.

Endocrine secretion from the gut and gut related organs

The adaptation to extra-uterine nutrition involves many changes in gastro-intestinal function. There is considerable evidence that hormones, particularly gut hormones, are involved in these processes. It is clear from studies in experimental animals that gastrin and enteroglucagon may stimulate growth of the gastro-intestinal mucosa and that pancreatic polypeptide, gastrin and cholecystokinin may stimulate growth of the exocrine pancreas. Recently, surges in the release of many gut hormones have been described in both preterm and term infants, (Lucas et al 1979, 1980a,b). During the first 24 days of life, whilst receiving oral milk feeds, the surges in enteroglucagon and motilin were particularly marked. In a group of preterm infants who were fed by TPN, no such postnatal surges were seen (Lucas et al 1980a,b). Clearly it is possible that gut hormones have a role in the adaptive changes which occur following the start of oral feeding. Cyclical changes in plasma motilin concentrations have been shown to be closely associated with the presence of MMC's (Ruppin et al 1976). In experimental animals, circulating enteroglucagon has been found to be elevated in proportion to the degree of adaptation occurring after intestinal resection. In preterm infants, the plasma level of enteroglucagon is in proportion to the postnatal volume of milk consumed (Figure 1.3) (Lucas, personal communication). It is of particular interest that only 15 ml/kg body weight of milk promoted a threefold rise in enteroglucagon, suggesting that even subnutritional quantities of food may be useful in inducing a postnatal adaptive response. Sagor et al (1982) have shown that the major distribution of enteroglucagon in man lies in the ileum and colon; this may explain many of the earlier observations regarding resections. There is thus considerable evidence that enteroglucagon is trophic to gastro-intestinal mucosa, and that cholecystokinin and pancreatic polypeptide are trophic to the exocrine pancreas.

Clinical implications

With the easy availability of TPN, infants with gastro-intestinal disease may be deprived of oral nutrition as part of their management: Such practices need to be reviewed in the light of our current knowledge regarding the development of intestinal function. It is clear that luminal nutrients play an important role in the development and maintenance of normal digestive and absorptive function, and, even in minimal amounts, may have a therapeutic as well as a biological role.

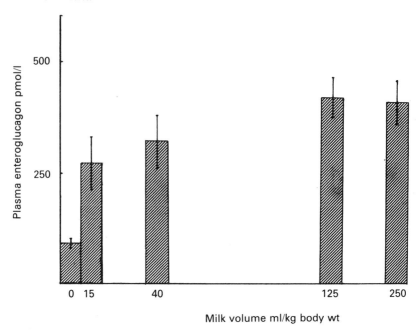

Figure 1.3. Plasma enteroglucagon concentration and volume of milk consumed by preterm infants after birth. Data from Lucas (personal communication).

REFERENCES

Ahn C I & Kim Y J (1963) Acidity and volume of gastric contents in the first week of life. *Journal of the Korean Medical Association* **6**: 948.

Altman G G (1971) Influence of bile acid and pancreatic secretion on the size of the intestinal villi in the rat. *American Journal of Anatomy* **132**: 167–168.

Bueno L & Ruchebusch Y (1979) Perinatal development of intestinal myoelectrical activity in dogs and sheep. *American Journal of Physiology* **237**: E61–67.

Cavell B (1981) Gastric emptying in infants with congenital heart disease. *Acta Paediatrica Scandinavica* **70**: 517–520.

Dembinski A, Gregory H, Konturek S J & Polanski M (1982) Trophic action of epidermal growth factor on the pancreas and gastro-duodenal mucosa in rats. In Robinson J W L, Dowling R & Riecken E O (eds) *Mechanisms of Intestinal Adaptation* Lancaster: MTP Press.

Ducker D A, Hughes C A, Warren I & McNeish A S (1980) Neonatal gut function measured by the one hour blood D(+) xylose test: influence of gestational age and size. *Gut* **21**: 133–136.

Field M (1978) Corticosteroids Na$^+$-K$^+$–ATPase and intestinal water and electrolyte transport. *Gastroenterology* **75**: 317–325.

Grand R J, Torti F M & Jaksina S (1973) Development of intestinal adenyl cyclase and its response to cholera enterotoxin. *Journal of Clinical Investigation* **52**: 2053–2059.

Grand R J, Watkins J B & Torti F (1976) Development of the human gastrointestinal tract. A review. *Gastroenterology* **70**: 790–810.

Gupta B L, Hall T A & Naftalin R J (1978) Microprobe measurements of Na, K and Cl concentration profiles in epithelial cells and intercellular spaces of rabbit ileum. *Nature* **272**: 70–73.

Heath A & Milla P J (1983) Development of colonic transport in early childhood: implications for diarrhoeal disease. *Gut* **24**: A977.

Holmberg C, Perheentupa J, Launiala K & Hallman N (1977) Congenital chloride diarrhoea. *Archives of Disease in Childhood* **52**: 255–267.

Hughes C A & Dowling R H (1980) Speed of onset of adaptive mucosal hypoplasia and hypofunction in the intestine of parenterally fed rats. *Clinical Science* **59**: 317–327.

Hughes C A & Ducker D A (1982) The effect of enteral nutrition on the gut and pancreas after total parenteral nutrition. In Robinson J W L, Dowling R H & Riecken E O (eds) *Mechanisms of Intestinal Adaptation*, pp 173–174. Lancaster: MTP Press.

Hughes C A, Ducker D A, Warren I F & McNeish A S (1979) Effect of pancreaticobiliary secretions on mucosal structure and function of self-emptying jejunal blind loops in rats. *Gut* **20**: 924–925 (Abstract).

Hughes C A, Breuer R S, Ducker D A, Hatoff D E & Dowling R H (1982) The effect of cholecystokinin and secretin on intestinal and pancreatic structure and function. In Robinson J W L, Dowling R & Riecken E O (eds) *Mechanisms of Intestinal Adaptation*, pp 435–450. Lancaster: MTP Press.

Husband J & Husband P (1969) Gastric emptying of water and glucose solutions in the newborn. *Lancet* **2**: 409–411.

Koldovsky O, Heringova A, Jirsova V, Jirasek J E & Uher J (1965) Transport of glucose against a concentration gradient in everted sacs of jejunum and ileum of human fetuses. *Gastroenterology* **48**: 185–187.

Lebenthal E & Lee P C (1980) Glucoamylase and disaccharidase activities in normal subjects and in patients with mucosal injury of the small intestine. *Journal of Pediatrics* **97**: 389–393.

Lebenthal E, Lee P C & Heitlinger L A (1983) Impact of development of the gastrointestinal tract on infant feeding. *Journal of Pediatrics* **102**: 1–9.

Levin R J, Koldovsky O, Hoskova J & Jirsova A (1968) Electrical activity across human foetal small intestine associated with absorption processes. *Gut* **9**: 206–213.

Lichtenberger L & Johnson L R (1977) Gastrin in the ontogenic development of the small intestine. *American Journal of Physiology* **227**(2); 390–395.

Lindberg T (1966) Intestinal dipeptidases in the human foetus. *Clinical Science* **30**: 505–515.

Lloyd J R & Clatworthy H W (1958) Hydramnios as an aid to the early diagnosis of congenital obstruction of the alimentary tract: a study of the maternal and fetal factors. *Pediatrics* **21**: 903–909.

Lucas A, Adrian T, Bloom S R & Aynsley Green A (1979) Gut hormones in the neonate. *Proceedings of European Society for Paediatric Research*, A72.

Lucas A, Adrian T, Christofides N D, Bloom S R & Aynsley Green A (1980a) Plasma motilin, gastrin and enteroglucagon and feeding in the human newborn. *Archives of Disease in Childhood* **55**: 673–677.

Lucas A, Bloom S R, & Aynsley Green A (1980b) The development of gut hormone response to feeding in neonates. *Archives of Disease in Childhood* **55**: 678–682.

McLain C R (1963) Amniography studies of the gastrointestinal motility of the human fetus. *American Journal of Obstetrics and Gynecology* **86**: 1079–1087.

McNeish A S, Ducker D A, Warren I F, et al (1979) The influence of gestational age and size on the absorption of D-xylose and D-glucose from the small intestine of the human neonate. In *Development of Mammalian Absorptive Processes: Ciba Foundation Symposium* **70**: pp 267–275. Amsterdam: Excerpta Medica.

Mayne A J, Ducker D A, Aucott G, Hughes C A & McNeish A (1982) Functional development of the neonatal gut as measured by electrogenic glucose absorptive. *Gut* **23**: A925.

Milla P J (1983) Aspects of fluid and electrolyte absorption in the newborn. *Journal of Paediatric Gastroenterology and Nutrition* **2**: 272–276.

Milla P J, Fenton T R, Harries J (1982) Fetal secretory diarrhoea: a new congenital intestinal transport defect. Gut **23**: A925.

Morin C L, Grey V L & Garofalo C (1982) Influence of lipids on intestinal adaptation after resection. In Robinson J W L, Dowling R H & Riecken E O (eds) *Mechanisms of Intestinal Adaptation* pp 175–184. Lancaster: MTP Press.

Moxey P C & Trier J S (1978) Specialized cell types in the human fetal small intestine. *Anatomical Record* **191**: 269–286.

Phillips S & Giller J E (1973) The contribution of the colon to electrolytes and water conservation in man. *Journal of Laboratory and Clinical Medicine* **81**: 733–746.

Pritchard J A (1966) Fetal swallowing and amniotic fluid volume. *Obstetrics and Gynecology* **28**: 606–610.

Rosenberg I H (1966) Development of fetal guinea-pig small intestine: Amino-acid transport and sodium-potassium dependent ATPase (Na-K ATPase). *Federation Proceedings* **25**: 456, A1490.

Ruppin H, Sturm G, Westhoff D et al (1976) Effect of B NLe motilin on small intestinal transit time in healthy subjects. *Scandinavian Journal of Gastroenterology (Suppl)* **11** (39): 85–88.

Sackin H & Boulpaep E L (1975) Models for coupling of salt and water transport. *Journal of General Physiology* **66**: 671–733.

Sagor G R, Almukhtar M Y T, Ghatei M A, Wright N A & Bloom S R (1982) The effect of altered luminal nutrition on cellular proliferation and plasma concentrations of enteroglucagon and gastrin after small bowel resection in the rat. *British Journal of Surgery* **69**: 14–18.

Savage M O, Jefferson I G, Dillon M J, et al (1982) Pseudohypoaldosteronism: severe salt-wasting in infancy caused by generalised mineralocorticoid unresponsiveness. *Journal of Pediatrics* **101**: 239–242.

Schmitz J, Rey F, Bresson J L, Ricour C & Rey J (1980) Etude par perfusion intestinale de l'absorption des sucres après résection étendue du grêle. *Archives Françaises de Pédiatrie* **37**: 491–495.

Stoddart R W & Widdowson E W (1976) Changes in the organs of pigs in response to feeding for the first 24 hours after birth. III. Fluorescence histochemistry of carbohydrates of the intestine. *Biology of the Neonate* **29**: 18–27.

Tanner M S & Stocks R J (eds) (1983) *Neonatal Gastroenterology*. Newcastle, England: Intercept Ltd.

Werner B (1948) Peptic and tryptic capacity of the digestive glands in newborns. *Acta Paediatrica Scandinavica* **35** (Suppl. VI): 1–80.

Williamson R C N (1982) Intestinal adaptation: Factors that influence morphology. *Scandinavian Journal of Gastroenterology* **17** (Suppl. 74): 21–29.

Wozniak E, Fenton T R & Milla P J (1983) The development of fasting small intestinal motility in the human neonate. In Roman C (ed) *Gastrointestinal Motility*, pp 265–284. Lancaster: MTP Press.

Yu V Y H (1975) Effect of body position on gastric emptying in the neonate. *Archives of Disease in Childhood* **50**: 500–504.

Zoppi G, Andreotti G, Pajno-Ferrara F A, Njai D M & Gaburro D (1972) Exocrine pancreas function in premature and full term neonates. *Pediatric Research* **6**: 880–886.

Chapter 2
The Effect of Food on Gut Hormones

T. E. Adrian and S. R. Bloom

The workings of the bowel are still a mystery to us. There are several circulating peptides which have been found to play a role in the control of gastro-intestinal function. These hormonal peptides are released into the bloodstream following the ingestion of food and stimulate the secretory and motor responses required for digestion, absorption and subsequent assimilation of nutrients. By controlling the rate of gastric emptying, and therefore the absorption of nutrients, these regulatory peptides can also have an indirect effect on metabolism. The pattern of hormone release is closely dependent on the size and type of meal ingested. This is important in ensuring that the appropriate digestive responses are triggered; that is, sufficient to cope with the ingested load without over-stimulation. In recent years, there has been considerable interest in the physiological role played by each individual hormonal peptide, as well as on its mechanism of release by the different components of a meal. There is now a fair insight into the ways in which the release of gastro-intestinal hormones may be altered in various alimentary diseases. Abnormal release occurs from the area of bowel affected by the disease, and secondary adaptive changes in other parts of the bowel tend to compensate for the resulting loss of gut function. Study of the ways in which dietary manipulations influence these control processes may reveal the role which they play in the aetiology of gastro-intestinal disease, and also provide information for future therapeutic manoeuvres.

HORMONES OF THE GASTRO-INTESTINAL TRACT

There are now nine peptides which are thought to act as circulating gastro-intestinal hormones (Table 2.1). The release and action of these are considered in turn.

Gastrin

Gastrin, together with the vagal innervation and locally acting histamine, is reponsible for the stimulation of gastric acid secretion (Walsh and Grossman 1975). Gastrin circulates in two major molecular forms, a 17 amino acid molecule (little gastrin) and a 34 amino acid peptide (big gastrin), which has the sequence of little gastrin in its C-terminal end. In man, about half the gastrins are sulphated, although this has no influence on biological activity which resides in the C-terminal pentapeptide of the molecules. Gastrin is released by the presence of partially digested proteins in the stomach, by

13

Table 2.1. Circulating regulatory peptides of the gut.

Hormone	Location	Actions	Release
Gastrin	Antrum	Stimulates gastic acid, trophic to gastric mucosa	Food in stomach, distension and peptides
Secretin	Duodenum and jejunum	Stimulates pancreatic bicarbonate	Low duodenal pH
Cholecystokinin (CCK)	Duodenum and jejunum	Stimulates pancreatic enzymes	Protein and fat
Gastric inhibitory peptide (GIP)*	Small intestine	Contracts gall-bladder, potentiates insulin release	Carbohydrate and fat
Motilin	Small intestine	Stimulates gastric emptying, stimulates bowel motility	Fat releases (carbohydrates and protein inhibit)
Pancreatic polypeptide (PP)	Pancreas	Inhibits pancreatic secretion, relaxes gall-bladder	Protein and fat
Neurotensin	Ileum	Inhibits gastric acid and gastric emptying, stimulates pancreatic bicarbonate	Fat
Enteroglucagon	Ileum and colon	Trophic to small intestinal mucosa	Fat and carbohydrate
Peptide tyrosine tyrosine (PYY)	Ileum and colon	Inhibits acid secretion, slows gut transit	Fat, protein and carbohydrate

*Also known as 'glucose dependent insulinotrophic peptide'.

neural influences and by gastric distension (Figure 2.1). Acid in the stomach inhibits gastrin release, a negative feedback mechanism which prevents over-stimulation of acid (Walsh and Grossman 1975). In addition to stimulation of gastric acid secretion, gastrin is trophic to the gastric mucosa.

Gastrin levels are grossly elevated in any condition associated with achlorhydria such as pernicious anaemia or atrophic gastritis (Ganguli et al 1971). In duodenal ulcer, basal gastrin concentrations are normal but postprandial secretion is moderately increased (Dockray 1978).

Secretin

Secretin is the hormone of the small intestine responsible for the postprandial secretion of water and bicarbonate from the pancreas (Jorpes and Mutt 1966). Secretin is released by acid in the duodenum. In the postprandial state, duodenal pH only falls transiently and the increase in plasma secretin concentrations is likewise small and transient (Schaffalitzky De Muckadell et al 1979).

In contrast, however, the secretin response to the ingestion of commercial soft drinks is much more marked (Hacki 1978). These drinks often have a pH well below the threshold level of 4.5, due to the addition of phosphoric or citric acid. The secretin response is important for neutralising this exogenous acid load which can be substantial (soft drinks may contain more than 150

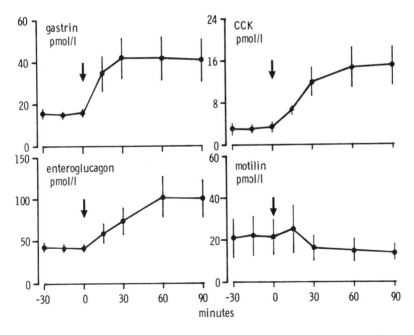

Figure 2.1. The effect of meal ingestion on circulating concentrations of gastrin, cholecystokinin (CCK), enteroglucagon and motilin in six young fasting pigs.

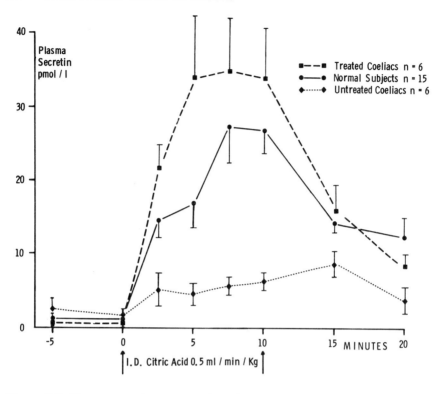

Figure 2.2. Plasma secretin concentrations following an intraduodenal infusion of citric acid in a group of children with active coeliac disease, a group successfully treated with a gluten-free diet, and normal controls. A greatly reduced secretin response is seen in patients with sub-total villous atrophy. From Besterman et al (1978), with kind permission of the authors and the editor of *Lancet*.

mmol/l titratable acid). Secretin levels are reduced in conditions associated with small intestinal mucosal atrophy such as coeliac disease (Besterman et al 1978) (Figure 2.2).

Cholecystokinin

Cholecystokinin (CCK) is responsible for stimulation of pancreatic enzyme secretion and gall bladder contraction in response to the presence of chyme in the duodenum (Jorpes and Mutt 1973). CCK also potentiates the effect of secretin on bicarbonate secretion and has potent trophic effects on the pancreas (Mainz et al 1974). CCK is released by fat and protein in the small intestine and circulates in several molecular forms which appear to have similar biological potency (Figure 2.1). CCK levels, like those of secretin, are reduced in coeliac disease, due to inflammation of the intestinal mucosa (Calam et al 1982). It is failure of hormone secretion in the small intestine that is responsible for the poor pancreatic exocrine function seen in that disease, as the pancreas responds normally to exogenous CCK and secretin.

Pancreatic polypeptide

Although pancreatic polypeptide (PP) is localised to the pancreas, it behaves as a gut hormone. Its actions include inhibition of pancreatic secretion and inhibition of gall bladder contraction (Greenberg et al 1978). The PP response to food involves a complex mechanism in which both the cholinergic innervation and circulating gut hormones appear to play a role (Adrian et al 1977, 1979a). This indirect signal for PP release has been called the extero-PP-axis. Protein and fat are nutrients which evoke the largest PP response although carbohydrate, gastric distension and even sham feeding cause some release (Adrian 1980) (Figure 2.3).

Low plasma PP concentrations are seen in patients with steatorrhoea due to chronic destructive pancreatitis (Figure 2.4) and moderate elevations are seen in many conditions including stress, infective diarrhoea, diabetes, chronic inflammatory disorders, some infections and alcohol abuse (Adrian et al 1979b, Besterman et al 1983; Fink et al 1983).

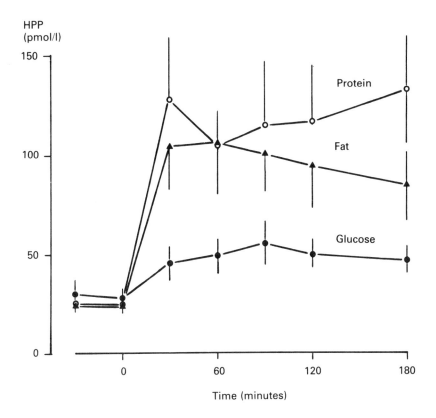

Figure 2.3. Plasma concentration of pancreatic polypeptide (PP) during ingestion of isocaloric amounts of protein (steamed cod), fat (cream) and glucose in six healthy subjects. From Adrian et al (1978), with kind permission of the authors and the publisher, Churchill Livingstone.

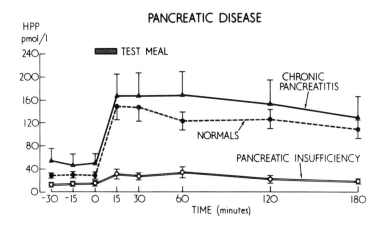

Figure 2.4. Plasma pancreatic polypeptide (PP) response to food in patients with chronic pancreatitis and in healthy controls; the postprandial PP response is greatly obtunded in patients with steatorrhoea due to chronic pancreatitis. From Adrian et al (1979b), with kind permission of the authors and the editor of *Gut*.

Motilin

Motilin is a hormone of the small intestine which has powerful actions on gastro-intestinal motility (Brown et al 1973). For example, motilin can initiate the interdigestive myoelelectric complexes (intestinal housekeeping waves) which sweep the intestine clear of debris and undigested food in the interprandial period (Vantrappen et al 1979). Motilin also increases the rate of gastric emptying and therefore speeds the rate of nutrient entry into the bloodstream (Christofides et al 1979b). When motilin is infused during the ingestion of a carbohydrate rich meal, it results in a more rapid and greater insulin response than is seen when saline is infused. This is an example of how a peptide, which has its primary action on gastro-intestinal motility, can have a profound secondary influence on metabolism. Motilin is released by fat and acid in the duodenum in man whereas oral glucose reduces plasma motilin levels (Christofides et al 1979a) (Figure 2.1).

High motilin concentrations have been observed in patients with diarrhoea (Figure 2.5), whereas patients with constipation tend to have low levels (Besterman et al 1983).

Gastric inhibitory peptide

The physiological role of gastric inhibitory peptide (GIP) is uncertain. The biological actions of this peptide, however, include the inhibition of gastric acid secretion and potentiation of glucose-stimulated insulin release (Dupré et al 1973). The action on acid secretion was subsequently shown to be pharmacological, whereas the insulin releasing action was more likely to be physiological (Figure 2.6). It is well established that oral glucose ingestion causes a far greater insulin reponse than the same amount of glucose given intravenously, and it was postulated that a gut factor 'incretin' potentiated the

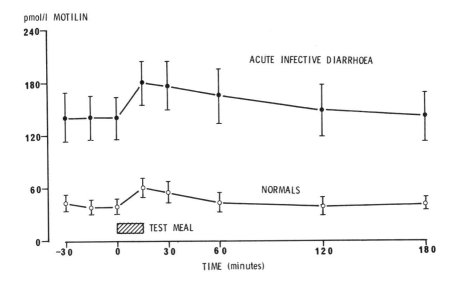

Figure 2.5. Plasma motilin concentrations in patients recovering from acute infective diarrhoea and in healthy controls. After Besterman et al (1983), with kind permission of the authors and the editor of *Gut*.

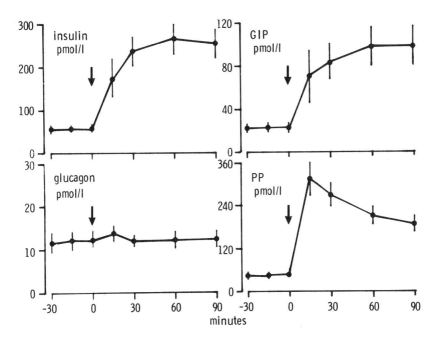

Figure 2.6. The effect of meal ingestion on circulating concentrations of insulin, glucose dependent insulinotrophic peptide (GIP), glucagon and pancreatic polypeptide (PP) in six young fasting pigs.

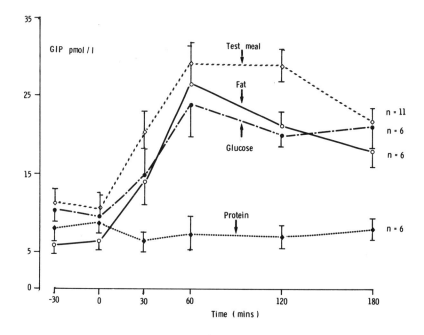

Figure 2.7. Plasma GIP concentrations during ingestion of isocaloric amounts of protein (steamed cod), fat (cream), glucose and a mixed meal in six healthy fasting subjects. From Sarson et al (1981), with kind permission of the authors and the publisher, Churchill Livingstone.

release of insulin in response to oral glucose (McIntyre et al 1964). Several gut hormones have been implicated as possible 'incretins', but of those studied to date, GIP is the most likely candidate. Because of the importance of the postprandial insulin response, it is probable that other circulating and neural factors also influence insulin release (Sarson et al 1982). Plasma GIP concentrations rise in response to ingested nutrients, particularly glucose and fat, but some amino acids also evoke a response (Figure 2.7). It would appear that nutrient digestion and absorption is required in order to stimulate GIP release. Because of its role in insulin release, GIP has now been re-named glucose-dependent insulinotrophic peptide.

GIP and insulin responses are reduced in parallel in malabsorption states, such as coeliac disease and tropical sprue, and also in patients who have undergone jejuno-ileal bypass for morbid obesity (Besterman et al 1978, 1979, Bloom and Polak 1980). Similar blunted responses of both hormones follow the use of non-absorbable carbohydrates such as guar and pectin, or sucrase inhibitors such as acarbose (Jenkins et al 1979).

Neurotensin

As well as acting as a neurotransmitter in the central nervous system, neurotensin is also present in endocrine cells of the ileal mucosa (Polak et al

1977). Neurotensin is released into the circulation and it exhibits several biological effects on the gastro-intestinal tract. These include inhibitory actions on both the motor and secretory functions of the stomach and also stimulation of pancreatic bicarbonate secretion (Blackburn et al 1980b; Fletcher et al 1981). Fat appears to be the major stimulus for the release of neurotensin, although carbohydrate will also evoke a response if it reaches the terminal ileum. Thus neurotensin levels are grossly elevated in patients with the dumping syndrome following gastric surgery, and in malabsorption states where undigested food passes into the ileum (Besterman et al 1979; Blackburn et al 1980a).

Enteroglucagon

Enteroglucagon is a peptide predominantly localised to the terminal ileum and colon, which appears to be trophic to the mucosa of the small intestine and slows intestinal transit (Bloom 1972; Sagor et al 1983). Plasma enteroglucagon levels rise substantially following the ingestion of fat (particularly long chain triglycerides) or carbohydrate, although the response to a small mixed meal is usually mediocre (Ghatei and Bloom 1981). This reflects the distribution of the cells in the ileum and colon, which normally receive little stimulation, as most nutrients are absorbed in the proximal small intestine. Large increases in plasma enteroglucagon levels are seen in malabsorption states (Figure 2.8) and following bypass or resection of the small intestine. This adaptive response is quite appropriate as enteroglucagon appears to increase absorptive surface area and slow intestinal transit (Besterman et al 1978, 1979, 1982; Bloom and Polak 1980).

Peptide YY

Peptide YY (PYY) is a 36 amino acid, straight chained polypeptide, which was recently isolated from porcine small intestine (Tatemoto 1982); PYY shares considerable sequence homology with PP from the pancreas and neuropeptide Y from the central nervous system.

The PYY molecule has a tyrosine residue at each end and it is these which gives PYY its name as Y represents tyrosine in the new peptide nomenclature. PYY circulates in plasma and its concentrations rise in response to food. Fat is the most potent stimulus for PYY but protein and carbohydrate also elicit a response. Like neurotensin and enteroglucagon, PYY is released whenever nutrient reaches far down into the intestine since this peptide is localised to the distal bowel (Adrian et al 1985).

Plasma PYY concentrations show little response to a small mixed meal but much larger rises occur after large fatty or liquid meals. Cream, for example, is a potent stimulus (Figure 2.9). Recent infusion studies in man have shown that PYY inhibits gastric acid secretion and slows the speed at which the stomach empties after food (Adrian et al 1983; Allen et al 1984). These effects are seen at doses which cause increments in plasma PYY concentrations similar to those seen after food, suggesting that they are physiological. Plasma PYY concentrations are grossly elevated in malabsorption states and after intestinal resection (Adrian et al 1984). They are also high in patients with inflammatory bowel disease or infective diarrhoea.

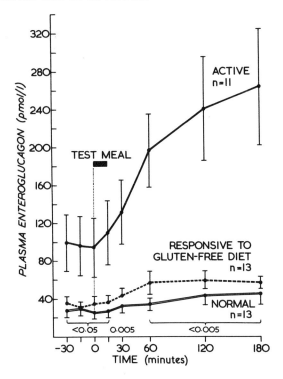

Figure 2.8. Plasma enteroglucagon concentrations during breakfast in patients with active coeliac disease, in a group successfully treated with a gluten-free diet and in healthy controls. Enhanced enteroglucagon secretion in patients with malabsorption is shown. From Besterman et al (1978), with kind permission of the authors and the editor of *Lancet*.

INFLUENCE OF FOOD ON CIRCULATING GUT HORMONES

The release of individual hormonal peptides may be influenced by the size and nature (solid or liquid) of the meal, the form of nutrient present, and by the presence of inhibitors of digestive enzymes.

Size of meal

In general, the amounts of hormone released into the bloodstream, and therefore the circulating plasma levels, increase with increasing meal size. This increase may be mediocre as is seen, for example, with PP, where plasma levels after a 5000 calorie meal are only two-fold higher than after a 500 calorie meal. In contrast the increase in peptides from the distal bowel may be profound: a ten-fold increase in circulating levels of PYY follows a similar increase in meal size (Adrian et al 1985). The effect of meal size on the hormones of the small intestine falls somewhere in between. These observations would suggest that hormones from the ileum and colon respond mainly to large meals where a proportion of nutrients reach the distal gut un-

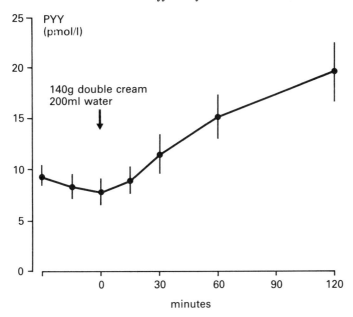

Figure 2.9. Plasma PYY concentrations during the ingestion of cream in six healthy fasting subjects.

absorbed. A similar large response in neurotensin, PYY and enteroglucagon is seen after liquid meals, where transit through the gut is more rapid (Read et al 1984).

Type of nutrient

The pattern of hormones released from the gut after food depends very much on the type of nutrient present. For example, a carbohydrate-rich meal will release GIP and enteroglucagon but will have little effect on gastrin, CCK or neurotensin and will inhibit the release of motilin. In contrast, a fatty meal will release CCK, neurotensin and motilin as well as GIP and enteroglucagon. Gastrin secretin is predominantly triggered by protein, which will also release CCK, PP and PYY. However, GIP, motilin, neurotensin and enteroglucagon do not respond well to ingested protein and peptides.

Form of nutrient

It is well known that complex macromolecules require digestion before absorption whereas simple sugars, short peptides and medium chain triglycerides can be absorbed without modification. The effect of different forms of nutrients on the release of gastro-intestinal hormones is, however, more complex. For example, cholecystokinin is predominantly released by long chain triglycerides (LCT), whereas medium chain triglycerides are relatively ineffective (Isaacs et al 1983). The cholecystokinin contracts the gall bladder and releases the pancreatic lipase which is required for digestion of the

LCT's. In contrast, however, GIP is released only by absorbable simple sugars such as glucose, whereas complex carbohydrates require prior digestion. Thus the GIP and insulin responses to complex carbohydrate are prolonged and attenuated; if GIP is an important factor in the postprandial secretion of insulin, then this release pattern appears useful, as insulin is required only when nutrients are absorbed (Cataland 1978). Indeed, the release of insulin by non-absorbed nutrients would result in inappropriate hypoglycaemia.

Amino acid mixtures, particularly the essential amino acids, can release gastrin and cholecystokinin but they are not nearly as effective as peptides in this respect.

Complex carbohydrates, which are broken down by the microflora of the large bowel, will elicit a substantial response of the lower intestinal hormones, such as enteroglucagon; they have less effect on hormones of the upper small intestine, such as GIP (Jenkins et al 1982). Although it is not clear what role this enhanced release of hormones plays in the slower intestinal transit associated with high fibre diets, the physically larger bulk of such diets delays transit due to the slower rate of gastric emptying.

EFFECT OF DIGESTIVE ENZYME INHIBITORS

Inhibitors of the major digestive enzymes can have a profound effect on gastro-intestinal function and, perhaps not surprisingly, on intestinal hormone secretion. Amongst those which have been extensively investigated there are the alpha-glucosidase inhibitor (acarbose), which induces carbohydrate maldigestion, and several naturally occurring trypsin inhibitors (such as that found in soya beans) which prevent protein digestion.

Effect of acarbose on gastro-intestinal hormones

Acarbose is a competitive inhibitor of alpha-glucosidase, the enzyme which hydrolyses sucrose and starch-derived dextrins. Because acarbose induces carbohydrate malabsorption and dramatically reduces postprandial glycaemia, it has been used to treat patients with the dumping syndrome after gastric surgery and also patients with diabetes mellitus (Gerard et al 1981; Sachse et al 1981; Taylor et al 1981). When given acutely to diabetics, acarbose had a profound effect in reducing the postprandial glucose increment, following a test breakfast, to 24% of control values. This was accompanied by a similar reduction in insulin (33% of control) and GIP levels (32% of control) (Uttenthal et al 1983). Enteroglucagon concentrations were dramatically increased by acarbose in response to the presence of non-absorbed nutrients in the terminal ileum. Thus the response of GIP and enteroglucagon to acarbose reflects the shift of carbohydrate absorption from the upper to the lower small intestine. Acarbose at high doses, however, sometimes causes intestinal hurry due to fermentation in the large bowel.

In healthy subjects, a low dose of acarbose (50 mg), combined with a small amount of guar gum (14.5 g), caused a 70% reduction in peak glucose in response to breakfast (Jenkins et al 1979). There was no evidence of carbohydrate malabsorption, assessed by breath hydrogen, with this low dose of acarbose. This combination of acarbose with guar also causes a great reduction in the postprandial insulin and GIP responses. In contrast, acarbose alone caused troublesome symptoms in some volunteers, and the postprandial glucose peak was only reduced by 28%. Thus the combination of acrabose and guar reduced the rate of carbohydrate absorption without increasing the side effects. Slowing of intestinal transit following acarbose is likely to be mediated by increased release of hormones from the lower intestine (Read et al 1984).

Effect of trypsin inhibitors on gastro-intestinal hormones

When rats are fed with raw soya flour, marked pancreatic hypertrophy and hyperplasia occur (Mainz et al 1974). This effect is thought to be due to the trophic action of increased circulating concentrations of CCK on the pancreas. Increased release of CCK occurs in response to ingestion of trypsin inhibitors, such as that found in soya beans (Brand and Morgan 1981; Adrian et al 1982) (Figure 2.10). This suggests that in the rat, CCK release is controlled by intestinal trypsin levels and the removal of trypsin, due to its binding to an inhibitor, is thought to produce an increased release of CCK. A general enlargement of the gland first takes place, but soon foci of abnormal growth occur which become autonomous adenomata and then carcinomas

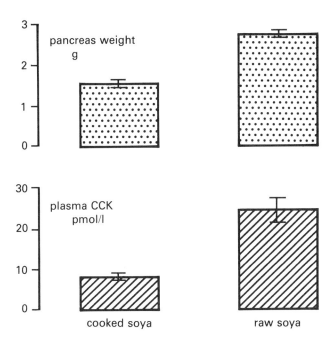

Figure 2.10. Pancreatic wet weight and plasma cholecystokinin (CCK) concentrations in 30 rats fed with raw soya flour (containing active trypsin inhibitor) for 21 days and 30 controls fed on heat inactivated soya flour.

(McGuinness et al 1982). About one in six rats fed raw soya flour develops pancreatic cancer. In addition, raw soya feeding potentiates the effects of sub-threshold doses of carcinogens (such as azoserine) (Morgan et al 1977). The raw soya diet appears therefore to promote the effect of a genotoxic (initiating) carcinogen.

The trophic action of CCK has not been investigated in man. It has been observed, however, that large doses of oral pancreatic enzyme supplements reduce trypsin output in pancreatic fistulae. This suggests that a similar control mechanism, with feedback inhibition by luminal tryptic activity on pancreatic secretion, may exist in man.

Naturally occurring trypsin inhibitors are found in many food-stuffs, for example, peas, beans and potatoes, although these should be rendered inactive by adequate cooking, as are those in soya derived products. The increasing incidence of pancreatic cancer in the Western world makes the study of these mechanisms a matter of considerable importance.

CONTROL OF GUT FUNCTION

In addition to the hormonal peptide control, the gut is supplied by an extensive network of intrinsic nerve fibres which appear to be involved in normal secreto-motor responses. Several active neuropeptides are localised in these nerves in the gut wall. Sometimes a peptide neurotransmitter is co-localised with a classical neurotransmitter, for example, vasoactive intestinal peptide (VIP) with acetylcholine, or neuropeptide Y (NPY) with noradrenaline. In addition, regulators such as histamine, somatostatin and prostaglandins appear to function as paracrine (local) hormones. These are released into the interstitial fluid and have major actions on other cells in the immediate vicinity. Overall control of gastro-intestinal function is therefore brought about by a combination of these different regulators, acting in concert.

CONCLUSIONS

The pattern of release of the gastro-intestinal hormones after the ingestion of food thus reflects the type, size and composition of the meal. Manipulation of nutrient intake, either by diet or by the use of specific digestive enzyme inhibitors, can result in changes in the release pattern of regulatory peptides which is reflected in the physiological function of the gut. The hormone profile also changes in the common gastro-intestinal diseases, with a pattern characteristic of each particular disorder. Changes in regulatory peptide release may reflect the diseased area of bowel and also the adaptive changes in other areas of gut which tend to compensate for the disease process. Measurement of gut hormone profiles after a simple test meal is useful in the diagnosis of alimentary disease and also in monitoring the effectiveness of therapy. Measurement of gut hormone profiles is also of value in monitoring the effects of dietary manipulation when used, for example, to treat obesity, diabetes mellitus, or the dumping syndrome after gastric surgery. Much more work is required to assess more particular aspects of our diet and their physiological results. Gut hormone measurement is a relatively simple and non-invasive way to do this. Perhaps the 'PYY response to quail's eggs' or 'Bombesin suppression by port' will form the titles of tomorrow's articles on nutrition.

REFERENCES

Adrian T E (1980) Pancreatic polypeptide. *Journal of Clinical Pathology* **33** (Suppl. 8): 85–91.
Adrian T E, Bloom S R, Besterman H S, et al (1977) Mechanism of pancreatic polypeptide release in man. *Lancet* **1**: 161–163.
Adrian T E, Bloom S R, Besterman H S & Bryant M G (1978) Pancreatic polypeptide. In Bloom S R (ed) *Gut Hormones*, pp 254–260. Edinburgh: Churchill Livingstone.
Adrian T E, Besterman H S & Bloom S R (1979a) Importance of cholinergic tone in the release of pancreatic polypeptide by gut hormones in man. *Life Sciences* **24**: 1989–1994.
Adrian T E, Besterman H S, Mallinson C N, Garalotis C & Bloom S R (1979b) Imparied pancreatic polypeptide release in chronic pancreatitis with steatorrhoea. *Gut* **20**: 98–101.
Adrian T E, Pasquali C, Pescosta F, Bacarese–Hamilton A J & Bloom S R (1982) Soya induced pancreatic hypertrophy and elevation of circulating cholecystokinin. *Gut* **23**: A889.
Adrian T E, Sagor G R, Savage A P et al (1983) Low dose PYY inhibits gastric secretion in man. *Gut* **24**: A479.
Adrian T E, Bacarese–Hamilton A J, Savage A P, et al (1984) Plasma PYY in gastrointestinal diseases. *Digestive Diseases and Sciences* **29** (Suppl.): 3S.
Adrian T E, Bacarese–Hamilton A J, Ferri G-L, Polak J M & Bloom S R (1985) Human distribution and release of a putative new gut hormone, peptide YY (PYY). *Gastroenterology* In press.
Allen J M, Fitzpatrick M L, Yeats J C, et al (1984) Effects of peptide YY and neuropeptide Y on gastric emptying in man. *Digestion* **30**: 255–262.
Besterman H S, Bloom S R, Sarson D L, et al (1978) Gut hormone profile in coeliac disease. *Lancet* **1**: 785–788.
Besterman H S, Cook G C, Sarson D L, et al (1979) Gut hormones in tropical malabsorption. *British Medical Journal* **2**: 1252–1255.
Besterman H S, Adrian T E, Bloom S R, et al (1982) Gut hormone release following intestinal resection. *Gut* **23**: 854–861.
Besterman H S, Christofides N D, Welsby P D, et al (1983) Gut hormones in acute diarrhoea. *Gut* **24**: 665–671.
Blackburn A M, Christofides N D, Ghatei M A et al (1980a) Elevation of plasma neurotensin in the dumping syndrome. *Clinical Science* **59**: 237–243.
Blackburn A M, Fletcher D R, Bloom S R, et al (1980b) Effect of neurotensin on gastric function. *Lancet* **1**: 987–989.
Bloom S R (1972) An enteroglucagon tumour. *Gut* **13**: 520–523.
Bloom S R & Polak J M (1980) Plasma hormone concentrations in gastrointestinal disease. *Clinics in Gastroenterology* **93**: 785–798.
Brand S J & Morgan R G H (1981) The release of rat intestinal cholecystokinin after oral trypsin inhibitor measured by bioassay. *Journal of Physiology* **319**: 325–343.
Brown J C, Cook M A & Dryburgh J R (1973) Motilin, a gastric motor activity stimulating polypeptide: the complete amino acid sequence. *Canadian Journal of Biochemistry* **51**: 533–537.
Calam J, Ellis A & Dockray G. J (1982) Identification and measurement of molecular variants of cholecystokinin in duodenal mucosa and plasma. *Journal of Clinical Investigation* **69**: 218–225.
Cataland S (1978) Physiology of GIP in man. In Bloom S R (ed) *Gut Hormones*, pp 288–293. Edinburgh: Churchill Livingstone.
Christofides N D, Bloom S R, Besterman H S, Adrian T E & Ghatei M A (1979a) Release of motilin by oral and intravenous nutrients in man. *Gut* **20**: 102–106.
Christofides N D, Modlin I M, Fitzpatrick M L & Bloom S R (1979b) Effect of motilin on the rate of gastric emptying and gut hormone release during breakfast. *Gastroenterology* **76**: 903–907.

Dockray G J (1978) Gastrin overview. In Bloom S R (ed) *Gut Hormones*, pp 129–139. Edinburgh: Churchill Livingstone.

Dupré J, Ross S A, Watson D & Brown J C (1973) Stimulation of insulin secretion by gastric inhibitory peptide in man. *Journal of Clinical Endocrinology* 37: 826–828.

Fink R S, Adrian T E, Margot D H & Bloom S R (1983) Increased plasma pancreatic polypeptide in chronic alcohol abuse. *Clinical Endocrinology* 18: 417–421.

Fletcher D R, Blackburn A M, Adrian T E, Chadwick V S & Bloom S R (1981) Effect of neurotensin on pancreatic function in man. *Life Sciences* 29: 2157–2161.

Ganguli P C, Cullen D R, Irvine W J (1971) Radioimmunoassay of plasma gastrin in pernicious anaemia, achlorhydria without pernicious anaemia, hypochlorhydria, and in controls. *Lancet* 1: 155–158.

Gerard J, Luyckx A S & Lefebre P J (1981) Two months treatment with acarbose in type 1 diabetics. In Creutzfeldt W (ed) *Proceedings of the First International Symposium on Acarbose*, pp 406–416. Amsterdam: Excerpta Medica.

Ghatei M A & Bloom S R (1981) Enteroglucagon in man. In Bloom S R & Polak J M (eds) *Gut Hormones*, Vol. 2, pp 332–338. Edinburgh: Churchill Livingstone.

Greenberg G R, McCloy R F, Adrian T E, et al (1978) Inhibition of pancreas and gall bladder by pancreatic polypeptide. *Lancet* 2: 1280–1282.

Hacki W H, Greenberg G R & Bloom S R (1978) Role of secretin in man I. In Bloom S R (ed) *Gut Hormones*, pp 182–192. Edinburgh: Churchill Livingstone.

Isaacs P E T, Ladas S, Forgacs I, Adrian T E & Ellam S (1983) Human gallbladder and gut hormone responses to ingested medium chain triglyceride (MCT) and long chain triglyceride LCT. *Clinical Science* 64: 54.

Jenkins D J A, Taylor R H, Nineham R, Goff D V et al (1979) Combined use of guar and acarbose in reduction of postprandial glycaemia. *Lancet* 2: 924–927.

Jenkins D J A, Wolever T M S, Taylor R H et al (1982) Slow release dietary carbohydrate improves second meal tolerance. *American Journal of Clinical Nutrition* 35: 1339–1346.

Jorpes J E & Mutt V (1966) On the biological assay of secretin. The reference standard. *Acta Physiologica Scandinavica* 66: 316–325.

Jorpes J E & Mutt V (1973) Secretin, cholecystokinin (CCK). In Jorpes J E & Mutt V (eds) *Secretin, Cholecystokinin, Pancreozymin and Gastrin*, pp 1–144. Berlin: Springer-Verlag.

Mainz D L, Black O & Webster P D (1974) Hormonal control of pancreatic growth. *Journal of Clinical Investigation* 52: 2300–2304.

McGuinness E E, Hopwood D & Wormsley K G (1982) Further studies of the effects of raw soya flour on the rat pancreas. *Scandinavian Journal of Gastroenterology* 17: 273–277.

McIntyre N, Holdsworth C D & Turner O S (1964) New interpretation of oral glucose tolerance. *Lancet* 2: 20–21.

Morgan R G H, Levinson D A, Hopwood D, Saunders J H B & Wormsley K G (1977) Potentiation of the action of azoserine on the rat pancreas by raw soya bean flour. *Cancer Letters* 3: 87–90.

Polak J M, Sullivan S N, Bloom S R et al (1977). Neurotensin in human intestine: radioimmunoassay and specific localisation in the N cell. *Nature, London* 270: 183–185.

Read N W, McFarlane A, Kinsman R I, et al (1984) Effect of infusion of nutrient solutions into the ileum on gastrointestinal transit and plasma levels of neurotensin and enteroglucagon. *Gastroenterology* 86: 274–280.

Sachse G, Moses E, Laube H & Federlin K (1981) Effect of long term acarbose therapy on the metabolic situation of sulphonylurea treated diabetics. In Creutzfeldt W (ed) *Proceedings of the First International Symposium on Acarbose*, pp 298–304. Amsterdam: Excerpta-Medica.

Sagor G R, Ghatei M A, Al-Mukhtar Y T, Wright N A & Bloom S R (1983) Evidence for a humoral mechanism after small intestinal resection. *Gastroenterology* 84: 902–906.

Sarson et al (1981) Physiology of GIP. In Bloom S R & Polak J M (eds) *Gut Hormones II*, p 101 Edinburgh: Churchill Livingstone.

Sarson D L, Wood S M, Holder D & Bloom S R (1982) The effect of glucose-dependent insulinotrophic polypeptide infused at physiological concentrations on the release of insulin in man. *Diabetologia* 22: 33–36.

Schaffalitzky de Muckadell O B, Fahrenkrug J & Rune S J (1979) Physiological significance of secretin in the pancreatic bicarbonate secretion: 1. Responsiveness of the secretin-releasing system in the upper duodenum. *Scandinavian Journal of Gastroenterology* 14: 79–83.

Tatemoto K (1982) Isolation and characterisation of peptide YY (PYY), a candidate gut hormone that inhibits pancreatic exocrine secretion. *Proceedings of the National Academy of Sciences, USA* 79: 2514–2518.

Taylor R H, Jenkins D J A & Barker H M (1981) Low dose acarbose and the dumping syndrome. In Creutzfeldt W (ed) *Proceedings of the First International Symposium on Acarbose*, pp 527–529. Amsterdam: Excerpta Medica.

Uttenthal L O, Ukponmwan O O, Ghatei M A & Bloom S R (1983) Acute and short term effects of intestinal alpha-glucosidase inhibition on gut hormone responses in man. *Gut* **24**: A461.

Vantrappen G, Janssens J, Peeters T L et al (1979) Motilin and the interdigestive migrating motor complex in man. *Digestive Diseases and Sciences* **24**: 497–500.

Walsh J H & Grossman M I (1975) Gastrin. *New England Journal of Medicine* **292**: 1377–1384.

Chapter 3
Intestinal Permeability

T. J. Peters and I. Bjarnason

There is considerable current interest in the concept of enhanced intestinal permeability and its possible role in the pathogenesis and pathophysiology of a variety of intestinal and extra-intestinal disorders. This review will consider briefly, from a historical viewpoint, how the techniques and concepts of intestinal permeability have developed and will review some current applications of these techniques.

ASSESSMENT OF PERMEABILITY

There have been essentially three eras in the development of ideas and techniques for assessing intestinal permeability in man: (i) studies by Menzies and colleagues on sugar permeability which have been extended more recently by various other groups, (ii) the introduction and application of poly(ethylene glycol) polymers by Chadwick and colleagues, and (iii) the use of in vitro techniques for measuring permeability and the introduction of ^{51}Cr-EDTA as a permeability probe by Bjarnason and colleagues (Table 3.1).

Table 3.1. Comparison of in vitro probes for assessing intestinal permeability in man.

	Sugars	Poly(ethylene glycol)	^{51}Cr-EDTA
Cost of probes	50 p	50 p	30 p – £3.00
Assay procedure	3–6 month training, 18 h/assay	3–6 month training, 18 h/assay	1–2 min γ counting
Patient acceptability	Frequently nausea, abdominal discomfort and diarrhoea	Nausea	Palatable, no side-effects
Sensitivity	Adequate	Limited	Highly sensitive
Bacterial degradation	+++	(+)	(−)
Endogenous excretion	+	−	−

Sugar probes

The fundamental concept behind the sugar tests is easily comprehensible but widely misunderstood, largely because of lack of historical perspective. Originally it was found that patients with coeliac disease excreted significant amounts of sucrose and lactose (Weser and Sleisenger 1965) and peptides (Kowlessar et al 1964) in their urine. It was unclear, however, whether this increased urine excretion was due to increased mucosal permeability, decreased brush border hydrolase activities, or both. Because of the apparent successful and widespread use of the xylose test, which shows markedly reduced absorption in coeliac disease, these observations remained largely unnoticed until 1974 when Menzies introduced and advocated the use of non-hydrolysable di- and tri-saccharides as test substances for assessing intestinal permeability (Menzies 1974). This study showed, not only that intestinal permeability to poorly absorbed test substances is markedly elevated in untreated patients with coeliac disease, but also that when the test solution was made hypertonic, many well-treated patients showed persistent abnormalities (Menzies et al 1979).

In this study patients were given various sugar mixtures either singly or in combination, with or without osmotic fillers, and urine was collected for a short period, usually 5 hours. Clearly the possible combinations of mono-, di-, or tri-saccharides, their amount and tonicity, have led to a confusion of tests with little attempt at standardisation. In addition, the use of combinations of mono- and oligo-saccharides with the determination of urine excretion ratios has also led to a certain degree of confusion in interpretation of the results. This has occurred because certain sugars, e.g. mannitol, are significantly absorbed (up to 20%) by normal subjects. Mucosal abnormalities, particularly those leading to a decrease in surface area in either macroscopic or microscopic terms, will lead to decreased absorption of these substances. Conversely, larger molecules which are not absorbed by normal subjects will show increased absorption if permeability is increased, but their absorption will not be significantly affected by alterations in mucosal surface area. Thus, expressing the permeability in terms of a urinary ratio of the two types of sugars may be grossly misleading. Similarly, sequential studies in which there are significant alterations in mucosal morphology, for example in coeliac disease, may lead to confusing conclusions.

The use of various sugar compounds has also led to a proliferation of analytical methods. The method employed by Menzies and colleagues uses thin-layer chromatography combined with quantitative densitometry. This is a demanding technique, and others have failed to achieve the necessary degree of accuracy and precision: this has led to the development of complex high-performance liquid chromatographic (HPLC) and gas–liquid chromatographic (GLC) techniques. Chemical and enzymatic methods are now available for certain of the sugars. Although the sugars are claimed to be inert, some, for example cellobiose, are undoubtedly partially hydrolysed by the mucosal cells of the gastro-intestinal tract. Others, for example mannitol, are to a small but variable extent endogenous metabolites and may be detected in the urine of fasted subjects (Laker et al 1982). Another disadvantage of the sugar tests, which may be relevant in certain intestinal disorders, is that the sugars are subject to extensive bacterial degradation.

This clearly limits their use to the upper small intestine in normal subjects; situations where upper gastro-intestinal bacterial overgrowth occurs may lead to confusing results.

Routinely, urine collections are performed over the 5 hours following oral administration of the sugars but it is uncertain whether this is an adequate time to ensure complete renal excretion of the various sugars, some of which (particularly the disaccharides) may be hydrolysed by the renal brush border enzymes. Nevertheless, the various sugar permeability tests have been used fairly extensively, with reasonable agreement being achieved between workers, and in comparison with other permeability probes.

Poly(ethylene glycol) (PEG)

High molecular weight (~4000) poly(ethylene glycol) polymers have been used extensively, in both man and experimental animals, as faecal markers and as extracellular markers in perfusion studies. Therefore the introduction of low molecular weight (~400) PEG's as indicators of intestinal permeability was potentially of interest. The format of the test is similar to that of the sugar tests in that the fasted patient consumes approximately 5 g of the mixed polymers and the urine is collected for 5–8 hours and assayed for the various glycols. Because of the heterogeneity of commercially available poly(ethylene glycol)s, ranging from 300 to 700 molecular weight for supposedly PEG 400, there was also the opportunity to investigate the gradation of permeability over this range by comparing the ratios of the various glycols in the oral dose and in urine. Measurements of the various polymers in the urine is technically difficult, requiring either HPLC methods or the preparation of volatile derivatives for their subsequent GLC (Chadwick et al 1977a).

The initial results of Chadwick and colleagues (1977b) showed that the low molecular weight fractions of PEG 400 were absorbed to a greater extent than the high molecular weight fractions. Patients with symptomatic coeliac disease excreted less PEG 400 than either normal controls or asymptomatic patients with coeliac disease. The same patients had, in addition, abnormal urinary ratios of high to low molecular weight polymers. Nothing is known for certain, however, about the absorption pathway of PEG 400 or its polymers. Despite their molecular weight range of 200–500, more than 20% is absorbed and excreted in 5 hours by normal subjects, which contrasts sharply with that of the disaccharides and ^{51}Cr-EDTA (molecular weight $\simeq$ 340) which are poorly absorbed (<1% in 5 hours). The size of PEG 400 excludes its absorption from the 'small pore pathway' for monosaccharides (upper molecular weight of probes using this pathway approximately 180). It is therefore suggested that PEG 400 is primarily absorbed through the lipophilic portion of the brush border, which is in keeping with the much higher lipid-to-water partition coefficient of PEG, compared with the disaccharides or ^{51}Cr-EDTA.

There are also considerable supplier and batch variations in the composition of the various polymer mixtures, and the completeness of urinary excretion of absorbed PEG polymers has not been adequately tested. Nevertheless, the introduction of PEG tests for intestinal permeability stimulated considerable interest and much work has since been carried out using this probe, particularly by a Swedish group who found that, in various disease conditions, PEG almost invariably gives a different result to that of the sugar tests and ^{51}Cr-EDTA (see Magnusson and Sundqvist 1984). PEG 400 is little used at present and appears to have failed to live up to the initial claims that it was an ideal probe for assessing intestinal permeability.

^{51}Cr-EDTA tests in vitro and in vivo

The introduction of this probe resulted from in vitro measurements of intestinal permeability in man (Bjarnason and Peters 1984). It was apparent that the in vivo measurements of permeability were dependent on gastric emptying, intestinal transit, mucosal surface area, mucosal blood, and possibly lymphatic, flow. In an attempt to resolve some of the paradoxes concerning altered permeability in coeliac and other diseases, in particular the apparent reduced permeability to low molecular weight probes in coeliac patients in relapse, we developed this in vitro technique.

Using short term (3–10 min) uptake by fragments (2–5 mg) of Crosby capsule biopsy samples, permeability to three probes of molecular weight 340, 1240 and 5200 was assessed. The technique has been extensively used for assessing absorption of Fe^{3+}, Ca^{2+}, glucose and other nutrients in man and experimental animals (Cox and Peters 1979; Scott and Peters 1983; Duncombe et al 1984; Raja et al 1985). These probes are essentially non-absorbable by normal mucosa and have all been validated as extra-cellular fluid markers (e.g. Russell et al 1970). The results clearly showed that uptake is inversely related to the log molecular weight of the probe, both in control subjects and in patients with coeliac disease in relapse and remission (Figure 3.1). In coeliac disease in remission, permeability is still enhanced. This observation may have pathogenic implications and is discussed below.

This in vitro technique has clearly clarified the concept of intestinal permeability and indicated that ^{51}Cr-EDTA is a suitable probe for in vivo use in man. The in vitro technique is used for research, rather than for routine purposes, and can be used on biopsy samples from other regions of the gastro-intestinal tract. It is also noteworthy that a recent report uses the in vitro technique to validate the use of sugars in permeability studies (Dawson et al 1984).

Because whole tissue fragments are used, it has been suggested that this technique will measure tissue uptake through the cut surfaces of the biopsy rather than via the luminal surface. Undoubtedly, some entry of the probe will occur via the serosal surface and some of the medium will remain adherent to the under surface. However, the surface area of the luminal aspect is many times greater than that of the cut surface. In addition, recent experimental studies comparing iron uptake by tissue fragments and the whole animal show excellent agreement between the two techniques (Peters et al 1984). Furthermore the in vivo and in vitro ^{51}Cr-EDTA absorption results are similar, both qualitatively and quantitatively. These findings all validate the use of this in vitro uptake technique.

The ^{51}Cr-EDTA test represents a useful clinical test which has gained widespread acceptance. Table 3.2 lists some of the applications. The main virtue of the test is its simplicity: it can readily be carried out on an out-patient

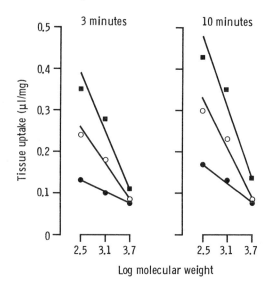

Figure 3.1. In vitro tissue uptake of three probes by control subjects (●), patients with coeliac disease in relapse (■), and patients in remission (○). Data show mean values for 3 and 10 min incubations. From Bjarnason and Peters (1984), with kind permission of the editor of *Gut*.

basis and may be combined with the Schilling test. The radioactive dose is trivial (0.1 m Sieverts) with a risk of malignancy equivalent to a lifetime consumption of two cigarettes!

The test is highly sensitive and certain precautions are necessary. Thus the ^{51}Cr-EDTA test shows increased permeability in alcohol abusers (Bjarnason et al 1984e). Even heavy social drinkers will show increased permeability which, however, returns to normal with two weeks abstinence. Similarly,

Table 3.2. Applications of the ^{51}Cr-EDTA permeability test.

Coeliac disease (Bjarnason et al 1983b)
Crohn's disease (Bjarnason et al 1983a; Jenkins et al 1984; O'Morain et al 1984)
Differential diagnosis of ileal disorders (Bjarnason et al 1984a)
Investigation of irritable bowel syndrome (I. Bjarnason, unpublished results)
Alcoholic enteropathy (Bjarnason et al 1984d)
Parenteral nutrition (G. Neale, unpublished results)
Intestinal graft versus host disease (Selby et al 1984)
Cytotoxic enteropathy (Selby et al 1984)
Joggers enteropathy (I. Bjarnason, unpublished results)
NSAID enteropathy (Bjarnason et al 1984e)
Investigation of miscellaneous disorders claimed to show enhanced permeability, e.g.
  rheumatoid arthritis (Bjarnason et al 1984f), atopic eczema (Bjarnason et al 1985),
  schizophrenia (Bjarnason et al 1984b), dermatitis herpetiformis (Bjarnason et al
  1984b)

certain drugs, particularly non-steroidal anti-inflammatory drugs (NSAID), can cause an increase in permeability and thus careful clinical documentation of the patients is necessary.

The ^{51}Cr-EDTA test essentially measures small bowel permeability. Gastritis due to various causes, including pernicious anaemia, alcohol and even severe gastritis with protein-losing enteropathy is not, on its own, associated with increased permeability (I. Bjarnason, unpublished results). Similarly, pancreatic insufficiency and biliary tract or hepatic diseases are not accompanied by enhanced permeability, although extensive studies of patients with these disorders have not been reported. It also seems that colonic inflammatory disease, with the exception of severe extensive ulcerative colitis, is not associated with increased ^{51}Cr-EDTA absorption.

ANATOMICAL AND BIOCHEMICAL BASIS OF THE INTESTINAL PERMEABILITY BARRIER

In spite of the extensive studies and widespread interest in various methods for measuring intestinal permeability in man, the nature of the 'barrier' under investigation is uncertain. It is widely quoted that the various monosaccharides, such as mannitol and rhamnose, pass via brush border pores, through the enterocytes and into the sub-mucosa. This would account for the significant absorption of these probes (approx. 15%) by normal subjects. However, the concept of the probe is a physiological one and has, as yet, no ultrastructural basis in the small intestine. The ability of certain monosaccharides, for example mannitol, to induce an osmotic gradient across the membrane of isolated intestinal brush border vesicles (Simpson and Peters 1984) argues against the existence of pores.

As discussed above, larger molecular weight (>250) probes are believed to pass between cells and thus are largely retarded by the various intercellular junctional complexes. PEG 400 would appear to be an exception to these generalisations as these polymers show significant absorption by normal subjects. However, they probably exist in solution as helical structures and thus their 'end-on' molecular radii are considerably less than that expected if a spherical structure is assumed. In addition, inspection of the molecular structure indicates a significant degree of hydrophobicity, so that the molecules may pass directly across cell membranes. The probes used in the in vitro studies probably assess cell-to-cell integrity of the enterocyte monolayer lining the gut lumen.

Although extensive ultrastructural studies of the epithelial cell junctional complexes in normal tissues have been made, little is known of their possible variation in disease. Reports of junctional complex alterations in untreated coeliac disease (Madara and Trier 1980; Madara et al 1980) probably reflect differences between the proliferative and non-proliferative zones of the villus. Nevertheless, the markedly increased permeability in untreated coeliac disease may be due to these differences. Clearly more detailed ultrastructural studies, particularly of the intercellular junctional complexes in patients with coeliac disease in apparently complete remission, are indicated.

It is also possible that the probes pass through regions of damaged or denuded enterocyte layer. Although this phenomenon is particularly prominent in the region of the villous tip, sub-epithelial cell bleb formations, typically described following ethanol-mediated damage (Millan et al 1980; Draper et al 1983), may also be associated with increased permeability. Studies aimed at correlating permeability in a variety of naturally occurring or experimentally induced mucosal lesions, with the extent of bleb formation, would be of interest. Cations also play an important role in maintaining mucosal integrity (Cassidy and Tidball 1967) and local depletion may contribute to permeability alterations.

It is postulated that cell-to-cell interactions may be stabilized by the formation of isopeptide bonds between adjacent cells (Folk 1980). These bonds are commonly formed between the ε-aminolysine residue of one polypeptide with the γ-carboxyglutamine residue of another and are synthesised by the enzyme transglutaminase. This activity has recently been demonstrated in the small intestine of both man (Bruce et al 1984a) and the rat (Bruce et al 1984b). Experimentally induced mucosal damage in the rat, produced by the acute administration of methotrexate, causes a marked, but transient, increase in permeability with a concomitant decrease in mucosal transglutaminase activity (Patel et al 1984). However, tissue localisation studies show that less than 2% of the activity is associated with the enterocytes or crypt cells and thus the causal relationship between the two phenomena is unclear.

The relationship between transglutaminase and coeliac disease is also of interest. Gluten, but not the deamidated non-toxic gluten, is an excellent substrate for intestinal transglutaminase; this enzyme might therefore be involved in the binding of gluten to various cell membranes, initiating the mucosal inflammatory reaction. It is therefore of particular interest that the mucosal activity of transglutaminase is increased in coeliac disease (Bruce et al 1984a). However, the importance of mucosal transglutaminase in maintaining the intestinal permeability barrier remains to be determined.

Our recent finding that NSAID's can rapidly, reversibly, but selectively increase intestinal permeability (Bjarnason et al 1984f), has implicated prostanoids in the maintenance of the permeability barrier. Prostanoids have long been implicated as mucosal cytoprotective agents (Ligumsky et al 1982) and the ^{51}Cr-EDTA absorption test may therefore be reflecting this function. A single dose of indomethacin or some other NSAID can transiently increase permeability in man (Figure 3.2). This is not a local effect, as similar results are obtained following rectally administered indomethacin.

It is of particular interest that indomethacin causes small bowel ulceration in experimental animals (Kent et al 1969; Wax et al 1970). The pathogenesis of the lesion is not certain, but it appears that the inhibition of prostanoid synthesis somehow causes a susceptibility to mucosal bacterial invasion, since the lesions are inhibited by prior antibiotic or prostaglandin adminstration (Robert and Asano 1977; Saton et al 1983). Whether a similar mechanism occurs in man is uncertain, but we are currently investigating whether exogenous prostaglandin adminstration inhibits the NSAID-induced permeability increase.

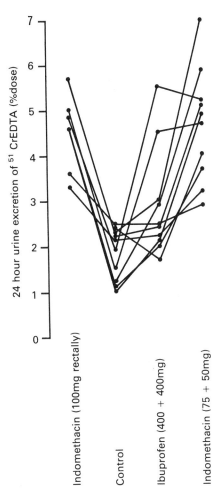

Figure 3.2. Urinary excretion (24 h) of ^{51}Cr-EDTA in control subjects after treatment with indomethacin either orally or rectally or after ibuprofen.

ALTERED PERMEABILITY IN INTESTINAL DISEASE

An extensive review of gastric intestinal disease associated with altered permeability is not appropriate in this chapter and the references listed in Table 3.2 provide suitable sources. However, certain diseases are worthy of mention, particularly since they are believed to be precipitated or perpetuated by dietary components.

Coeliac disease

The pathogenic role of gluten is well established, but the mechanism of tissue injury has still not been clarified. Permeability measurements have shown, both in vitro (Figure 3.3) and in vivo (Figure 3.4), that the mucosa of these patients is more permeable to low molecular weight probes than is normal mucosa. This abnormality persists in over 80% of patients, even after treatment for many years, with restoration of the mucosa to histological normality (Bjarnason et al 1984e). The in vitro studies suggest this increased permeability is selective for probes of molecular weight <1000. This is of interest, as the smallest toxic fragment of gluten that has been identified has a similar molecular weight range (Bronstein et al 1966; Offord et al 1978) and therefore, if enhanced permeability is a primary event in coeliac disease, entry of toxic gluten fragments could initiate the lesion, possibly by being selectively trapped by mucosal transglutaminase activity (Peters and Bjarnason 1984).

Inflammatory bowel disease

The ^{51}Cr-EDTA test clearly distinguishes between small and large bowel disease (Figure 3.5). Permeability is essentially normal in most cases of

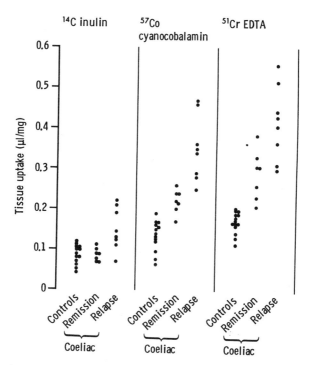

Figure 3.3. In vitro tissue uptake of three probes by control subjects and patients with coeliac disease. Each point represents mean of duplicate uptake experiments for each patient for 10 min incubations. From Bjarnason and Peters (1984), with kind permission of the editor of *Gut*.

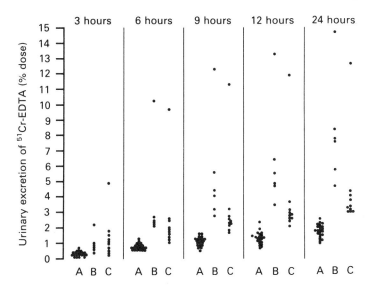

Figure 3.4. Cumulative urine secretion of ^{51}Cr-EDTA after oral ingestion by control subjects and patients with coeliac disease. A, control subjects; B, coeliac patients in relapse; C, coeliac patients in remission. From Bjarnason et al (1983b), with kind permission of the editor of *Lancet*.

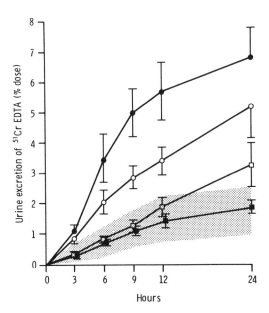

Figure 3.5. Cumulative urinary excretion of ^{51}Cr-EDTA after oral administration. The shaded area represents control subjects. The mean ($\pm$SE) excretion for small bowel Crohn's disease ($\bullet$), ileo-caecal Crohn's disease ($\circ$), colonic Crohn's disease ($\square$), and ulcerative colitis ($\blacksquare$), is shown.

typical ulcerative colitis, but is significantly increased in patients with small bowel Crohn's disease (Bjarnason et al 1983a). Patients with apparent Crohn's colitis may show enhanced ^{51}Cr-EDTA absorption (Figure 3.6), but where these patients have been carefully reinvestigated, many show evidence of small bowel involvement.

The relationship of the increased permeability to the pathogenesis of the intestinal lesion is uncertain. It is unlikely to be a primary event as patients with quiescent disease, particularly if they have had gut resections, may show normal permeability: permeability roughly correlates with extent and severity of the disease. Enhanced permeability, however, may perpetuate the inflammatory process by allowing entry of foreign proteins (probably bacterial and possibly dietary) into the mucosa. This is consistent with the observations

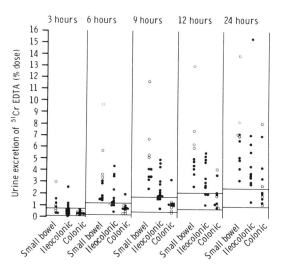

Figure 3.6. Cumulative urinary excretion of ^{51}Cr-EDTA by patients with Crohn's disease at different times after oral administration. The horizontal lines indicate the upper limit for normal subjects. Patients with active disease (○), patients with inactive disease (●). Reprinted by permission of Elsevier Science Publishing Co., Inc. from Bjarnason et al (1983a). Copyright 1982 by The American Gastroenterological Association.

tions that antibiotics may induce a remission, and with the precipitating effect of NSAID (Rampton et al 1983). Enhanced permeability may also contribute to the extra-intestinal manifestations of Crohn's disease, including hepatic damage, arthritis and other immune-complex phenomena. Development of drugs, dietary regimes, etc, aimed at reducing mucosal permeability, offer a potentially useful therapeutic approach.

Intestinal permeability in atopic eczema

Because of the possible role of dietary antigens, there have been several studies of intestinal permeability measurements in patients with eczema, but the results have often been conflicting. Thus Ukabam et al (1984) found increased permeability to lactulose, with normal permeability to mannitol, in contrast to Newton et al (1984) who found normal permeability to lactulose with reduced absorption of rhamnose. Du Mont et al (1984) have reported normal intestinal permeability in children with eczema.

Studies with poly(ethylene glycol)s (Jackson et al 1981) showed, paradoxically, that permeability to the smaller polymers (PEG 600) was normal but was increased to PEG 4000. However, these workers used an unvalidated turbidometric assay for measurement of urinary poly(ethylene glycol)s and their results can probably be discounted. Fälth–Magnusson et al (1984) have reported normal intestinal permeability to PEG in children with gastrointestinal allergy.

Our own studies (Bjarnason et al 1985), using the highly sensitive probe ^{51}Cr-EDTA for both in vitro and in vivo measurements of permeability, are shown in Figures 3.7 and 3.8, respectively. All but two of the 18 patients showed entirely normal permeability by both tests. One patient had previously undiagnosed gluten-sensitive coeliac disease and the other, with extensive eczema requiring systemic glucocorticoids, had minimal villous atrophy. This responded rapidly to the steroid therapy and the permeability rapidly and consistently returned to normal. It is therefore unlikely that, at least in adults, enhanced permeability is an important finding in eczema.

In children who more consistently show evidence of dietary sensitivity, permeability alterations may be contributory. However, in view of the

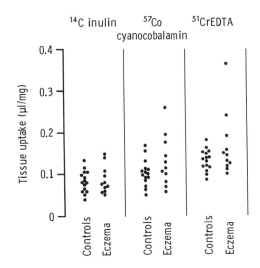

Figure 3.7. In vitro tissue uptake of three probes by jejunal mucosa from control subjects and patients with eczema. Each point represents mean of 2–4 uptake experiments for each patient for 3 and 10 min incubations. From Bjarnason et al (1985), with kind permission of the editor of *British Journal of Dermatology*.

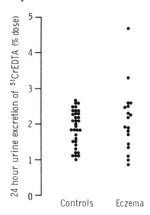

Figure 3.8. Total 24 h urinary excretion of ^{51}Cr-EDTA after oral ingestion by control subjects and patients with eczema. From Bjarnason et al (1985), with kind permission of the editor of *British Journal of Dermatology*.

frequent mucosal abnormalities found on intestinal biopsy in these children (McCalla et al 1980), permeability measurements alone would be unhelpful. Detailed sequential studies, correlating permeability with mucosal morphology and with degree and severity of skin involvement might be of interest, but it is unlikely that selectively increased intestinal permeability is an important aetiological factor in eczema.

CONCLUSIONS

This review compares and contrasts the three major approaches to assessing intestinal permeability. The ^{51}Cr-EDTA test is clearly the simplest and most sensitive test for routine clinical use and is rapidly gaining widespread acceptance. The in vitro test can be used to investigate further the site of the enhanced permeability; in patient studies some additional information can be gained by fractional urine collection. Permeability measurements have provided useful clues on the pathogenesis and aetiology of various intestinal and extra-intestinal disorders and have indicated potentially new and profitable lines of research. The ultrastructural and biochemical basis of the permeability changes remain an area where, as yet, little has been achieved.

REFERENCES

Bjarnason I & Peters T J (1984) In vitro determination of small intestinal permeability: demonstration of a persistent defect in patients with coeliac disease. *Gut* **25**: 145–150.
Bjarnason I, O'Morain C, Levi A J & Peters T J (1983a) Absorption of ^{51}Chromium-labelled ethylenediamine-tetraacetate in inflammatory bowel disease. *Gastroenterology* **85**: 318–322.
Bjarnason I, Peters T J & Veall N (1983b) A persistent defect in intestinal permeability in coeliac disease demonstrated by a ^{51}Cr-labelled EDTA absorption test. *Lancet* **1**: 323–325.

Bjarnason I, Levi A J, Wilkins R A & Peters T J (1984a) Ileal abnormalities and intestinal permeability. *Clinical Science* **67**: 10P.

Bjarnason I, Marsh M N, Levi A J et al (1984b) Intestinal permeability in coeliac sprue (CS), dermatitis herpetiformis (DH), schizophrenia (S) and atopic eczema (AE). *Gastroenterology* **86**: 1029.

Bjarnason I, Marsh M N, Levi A J, Price A & Peters T J (1984c) Mucosal recovery and permeability in gluten sensitive enteropathy. *Gut* **25**: A573.

Bjarnason I, Ward K & Peters T J (1984d) The leaky gut of alcoholism: possible route of entry for toxic compounds. *Lancet* **1**: 179–182.

Bjarnason I, Williams P, So A, Ansell B & Peters T J (1984e) Prostanoid inhibitors and intestinal permeability in man. *Gastroenterology* **86**: 1029.

Bjarnason I, Williams P, So A et al (1984f) Intestinal permeability and inflammation in patients with rheumatoid arthritis: effects of non-steroidal anti-inflammatory drugs. *Lancet* **ii**: 1171–1174.

Bjarnason I, Goolamali S K, Levi A J & Peters T J (1985) Intestinal permeability in patients with atopic eczema. *British Journal of Dermatology* **112**: 291–297.

Bronstein H D, Haeffner L J & Kowlessar O D (1966) Enzymatic digestion of glandin: the effect of the resultant peptides in adult coeliac disease. *Clinica Chimica Acta* **14**: 141–155.

Bruce S E, Bjarnason I & Peters T J (1984a) Jejunal transglutaminase: demonstration of activity, enzyme kinetics, substrate specificity and levels in patients with coeliac disease. *Clinical Science* **66**: 64P.

Bruce S E, Patel E & Peters T J (1984b) Transglutaminase activity of rat gastrointestinal tract. *Clinical Science* **66**: 64P.

Cassidy M M & Tidball C S (1967) Cellular mechanism of intestinal permeability alterations produced by chelation depletion. *Journal of Cell Biology* **32**: 685–698.

Chadwick V S, Phillips S F & Hofmann A F (1977a) Measurement of intestinal permeability using low molecular weight polyethylene glycols (PEG 400). I. Chemical analysis and biological properties of PEG 400. *Gastroenterology* **73**: 241–246.

Chadwick V S, Phillips S F & Hoffman A F (1977b) Measurements of intestinal permeability using low molecular weight polyethylene glycols (PEG 400). II. Application of normal and abnormal permeability states in man and animals. *Gastroenterology* **73**: 247–251.

Cox T M & Peters T J (1979) The kinetics of iron uptake in vitro by human duodenal mucosa: studies in normal subjects. *Journal of Physiology* **289**: 469–478.

Dawson D J, Barrow P C, Mahon M et al (1984) Validation of sugars as permeability probes in coeliac disease. *Clinical Science* **67**: 64P.

Draper L R, Gyuer L A, Hall J G & Robertson D (1983) Effect of alcohol on the integrity of the intestinal epithelium. *Gut* **24**: 399–404.

Duncombe V M, Watts R W E & Peters T J (1984) Studies on intestinal calcium absorption in patients with idiopathic hypercalcaemia. *Quarterly Journal of Medicine* **53**: 67–79.

DuMont G C L, Beach R C & Menzies I S (1984) Gastrointestinal permeability in food allergic eczematous children. *Clinical Allergy* **14**: 55–59.

Fälth-Magnusson K, Kjellman N I M, Magnusson K E & Sundqvist T (1984) Intestinal permeability in healthy and allergic children before and after sodium cromoglycate treatment assessed with different-sized polyetheylene glycols (PEG 400 and PEG 1000). *Clinical Allergy* **14**: 277–286.

Folk J E (1980) Transglutaminases. *Annual Review of Biochemistry* **49**: 517–531.

Jackson P G, Lessof M M, Baker R W R, Ferrett J & MacDonald D M (1981) Intestinal permeability in patients with eczema and food allergy. *Lancet* **1**: 1285–1286.

Jenkins R J, Goodacre R L, Rooney P R, Hunt R H & Bienstock J (1984) Intestinal permeability in inflammatory diseases. *Gut* **25**: A1166–1167.

Kent T H, Cardelli R M & Stamler F W (1969) Small intestinal ulcers and intestinal flora in rats given indomethacin. *American Journal of Pathology* **54**: 237–245.

Kowlessar O D, Haeffner L J & Bronstein H D (1964) Evidence for aminoaciduria and peptiduria in adult celiac disease. *Journal of Clinical Investigation* **43**: 1274.

Laker M F, Bull H J & Menzies I S (1982) Evaluation of mannitol for use as a probe marker of gastro-intestinal permeability in man. *European Journal of Clinical Investigation* **12**: 485–491.

Ligumsky M, Grossman M I P & Kauffman M L (1982) Endogenous gastric mucosal prostaglandins: their role in mucosal integrity. *American Journal of Physiology* **242**: G337–G341.

Madara J L & Trier J S (1980) Structural abnormalities of jejunal epithelial cell membranes in celiac sprue. *Laboratory Investigation* **43**: 254–264.

Madara J L, Trier J S & Neutra M R (1980) Structural changes in the plasma membrane accompanying differentiation of epithelial cells in human and monkey small intestine. *Gastroenterology* **76**: 963–975.

Magnusson K E & Sundqvist T (1984) Mathematical modelling for determining intestinal permeability using polyethylene glycol. *Gut* **25**: 428–429.

McCalla R, Saviahti E, Perkiö M, Kuitnen P & Backman A (1980) Morphology of the jejunum in children with eczema due to food allergy. *Allergy* **35**: 563–571.

Menzies I S (1974) Absorption of intact oligosaccharides in health and disease. *Biochemical Society Transactions* **2**: 1042–1047.

Menzies I S, Laker M F, Pounder R et al (1979) Abnormal intestinal permeability to sugars in villous atrophy. *Lancet* **1**: 1107–1109.

Millan M S, Morris G P, Beck I T & Henson J T (1980) Villous damage induced by suction biopsy and by acute ethanol intake in normal human small intestine. *Digestive Diseases and Sciences* **25**: 513–525.

Newton J A, Maxton D G, Bjarnason I et al (1984) Intestinal permeability in atopic eczema. *Clinical Science* **67**: 64–65P.

Offord R E, Anand B S, Piris J & Truelove S C (1978) Further subfractionation of digests of gluten. In McNicholl B, McCarthy C F & Fottrell P F (eds) *Perspectives in Coeliac Disease*, pp. 25–29. Lancaster: MTP Press.

O'Morain C, Cherva L R, Milstein D M & Das K M (1984) Chromium-51-EDTA and technetium-99m-DPTA for assessment of small bowel Crohn's disease. *Journal of Nuclear Medicine* **25**: P60.

Patel E, Bjarnason I, Smethurst P & Peters T J (1984) Intestinal permeability and transglutaminase alterations in methotrexate-induced enteropathy in the rat. *Clinical Science* **67**: 65P.

Peters T J & Bjarnason I (1984) Coeliac syndrome: biochemical mechanisms and the missing peptidase hypothesis revisited. *Gut* **25**: 913–918.

Peters T J, Raja K B & Simpson R J (1985) Comparison of in vitro and in vivo measurements of Fe^{3+} fluxes across mouse intestinal brush border membranes. *Journal of Physiology* **354**: 36P.

Raja, K B, Bjarnason I, Simpson R J & Peters T J (1985) In vitro measurement and adaptive response of Fe^{3+} uptake by mouse intestine. *American Journal of Physiology* in press.

Rampton D S, McNeil N I & Sarner M (1983) Analgesic ingestion and other factors preceding relapse in ulcerative colitis. *Gut* **24**: 187–189.

Robert A & Asano T (1977) Resistance of germ-free rats to indomethacin-induced intestinal lesions. *Prostaglandins* **14**: 333–341.

Russell R I, Misiewicz J J, Smith J A & Wiggins H S (1970) An assessment of the value of ^{51}Cr-EDTA and ^{51}CrCl$_3$ as non-absorbable intestinal markers by perfusion techniques. *Scottish Medical Journal* **15**: 236.

Saton H, Guth P H & Grossman M J (1983) Role of bacteria in gastric ulceration produced by indomethacin in the rat: cytoprotective action of antibiotics. *Gastroenterology* **84**: 483–489.

Scott J & Peters T J (1983) Protection of epithelial function in human jejunum cultured with hydrocortisone. *American Journal of Physiology* **244**: G532–540.

Selby P, McElwain T J, Crofts M, Lopes N & Mundy J (1984) ^{51}Cr-EDTA test for intestinal permeability. *Lancet* **2**: 39.

Simpson R J & Peters T J (1984) Studies of Fe^{3+} transport across isolated intestinal brush border membrane of the mouse. *Biochimica et Biophysica Acta* **772**: 220–226.

Ukabam S O, Mann R J & Cooper B T (1984) Small intestinal permeability to sugars in patients with atopic eczema. *British Journal of Dermatology* **110**: 649–652.

Wax J, Clinger W A, Vamer P, Bass P & Winder C V (1970) Relationship of the entero-hepatic cycle to ulcerogenesis in the rat small bowel with flufenamic acid. *Gastroenterology* **58**: 772–780.

Weser E & Sleisenger M H (1965) Lactosuria and lactose deficiency in adult celiac disease. *Gastroenterology* **48**: 571–578.

Chapter 4
Reduction of Postprandial Glycaemia by Dietary Manipulation

N. W. Read and I. McL. Welch

The diet of people living in the industrial countries of Western Europe, North America and Australasia includes large amounts of refined sugars and starches. These forms of carbohydrate are rapidly digested and absorbed, producing high postprandial blood glucose concentrations. In consequence, large amounts of insulin are released and the blood sugar drops rapidly to below fasting levels about 2 hours after a meal is ingested (Jenkins 1983). This rebound hypoglycaemia causes the person to feel hungry and eat more food. Release of large amounts of insulin is thought to lead to reduced sensitivity of insulin receptors and relative insulin resistance, a factor which may be crucial to the development of diabetes mellitus and obesity. Slowing the absorption of carbohydrate reduces the postprandial rise in plasma glucose and the secretion of insulin (Jenkins 1983), inducing a prolonged feeling of satiety (Krotkiewski, 1984); thus it is an effective way of treating diabetes mellitus and possibly obesity (Anderson and Ward 1978).

DELAY OF CARBOHYDRATE ABSORPTION

Carbohydrate absorption can be delayed by various simple modifications of the diet. These include the addition of viscous polysaccharides, the incorporation of foods that are either digested slowly or not at all by pancreatic enzymes (slow release carbohydrate), and the addition of fat and protein to carbohydrate foods. Cooking of food for shorter periods of time, and reduction in the mastication of food also reduce postprandial blood glucose levels.

The addition of viscous polysaccharides

The addition of viscous polysaccharides, such as guar gum, pectin, gum tragacanth, carboxymethyl cellulose, isphaghula and xanthan to drinks containing glucose reduces postprandial blood glucose levels (Jenkins et al 1978; Blackburn et al 1984a,b, 1985; Jarjis et al 1984). Plasma insulin levels are also lowered (Figure 4.1), in response partly to lower blood glucose levels and partly to the reduction in the release of glucose-dependent insulinotrophic peptide (GIP) from the duodenal and jejunal mucosae (Morgan et al 1979). The lower postprandial release of insulin suggests that the improvement in

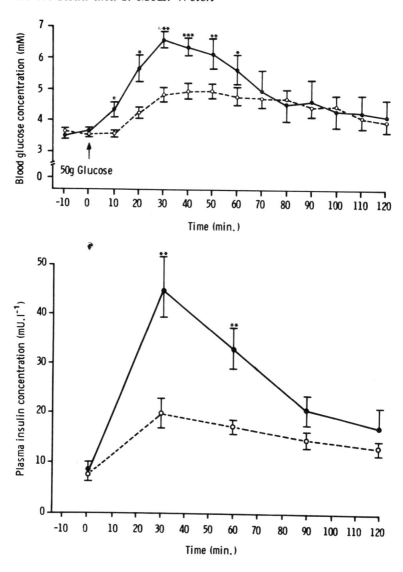

Figure 4.1. The effect of incorporating 14.5 g of guar (○) into a 250 ml drink of orange juice containing 50 g of glucose (●) on blood glucose and plasma insulin levels. Results are expressed as mean ± SEM of eight observations; *indicates significant differences between the pairs of data. From Blackburn et al (1984a), with kind permission of the authors and the editor of *Clinical Science*.

glucose tolerance caused by viscous polysaccharides is related to a delay in glucose absorption.

Similar effects have been observed if viscous polysaccharides are incorporated with a test meal (Jenkins et al 1976), but it is essential that the polysaccharide should be mixed intimately with the meal if any reduction in blood glucose is to be achieved (Jenkins et al 1979). If the viscous polysaccharide is given as a drink independently of the meal, there may well be little or no effect (Blackburn et al 1985).

Action of viscous polysaccharides

The effect of the different polysaccharides on the glycaemic response to a drink of glucose is directly related to the viscosity of the solution (Jenkins et al 1978). Increasing the viscosity of the gut contents reduces the rate of absorption, probably by impeding the access of nutrients to the absorptive epithelium. Viscous solutions resist the effect of gastro-intestinal contractions, inhibiting both propulsion and mixing; thus the emptying of food from the stomach (Leeds et al 1978; Holt et al 1979; Blackburn et al 1984a) and its transit along the intestine are delayed (Forman and Schneeman 1982; Blackburn et al 1984b) while the interactions between food and digestive enzymes (Dunaif and Schneeman 1981) and between the products of digestion and epithelium are also reduced. Studies of the action of viscous polysaccharides may therefore provide important insights into the role of intestinal motor activity in enhancing the absorption of food.

The reduction in postprandial glycaemia by viscous polysaccharides was originally thought to be dominated by their action in delaying the delivery of food from the stomach to the small intestine for, if given in sufficiently high concentrations, they delay gastric emptying (Leeds et al 1978; Holt et al 1979; Blackburn et al, 1984a,b). Moreover, if the delivery of gastric contents into the small intestine is slowed by propantheline, postprandial blood glucose levels are lower (Holt et al 1979). Despite these observations, we were unable to demonstrate any correlation between viscous polysaccharides and their effects on gastric emptying and blood glucose levels (Blackburn et al 1984a); administration of guar gum to a glucose drink can cause reductions in glucose tolerance in the absence of any change in gastric emptying, while another viscous polysaccharide, locust bean gum, may reduce blood glucose levels while actually accelerating gastric emptying (Blackburn et al, unpublished data). Thus while in some subjects, the delay in gastric emptying may contribute to the reduction in postprandial glycaemia induced by some viscous polysaccharides, the predominant action of these viscous substances is probably in the small intestine.

The addition of guar (Blackburn et al 1984a) or pectin (Flourie et al 1984) to solutions of saline and glucose used to perfuse segments of upper small intestine in human volunteers, reduces the rate of absorption of glucose (Figure 4.2), confirming that viscous polysaccharides have a direct action on the human small intestine. The mechanism of action of viscous polysaccharides on the small intestine has not been resolved. It seems likely that they act in the intestinal lumen to impede the access of glucose to the epithelium; the question then is whether this impeded access is caused by a resistance to mixing, or to inhibition of diffusion. We attempted to assess the relative importance of these two mechanisms by measuring the conductivity of solutions containing guar gum and different concentrations of saline (Edwards and Read, unpublished data). Addition of guar to achieve concentrations similar to those effective in man did not influence the conductivity of the

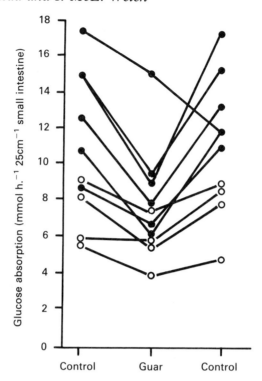

Figure 4.2. The effect of guar (6 g/l) on glucose absorption from the jejunum in 12 normal volunteers; (●) infusate containing glucose at 30 mmol/l, (○) infusate containing glucose at 15 mmol/l. From Blackburn et al (1984a), with kind permission of the authors and the editor of *Clinical Science*.

saline (Figure 4.3), suggesting that the effects observed in man were not related to impairment of diffusion. On the other hand, guar increased the time taken for a mixture of two solutions containing different concentrations of saline to achieve homogeneous conductivity (Figure 4.3). These observations suggest that guar impairs mixing rather than diffusion.

Viscous polysaccharides could also retard absorption in the small intestine by reducing the length of intestine exposed to luminal contents. Immediately after a meal is eaten, the head of the meal is spread along the intestine down as far as the ileum, coming into contact with a large number of absorptive sites (Jian et al 1984). Viscous polysaccharides resist the propulsion of food along the small intestine and slow small bowel transit (Forman and Schneemans 1982; Blackburn et al 1984b). However, studies on volunteers in which the distribution in the small intestine of a radiolabelled drink of glucose was mapped, using a gamma camera, showed that addition of 9 g of guar gum to the drink did not confine the solution to a shorter length of small intestine at the time of the peak glycaemic response (Blackburn et al 1984b). Moreover, when solutions containing glucose were confined to the upper 55 cm of intestine by the inflation of an intestinal balloon, the blood glucose levels

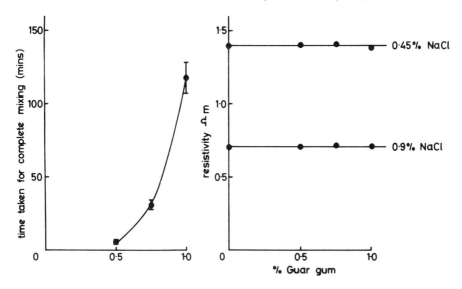

Figure 4.3. The effect of incorporating guar on the resistivity of two saline solutions and on the time taken for these solutions to attain homogeneous composition when mixed together. Mixing was achieved by removing a barrier between the high conductivity and low conductivity solutions and then rotating at 78 revolutions per min on a turntable.

were only slightly reduced when compared with those obtained from studies in which glucose solutions were allowed to flow freely down the small intestine (Blackburn et al 1984a). Thus, the reduction of the area of epithelium in contact with nutrients does not seem to be an important factor in explaining the action of guar gum on glucose tolerance, although it could possibly limit the absorption of nutrients from solid meals containing more complex carbohydrates.

'Second meal effect'

The ingestion of viscous polysaccharides not only reduces the blood glucose response following meals in which these substances are incorporated, but may also reduce the blood glucose response to the next meal (Jenkins et al 1980a). This is why long-term administration of food gums may aid diabetic control, even though the gums are not mixed with food. One explanation suggested for the 'second meal effect' is that viscous polysaccharides coat the epithelium of the small intestine providing a barrier to the diffusion of nutrients from the next meal (Blackburn and Johnson 1981; Johnson and Gee 1981). Epithelial coating has been observed in everted segments of rat small intestine pre-incubated with guar (J. M. Gee, personal communication). It is unlikely, however, that the same effect occurs in man; we found that absorption from a segment of human jejunum perfused with a glucose–electrolyte solution was unimpaired in the perfusion period following exposure to guar gum, and the thickness of the juxtamucosal diffusion barrier, the so-called 'unstirred layer', was unchanged (Blackburn et al 1984a).

An alternative explanation for the 'second meal effect' is that glucose absorption is delayed by the presence of nutrients in the ileum. Since viscous polysaccharides delay absorption, Jenkins (1983) has suggested that when these substances are ingested with food more nutrients reach the ileum. It is probable, therefore, that nutrients are still present in the lower small intestine as the next meal is being ingested. Infusion of nutrients, particularly fat, into the ileum reduces the postprandial glucose and insulin responses to ingestion of a meal of mashed potato (Figure 4.4) or a drink of glucose (Welch and Read, unpublished data). The mechanisms which underly these effects are discussed below.

Slow release carbohydrate

Ingestion of different foods which contain the same amounts of carbohydrate yield widely differing effects on blood glucose levels and insulin release (Crapo et al 1977, 1980; Jenkins et al 1981); root vegetables such as potato

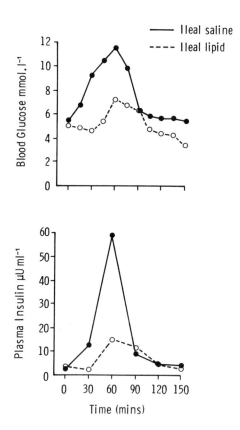

Figure 4.4. Plasma insulin and glucose responses to a carbohydrate meal during infusion of intralipid (○) or saline (●) into the ileum of one typical subject.

often give the largest, and legumes the smallest, effects. In general, the effect of a food is directly related to its digestibility by salivary and pancreatic amylases (Jenkins et al 1982a), although this relationship is not true for all substances. For example, ground lentils gave lower glucose and insulin responses than predicted by their in vitro digestibility (O'Dea and Wong 1983). Some legumes and other foods such as oats contain much of their carbohydrate in the form of non-starch polysaccharides, which cannot be digested by pancreatic enzymes. Some of these polysaccharides may form viscous mixtures in the small intestine and impair the absorption of other nutrients by virtue of their viscosity (Jenkins et al 1980b). Fructose, which is present in large amounts in some fruits, raises the blood glucose concentration less than glucose itself (Bohanum et al 1978). The ratio of straight chain amylose and branched amylopectin in different starches may be important; bean starch has a higher amylose/amylopectin ratio and is digested more slowly (Jenkins et al 1982b). Factors which may influence the digestibility of carbohydrate are listed in Table 4.1.

Table 4.1. Factors which may reduce the digestion and absorption of carbohydrate foods.

Presence of non-starch polysaccharides
Increased viscosity
Amylose/amylopectin ratio
Interactions with cell wall
Interactions with protein
Presence of fat
Presence of pharmacologically active substances
  (e.g. exorphins, tryptophan)
Phytates
Lectins
Amylase inhibitors
Large particle size
Shorter cooking times
Inadequate chewing

Interactions between polysaccharide and other components of food

Interactions between the carbohydrate and protein may impair digestibility; cake which is stiffened with egg white has a relatively low glycaemic index (46%) compared with wheat starch (80%) (Jenkins et al 1981).

The protection of carbohydrate by a cell wall composed of cellulose or lignin may also impair digestibility. Haber and his colleagues (1977) fed human subjects apple, apple purée and apple juice containing equivalent amounts of carbohydrate. They observed that plasma insulin responses were much less after whole apple than after apple juice and that there was less rebound hypoglycaemia after giving whole apple. Sweetcorn or legumes also have a waxy coat which needs to be chewed before the carbohydrate can be released.

Enzyme and transport inhibitors

Inhibitors of pancreatic amylase activity are found in some plant foods, such as wheat and red kidney beans (Folsch 1983). Some of these substances may be rapidly degraded by pepsin and trypsin, but an alpha-amylase inhibitor of microbial origin, acarbose, is very effective at reducing postprandial glucose and insulin levels (Caspary et al 1983; Folsch 1983) (see Chapter 2).

Apple pips contain phlorizin which is a competitive inhibitor of glucose absorption in the small intestine, but it is not known whether anybody has ever suffered carbohydrate malabsorption from eating apple cores!

Particle size

O'Dea and her colleagues (1980, 1981) found that ground rice or lentils produced greater insulin and glucose effects than whole rice. These changes were associated with increases in in vitro digestibility, and can be explained by increase in the surface area available for attack by digestive enzymes. Particle size will also influence gastric emptying; small particles will enter the small intestine more rapidly than large ones (Meyer et al 1979).

Effects of cooking and chewing

Cooking causes the starch granules to swell and burst increasing the surface area available to digestive enzymes. Plasma glucose and insulin responses to cooked corn starch are much greater than those to raw starch (Collings et al 1981) (Figure 4.5).

Chewing breaks up food into smaller particles, enhancing the delivery of food to the small intenstine and increasing its surface area so that it is more easily attacked by digestive enzymes; it also encourages the flow of saliva containing amylase, which will initiate carbohydrate digestion in the mouth and stomach. In a recent experiment, normal volunteers ingested two lots of 50 g samples of different carbohydrate foods; new potatoes and apples diced into 4 mm cubes, rice and sweetcorn. On one occasion the subject was instructed to chew the food thoroughly fourteen times; on the other occasion the subject was instructed to swallow the food whole. The rate of ingestion was the same in the two experiments. Swallowing the food whole caused large reductions in the glycaemic response to all four foods (Figure 4.6) (Read et al 1985).

The effect of other nutrients

We have recently shown that the infusion of lipid into the distal small intestine flattens the glycaemic responses to a starch or glucose drink and reduces postprandial insulin levels (Welch and Read, unpublished data) (Figure 4.4). The same stimulus also delays gastric emptying and small bowel transit time (Read et al 1984) and inhibits pancreatic secretion (Harper et al 1979). These responses have been collectively termed the 'ileal brake'. Similar effects on gastric emptying are obtained when fat is infused into the duodenum and jejunum. Thus the incorporation of fat in meals may reduce the absorption of carbohydrate by several mechanisms; pastry, for example,

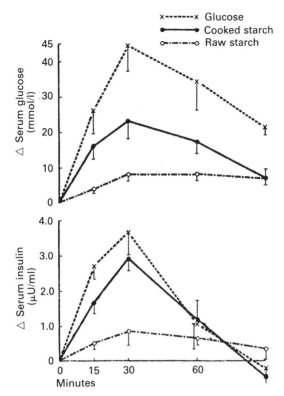

Figure 4.5. Plasma insulin and glucose concentrations after ingestion of glucose, raw starch and cooked starch. Results are shown as mean ± SEM. From Collings et al (1981), with kind permission of the authors and the editor of the *British Medical Journal*.

which contains a high proportion of fat, has a relatively low glycaemic index (59%) (Jenkins et al 1981). Since infusion of lipid into the ileum inhibits pancreatic secretion and delays small bowel transit, it seems likely that exposure of the ileum as well as the upper small intestine to nutrients will cause a more potent reduction in glucose and insulin responses than exposure of the upper small intestine alone. Infusion of lipid into the duodenum actually increases insulin secretin by release of GIP (Ebert and Creutzfeldt 1983).

The action of dietary fibre in delaying absorption may well result in more exposure of lower regions of the small intestine to nutrient material, especially when the next meal is being ingested. Thus the 'ileal brake' could account for the reduction in glycaemic response to the next meal eaten after the ingestion of viscous polysaccharide or slow release carbohydrate (Himsworth 1934; Jenkins 1983).

CONCLUSIONS

The dietary management of diabetes mellitus may have come full circle (Figure 4.7). Major dietary advice given to diabetics two decades ago was to

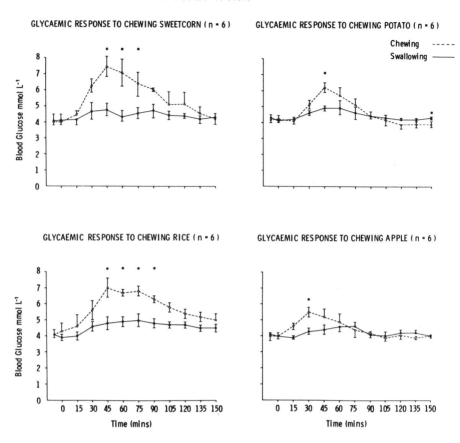

Figure 4.6. The effect of chewing on the plasma glucose responses to ingestion of four different carbohydrate foods; results shown as mean ± SEM.

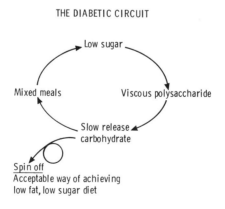

Figure 4.7. The diabetic circuit.

avoid sugars and other forms of carbohydrate. Then, with clearer understanding of the mode of action of certain forms of dietary fibre, viscous polysaccharides were advocated to slow the absorption of sugars. The knowledge that certain carbohydrate foods released sugars for absorption more slowly than other foods prompted the use of high legume diets; currently advocated in diabetic treatment. If it is established that the entry of fat into the small intestine may delay the absorption of the more rapidly absorbed forms of starch such as potato starch, we could again be back to advising diabetics to eat normal meals but to avoid sugars. It would be a mistake, however, to regard progression round the circuit as futile. Many diabetics are obese and it is essential for them to reduce intake of fat as well as sugar. The inclusion of a slow release carbohydrate in the diet, or the addition of viscous polysaccharides, offers a convenient and acceptable way of reducing the fat and sugar intake without reducing overall food intake.

REFERENCES

Anderson J W & Ward K (1978) Long term effects of high carbohydrate, high fibre diets on glucose and lipid metabolism; a preliminary report on patients with diabetes. *Diabetes Care* **1**: 77–82.

Blackburn N A & Johnson I T (1981) The effect of guar gum on the viscosity of the gastrointestinal contents and on glucose uptake from the perfused jejunum in the rat. *British Journal of Nutrition* **46**: 239–246.

Blackburn N A, Redfern J S, Jarjis H et al (1984a) The mechanism of action of guar gum in improving glucose tolerance in man. *Clinical Science* **66**: 329–336.

Blackburn N A, Holgate A M & Read N W (1984b) Does guar gum improve postprandial hyperglycaemia in humans by reducing small intestinal contact area. *British Journal of Nutrition* **52**: 197–204.

Bohanum N V, Karam J H & Forshan P H (1978) Advantages of fructose ingestion over sucrose and glucose in humans. *Diabetes* **27**: 438.

Caspary W F, Lembke B & Creutzfeldt W (1983) Delaying of carbohydrate absorption by glucosidase inhibitors. In Creutzfeldt W & Folsch U R (eds) *Delaying Absorption as a Therapeutic Principle in Metabolic Diseases,* pp. 87–96. Stuttgart: Georg Thieme Verlag.

Collings P, Williams C & Macdonald I (1981) Effects of cooking on serum glucose and insulin responses to starch. *British Medical Journal* **282**: 1032.

Crapo P A, Reaven G & Olefsky J (1977) Postprandial plasma glucose and insulin response to different complex carbohydrates. *Diabetes* **25**: 1178–1183.

Crapo P A, Kolterman O G, Waldeck N, Reaven G M & Olefsky J M (1980) Postprandial hormonal responses to different types of complex carbohydrate in individuals with impaired glucose tolerance. *American Journal of Clinical Nutrition* **33**: 1723–1728.

Dunaif G & Schneeman B O (1981) The effect of dietary fibre on human pancreatic enzyme activity in vitro. *American Journal of Clinical Nutrition* **34**: 1034–1035.

Ebert R & Creutzfeldt W (1983) Inhibition of absorption and impaired secretion of gastric inhibitory polypeptides (GIP). In Creutzfeldt W and Folsch U R (eds) *Delaying Absorption as a Therapeutic Principle in Metabolic Diseases,* pp 126–135. Stuttgart: Georg Thieme Verlag.

Flourie B, Vidon N, Florent C & Bernier J J (1984) Effect of pectin on jejunal glucose absorption and unstirred layer thickness in man. *Gut* **25**: 936–941.

Folsch U R (1983) Delaying of carbohydrate absorption by alpha-amylase inhibitors. In Creutzfeldt W & Folsch U R (eds) *Delaying Absorption as a Therapeutic Principle in Metabolic Diseases,* pp 78–85. Stuttgart: Georg Thieme Verlag.

Forman L P & Schneeman, B O (1982) Dietary pectins: effect on starch utilisation in rats. *Journal of Nutrition* **112**: 528–533.

Haber G B, Heaton K W, Murphy D & Burroughs L F (1977) Depletion and disruption of dietary fibre. Effects on satiety, plasma glucose and serum insulin. *Lancet* **2**: 679–682.

Harper A A, Hood A J C, Mushens J & Smy J R (1979) Inhibition of external pancreatic secretion by intracolonic and intraileal infusions in the cat. *Journal of Physiology* **292**: 445–454.

Himsworth H P (1934) Dietetic factors influencing the glucose tolerance and activity of insulin. *Journal of Physiology* **81**: 29–48.

Holt S, Heading R C, Carter D C, Prescott L F & Tothill P (1979) Effect of gel fibre on gastric emptying and absorption of glucose and paracetamol. *Lancet* **1**: 636–639.

Jarjis H, Blackburn N A, Redfearn J S & Read N W (1984) The effect of ispaghula (Fybogel and Metamucil) and guar gum on glucose tolerance in man. *British Journal of Nutrition* **51**: 371–378.

Jenkins D J A (1983) Fibre and delayed carbohydrate absorption in man: Lente carbohydrate. In Creutzfeldt W & Folsch U R (eds) *Delaying Absorption as a Therapeutic Principle in Metabolic Diseases*, pp. 45–56. Stuttgart: Georg Thieme Verlag.

Jenkins D J A & Wolever T M S (1981) Slow release carbohydrate and the treatment of diabetes *Proceedings of the Nutrition Society* **40**: 227–235.

Jenkins D J A, Leeds A R, Gassull M A et al (1976) Unabsorbable carbohydrates and diabetes decreased postprandial hyperglycaemia. *Lancet* **2**: 172–174.

Jenkins D J A, Wolever T M S, Leeds A R et al (1978) Dietary fibres analogues and glucose tolerance importance of viscosity. *British Medical Journal* **1**: 1392–1394.

Jenkins D J A, Nineham R & Craddock C (1979) Fibre and diabetes. *Lancet* **1**: 434–435.

Jenkins D J A, Wolever T M S, Nineham R et al (1980a): Improved glucose tolerance four hours afte taking guar with glucose. *Diabetologia* **19**: 21–24.

Jenkins D J A, Wolever T M S, Taylor R H, Barker H & Fielden H (1980b): Exceptionally low blood glucose response to dried beans: comparison with other carbohydrate foods. *British Journal of Medicine* **2**: 578–580.

Jenkins D J A, Wolever T M S, Taylor R H et al (1981) Glycaemic index of foods: a physiological basis for carbohydrate exchange. *American Journal of Clinical Nutrition* **34**: 362–366.

Jenkins D J A, Ghafari H, Wolever T M S et al (1982a): Relationship between the rate of digestion of foods and postprandial glycaemia. *Diabetologica* **22**: 450–455.

Jenkins D J A, Thorne M J, Camelan K et al (1982b) Effect of processing on digestibility and the blood glucose response: a study of lentils. *American Journal of Clinical Nutrition* **36** (6): 1093–1101.

Jian R, Nagean Y & Bernier J J (1984) Measurement of intestinal progression of a meal and its residue in normal subjects and patients with functional diarrhoea by dual isotope technique. *Gut* **25** 728–731.

Johnson I T & Gee J M (1981) Effect of gel forming gums on the intestinal unstirred layer and suga transport in vitro. *Gut* **22**: 398–403.

Krotkiewski M (1984) Effect of guar gum on body weight, hunger ratings and metabolism in obes subjects. *British Journal of Nutrition* **52**: 97–105.

Leeds A R, Ralphs D N, Boulas P et al (1978) Pectin and gastric emptying in dumping syndrome *Proceedings of the Nutrition Society* **37**: 23A.

Meyer J H, Thomson J B, Cohen M B, Shadcher A & Mandiola S A (1979) Sieving of solid food by th canine stomach and sieving after gastric surgery. *Gastroenterology* **76**: 804–813.

Morgan L M, Gaulder T J, Tsiolakis D, Marks V & Alberti K G M M (1979) The effect of unabsorbable carbohydrate on gut hormones. Modification of postprandial GIP secretion by guar. *Diabetolog* **17**: 85–89.

O'Dea K, Nestel P J & Antonoff L (1980) Physical factors influencing postprandial glucose and insuli responses to starch. *American Journal of Clinical Nutrition* **33**: 760–765.

O'Dea K, Snow P & Nestel P (1981) Rate of starch hydrolysis in vitro as a predictor of metaboli responses to complex carbohydrate in vivo. *American Journal of Clinical Nutrition* **34**: 1991–199⁷.

O'Dea K & Wong S (1983) The rate of starch hydrolysis in vitro does not predict the metabol responses to legumes in vivo. *American Journal of Clinical Nutrition* **38**: 382–387.

Read N W, McFarlane A, Kinsman R I & Bloom S R (1984) The effect of infusion of nutrient solution into the ileum on gastrointestinal transit and plasma levels of neurotensin and enteroglucagon *Gastroenterology* **86**: 274–280.

Read N W, Welch I McL, Austen C J, et al (1985) Swallowing food without chewing; a simple way reduce postprandial hyperglycaemia. (Submitted for publication.)

Welch I McL, Saunders K & Read N W (1985) The effect of ileal and intravenous infusion of f emulsions on feeding and satiety in human volunteers. *Gastroenterology* in press.

Chapter 5
Effect of Food on the Intestinal Microflora

Alison M. Stephen

The main focus of the effect of diet on the human intestinal microflora must be on those bacteria which inhabit the colon, since it is in the colon that the numbers of bacteria are particularly high, about 10^{11-12} per g compared with 10^4 per g in the stomach and 10^{5-7} per g in the small intestine. A new concept of the colonic microflora has developed in recent years, of a specialised organ weighing about 230 g (Banwell et al 1981) with a wide variety of functions. The effect of dietary components on this organ must therefore be considered seriously in any postulated mechanisms relating diet to disease.

The majority of the bacteria in the human colon, like those from the hind gut of other species, are obligately saccharolytic, that is, they require fermentable carbohydrate for growth (Salyers 1983). Many of our ideas about the human intestinal flora have been drawn from extensive research on the microbial population of the rumen, and although there are many similarities between these two systems in terms of the types of microbes and their metabolic activities, there remain several important differences (Table 5.1). The rumen is substrate-rich, receiving the total dietary intake of carbohydrate, whereas the human colonic flora is in an environment where sources of carbon and energy, in the form of carbohydrate, are limited. An organism growing in an environment with limited energy resources will not carry out reactions unless they are beneficial for its continued survival. The colon therefore imposes an economy on its flora which is not necessary in the rumen, nor in many in vitro systems, and this must always be taken into account when extrapolating microbial activities from such systems to the human large intestine.

Similar caution must be observed when comparing human bacterial metabolism and activity to other monogastrics, such as the rat or pig. Because of the difficulties of human experimentation much of the work on effects of diet on the intestinal microflora has been conducted on animals, particularly the rat. However, the hind gut microflora of the rat is vastly different from the human colonic microflora and, in addition, rats practise coprophagy, which presents a quite different source of nutrients to the animal. For example, B vitamins synthesised by the microflora almost certainly reach the animal following coprophagy, rather than by absorption following production (Haenel and Bendig 1975).

Table 5.1. Comparison between rumen and human colon.

Rumen	Human colon
Microflora	
Bacteria predominantly obligate anaerobes	Bacteria predominantly obligate anaerobes
Protozoa present	Protozoa absent
Bacteroides present in large numbers	Bacteroides present in large numbers
Bacteroides produce only succinate (B_{12} optional)	Bacteroides produce succinate and propionate (vitamin B_{12} required)
E. coli $10^{-5} - 10^{-6}$% of total viable count	*E. coli* 0.1–1.0% of total viable count
Methanogenic bacteria always present	<33% of individuals produce methane
Fermentation	
SCFA* major source of carbon and energy for metabolic activities	SCFA small contribution to total energy supply
Food protein converted to microbial protein — used by animal	Extent of degradation and absorption of microbial protein unknown
Microbial synthesis of B vitamins — essential for animal	Extent of microbial vitamin synthesis — unknown
Carbohydrate supply not usually limiting	Carbohydrate supply limiting
Nitrogen may be limiting	Nitrogen unlikely to be limiting
Branched-chain SCFA may be limiting	Role of branched-chain SCFA unknown
Cellulose degraded	Cellulose minimally degraded — long transits required

*SCFA = short chain fatty acids.

THE FAECAL FLORA

The human colon, particularly the right colon where microbial fermentation is at its most active, is almost inaccessible to direct observation. Intubation studies have been used on numerous occasions to study the terminal ileum and components entering the large intestine, but the strong absorptive forces in the colon and the resulting rapid reduction in water content following passage from the ileum (Debongnie and Phillips 1978), makes sampling from the colon through a multilumen tube virtually impossible. Hence investigators have been forced to examine the products of passage through the large intestine, namely stools. Much work on those species present in the human intestine, and of microbial interactions and effects on various substrates, has therefore been done using the faecal flora. In an effort to validate the use of faeces for such experiments Moore et al (1978) have examined the microflora of the colonic contents of victims of sudden death and have confirmed that the faeces contain a representative population of those bacteria present in the colon.

One major objective in examining the total bacterial content of stools has been the investigation of those factors which control faecal weight. Until recently, estimates of the bacterial content of stools were based on total bacterial counts and the size of typical bacteria, and these suggested that the microflora contributes 30–40% of faecal weight (Van Houte and Gibbons 1966; Moore and Holdeman 1975). In order to obtain a more direct estimate of bacterial mass, a gravimetric procedure based on methods from ruminant work was devised, and has now been used in a number of studies to estimate changes in microbial mass when colonic function has been modified by various means (Stephen and Cummings 1980a,b). Using this method it has been found that, for individuals on a typical western diet, bacteria contribute roughly 55% of dry stool weight (Stephen and Cummings 1980c). When converted to a wet weight, bacteria being about 80% water (Luria 1960) the faecal microflora account for 65–70% of stools, a far higher estimate than those obtained from bacterial counts. The reason for the difference between values using this method and previous indirect measurements may be related to differences in microbial composition which occur when bacteria are in a natural environment, rather than an artificial one. Bacteria in various habitats produce extracellular coats external to their outer membrane (Fletcher and Floodgate 1973; Costerton et al 1974; Patterson et al 1975). These are composed of polysaccharides or globular proteins and used to anchor the bacteria and stabilise their location, to adhere to food particles or other bacteria, or to protect the cell against predatory bacteria, antibodies, antibiotics or harmful molecules and ions. Many bacteria produce such coats in their normal environment, thus adding to their overall weight, but do not do so in culture (Shands 1966).

Starvation and low residue diets

In the colonic environment, without any dietary input of carbohydrate, the activity of the colonic microflora is severely restricted, but does continue, as shown by studies of starvation and low residue diets. Finegold and Sutter (1978) have reported that under total starvation, otherwise healthy individuals had bowel movements once every 30 days or so. Interestingly, the small amount of faeces produced contained the same types and numbers of bacteria as these subjects had on a normal diet. For individuals eating low residue diets, consisting of amino acids, glucose, oil, vitamins and electrolytes, where no dietary constituents would be anticipated to reach the large gut, stools are produced every 2–3 days, with an average daily output of 40–50 g (Winitz et al 1970; Kies and Fox 1976; McCamman et al 1977). In the absence of dietary residue in the stool, much of this small faecal output must be bacterial and a number of endogenous sources, such as the glycoproteins of intestinal mucus, sloughed epithelial cells and intestinal secretions, must supply the carbon and energy for this population. As far as is known, there is adequate nitrogen for the colonic microflora, largely in the form of ammonia, derived from the breakdown of urea from the circulation or from protein and peptides entering the colon from the upper gastrointestinal tract. Minerals and vitamins are also likely to be in adequate supply.

Of several investigations of the faecal flora of individuals on low residue diets, that of Winitz et al (1970) reported dramatic decreases in many bacterial species, such that only essentially three types, bacteroides, coliforms and enterococci remained. No subsequent study has confirmed such changes, finding only small decreases in one or two species. Attebery et al (1972) noted increased enterobacteria and clostridia while Crowther et al (1973) reported increased enterobacteria and decreased enterococci. However, Bornside and Cohn (1975) found no significant differences in bacterial species with such diets and it would appear that the overall bacterial profiles remain virtually unchanged in the absence of dietary input.

FOOD AND THE INTESTINAL MICROFLORA

Dietary constitutents can affect the colonic microflora either directly, by their passage through the upper gastrointestinal tract and into the large intestine, or indirectly, either by altering secretory processes in the upper gut with resultant changes in components entering the colon through the ileocaecal junction, or by affecting the physiological functions of the colon; the host metabolism may be modified in other ways, such that the requirements of the colonic microflora are affected.

There are various ways of looking at the effects of changes in diet on the colonic microflora: the traditional approach is to examine faecal bacterial profiles. Particular bacterial species carry out metabolic reactions which are different from those of other species, resulting in varying products; other species survive only under certain environmental conditions; still others grow only if necessary growth factors are available. Hence changes in bacterial species should indicate alterations in the colonic environment, and may be used to predict the likelihood of the development of disease, when compared with bacterial profiles in disease states or from population studies.

In recent years another approach has been used extensively in investigation of colonic microbial activity, namely the study of bacterial enzymes and their products. In particular, the observation that populations at high risk for cancer of the colon have a microflora with an increased ability to metabolise steroids and glucuronides, has led to many investigations of the enzymes which carry out such reactions. β-glucuronidase hydrolyses glucuronide conjugates, some of which may be conjugates of toxins or carcinogens excreted by the liver. High levels of β-glucuronidase may therefore indicate a risk for cancer through a reactivation of such carcinogens. Further evidence that β-glucuronidase is such an indicator comes from findings that activity of the enzyme is higher in, for example, the American population with a high risk of colonic cancer and very low in populations with a low risk, like the Japanese and Chinese (Reddy and Wynder 1973).

Similarly, faecal bile acids, particularly secondary bile acids, have been investigated in varying dietary conditions, as has 7-α-hydroxylase, the enzyme which produces the secondary acid. As with β-glucuronidase, faecal bile acids, particularly deoxycholic acid and lithocholic acid, are higher in populations with a high risk of colonic cancer (Hill and Aries 1971; Reddy and Wynder 1973). Bile acids, particularly deoxycholate, cause gross epithelial damage to the colonic musosa when applied experimentally in animals (Saunders et al 1975; Goerg et al 1982) and enhance tumour formation in carcinogen-treated animals (Reddy et al 1976).

A third and still more recent way of looking at the colonic microflora is to examine the overall mass of bacteria produced, as in the gravimetric method described earlier. Not only does this give an indication of overall bacterial growth and provision of substrate, but it also provides a sample of pure bacteria from the stool for investigation of changes in bacterial composition under different conditions. This approach gives more information on substrate utilization and the colonic environment than the other two methods, but little about particular reactions of interest. In order to gain an overall picture of how food affects the microflora, it is therefore necessary to consider each of these indicators of microbial function.

THE TYPICAL WESTERN DIET

The passage of nutrients into the colon of individuals on a typical Western diet, and the excretion of the major components in stools are shown in Figure 5.1. Alterations in diet may alter the content of one or more of these nutrients and thus affect the microflora and excretion in stools. The effects of each of the major nutrients, fat, protein and carbohydrate, will be considered in turn. Since carbohydrate is the major source of energy for the colonic microflora and therefore has the greatest influence on it, and since it modifies the effects of both fat and protein, it is considered last and in the greatest detail.

Fat

Little fat reaches the large intestine directly, only 1.5–3.8 g/day having been found in the ileostomy effluents of individuals on their normal diets (Kramer

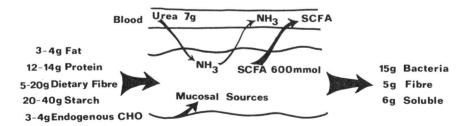

Figure 5.1. The daily supply of major nutrients to the colonic microflora from the upper gastro-intestinal tract and the circulation, and the excretion of major components of stools for a typical Western diet. SCFA = short chain fatty acids, CHO = carbohydrate, NH_3 = ammonia.

Table 5.2. Fat and bacterial species.

Reference	Dietary change	Bacterial profile
Glatzel (1963)	60% intake compared with normal	*Lactobacillus bifidus* ↓ Enterococci ↓ Bacteroides ↑
Reddy et al (1975)	High fat, high meat compared with meatless	Bacteroides ↑ *Bifidobacterium* ↑ Peptococci ↑ Lactobacilli ↑ Streptococci ↓ Staphylococci ↓ Bacilli ↑ Enterobacteria ↓
Drasar & Jenkins (1976)	+ 60 g olive oil + 60 g MCT*	No change
Cummings et al (1978b)	+ 90 g animal fat	No change

*Medium chain triglycerides.

et al 1962). This level can be markedly reduced by the omission of fat from the diet (Wiggins et al 1969), and therefore the amount passing into the colon depends in part on the content of fat in the diet.

The normal stool contains about 3 g of fat per day (Cummings et al 1978b). With estimates of bacterial fat content of 10–15% for pure cultures (Luria 1960) and 12–20% for mixed rumen populations (Czerkawski 1976), the faecal microflora accounts for over 70% of faecal fat output. Hence most of the faecal fat has been synthesised or modified by the bacteria, and this is confirmed by the composition of fatty acids in stools, which are predominantly saturated or have uneven numbers of carbon atoms, unlike the products of human metabolism (Webb et al 1963; Cummings et al 1978b). Fat not in bacteria is probably endogenous, derived from bile, the intestinal mucosa, or discarded epithelial cells, with a minimal proportion of unchanged fat being derived from the diet. The predominance of faecal fat in bacteria serves to explain normal excretion of fat in stools of individuals on fat-free diets (Lewis and Partin 1954).

Increases in dietary fat have been found to have no effect on faecal weight (Antonis and Bersohn 1962; Cummings et al 1978b) although they do result in increased excretion of fatty acids (Cummings et al 1978b). This, plus the observation of increased fatty acid excretion in patients with steatorrhea (Webb et al 1963), serves to demonstrate that the colonic microflora do not use fat as an energy source and, moreover, seem reluctant to degrade it.

Fat and bacterial species

In mixed microbial systems, such as in vitro culture or in the rumen, long chain fatty acids have an inhibitory effect on some bacteria, particularly gram positive organisms (Galbraith and Miller 1973; Maczulak et al 1981), but this effect has never been investigated using the human microflora.

Table 5.2 shows the results of several experiments to investigate changes in dietary fat on microbial species in human stools. Differences in dietary manipulation or bacteriological methods may explain the conflicting results although, in any case, the changes reported are small and fat appears to have little effect on bacterial profiles.

Fat and bacterial enzyme activity

Epidemiological studies have shown a close relationship between fat intake and incidence of colorectal cancer throughout the world (Armstrong and Doll 1975) and for this reason, numerous studies have been conducted on the effect of fat on the intestinal microflora, mainly on bacterial enzyme activities and products. However, there are several difficulties with the evidence obtained so far. Firstly, the close positive relationship between fat intake and colonic cancer is not shown for different areas within a country (Bingham et al 1979; Jensen et al 1982) nor was it demonstrated in a prospective study, where the fat intake of those who later developed colonic cancer was compared with that in matched controls (Stemmermann et al 1984). Secondly, much of the work on fat and enzyme activities which is said to substantiate the epidemiological findings has been conducted in animals, particularly the rat, and its relevance to the human colon is unknown. In this work, emphasis has been placed on the activity of β-glucuronidase, yet the importance of this enzyme has not been firmly established, nor has the significance of different levels of activity in man.

Studies in the rat have repeatedly found raised β-glucuronidase activity with increases in dietary fat and it has been suggested that this is mediated by increased bile acid concentrations, for β-glucuronidase activity has been found to increase when rat faecal microflora are treated with bile acids (Reddy et al 1977; Mallett et al 1983, 1984). However two human studies gave conflicting results. Reddy et al (1975) found that β-glucuronidase activity was raised on a high fat, high meat diet, compared with a meatless diet, whereas Cummings et al (1978b) found no change in β-glucuronidase when only fat in the diet was altered. It is therefore difficult, at present, to draw any conclusions about fat and β-glucuronidase in man and its importance in disease.

Fat and bile acid metabolism

Most of the 20–30 g of bile acids secreted daily are reabsorbed in the lower ileum, with only a small proportion (0.5–1.0 g/day) passing into the large intestine (Hayakawa 1973). Those bile acids which escape reabsorption in the terminal ileum enter the large intestine, where they are deconjugated and dehydroxylated by the intestinal microflora to form the secondary bile acids, deoxycholic acid and lithocholic acid. These derivatives are poorly absorbed and therefore appear in the stool. That this conversion is bacterial in nature is shown by the fact the germ-free animals have no ability to deconjugate or dehydroxylate bile acids, which remain in an absorbable form (Gustafsson 1983).

The relationship between fat and bile acid metabolism is clearer and more persuasive than that of β-glucuronidase. Epidemiological studies have shown higher faecal bile acid levels in those areas with a high incidence of colonic cancer, where those at risk also had the highest intakes of fat (Hill and Aries 1971; Reddy and Wynder 1973). Others have shown a reduced capacity for 7α-dehydroxylation in low risk populations (Mastromarino et al 1976). Diets supplemented with fat result in a greater concentration of bile acids in the stools, in both human (Cummings et al 1978b) and animal experiments (Redinger et al 1973). However, dietary fat does not appear to alter 7α-hydroxylase activity in man as would be expected on the basis of the epidemiological evidence (Cummings et al 1978b).

In summary, despite several contradictory findings, the weight of evidence points to a relationship between dietary fat, bile acids and colonic cancer, and in such a scheme, the colonic microflora would be likely to play a central role.

Protein

It is generally assumed that protein is not a major energy source for the intestinal microflora. Only a few species, notably the clostridia, are known to utilise proteins as their sole source of carbon and energy and since these are present in low numbers in the human large intestine, their utilisation of protein for growth is unlikely to make any substantial contribution to overall bacterial mass (Salyers 1983). In the absence of adequate carbohydrate substrate however, bacteria may adapt to using the carbon skeletons of proteins instead of those of carbohydrate and the abundance in the colon of nitrogen compounds would suggest such an adaptation might be ecologically beneficial. Very little work has been done in this field, which is worth further investigation.

Between 200 g and 500 g of protein enters the lumen of the upper small intestine daily, in the form of dietary intake, pancreatic and intestinal secretions, sloughed epithelial cells and mucus (Nasset 1965). Of this vast amount most is reabsorbed and only a tiny fraction escapes into the colon. In ileostomy patients, this has been estimated to be about 2 g of nitrogen per day, equivalent to 12–13 g of protein (Kramer et al 1962). In healthy subjects, intubation studies with aspiration from the terminal ileum have shown a fasting level of protein entering the colon of 261 mg/h equivalent to 6.3 g of protein per day. When the effect of three meals a day was taken into account, an extra 7.3 g protein per day was estimated to enter the colon, giving a total of 13.6 g as the average for seven normal individuals (Stephen, Haddad and Phillips, in preparation). Hence the presence of food increases the amount of protein reaching the colonic microflora directly, although it is not clear whether this is derived from the diet or whether it represents an increase in endogenous protein as a result of eating. Ileostomy studies also have shown that an increase in dietary protein brings about a greater excretion of protein in the ileostomy effluent (Gibson 1977).

On a typical Western diet, faecal nitrogen excretion is about 1–1.5 g/day (Cummings et al 1979a,b; Stephen 1980). Like fat, much of this excretion must be derived from the faecal microflora, since the nitrogen content of mixed populations of bacteria is about 7% (Tremolières et al 1961; Smith and

McAllan 1974) and, indeed, 70–80% of faecal nitrogen was found to be accounted for by its presence in bacteria (Stephen and Cummings 1980d). Faecal nitrogen excretion is unchanged by alterations in dietary protein (Cummings et al 1979b), which serves to confirm lack of utilisation of protein as an energy and carbon source for the colonic microflora as a whole.

Bacteria do, however, need a constant nitrogen supply and the colonic microflora obtains its nitrogen in two forms: (i) as preformed peptides and proteins which enter the colon from the upper gut or come from the mucosa of the colon itself or (ii) as ammonia, derived either from urea which diffuses into the colon from the circulation (Bown et al 1975; Wolpert et al 1971), or from the breakdown of those same proteins and peptides. The use of non-urea sources as precursors of ammonia has been demonstrated for both ruminant organisms (Pilgrim et al 1970) and the human faecal flora (Vince et al 1976). It is likely that ammonia is the major source of nitrogen for the human microflora since it has been shown to be so for bacteria in the rumen (Pilgrim et al 1970) and in the colon of pigs (Takahashi et al 1980). However, while some species require a certain proportion of amino acids and peptides in a preformed state, others will use preformed nitrogen sources if they are available, and ammonia if they are not (Salter et al 1978). That this may occur in the human colon has been indicated by a study where $^{15}NH_4$ was perfused into the large intestine of healthy individuals and the incorporation of marker into the faecal bacterial mass examined (Stephen et al 1983a). In those individuals where more protein passed through the ileocaecal junction, less of the marker was incorporated into bacterial cells compared with those where less protein entered the colon. Either the bacteria preferred the protein and peptides in the form they entered the colon, or they converted them to ammonia, diluting the pool of labelled ammonia. Regardless of the mechanism, it was clear that if more protein passes into the colon from the small intestine, less ammonia from other sources will be utilised.

Interest in protein in the diet and its effect on the intestinal microflora has grown with the epidemiological findings that dietary protein is related to the incidence of large bowel cancer (Armstrong and Doll 1975). It has been postulated that protein might affect bile acid metabolism, in a similar fashion to fat, but changes in protein in the diet have little (Cummings et al 1979c) or no effect (Hentges et al 1977) on faecal bile acid concentrations. Hence, if protein does predispose individuals to large bowel cancer, it is unlikely to be due to an effect on bile acid or steroid metabolism. Similarly, animal evidence indicates that changes in dietary protein have no effect on β-glucuronidase activity (Wise et al 1983). In studies where high meat diets have been compared to meatless ones and have shown changes in β-glucuronidase activity, the diets differed more with regard to fat than to protein content (Reddy et al 1974; Goldin et al 1978).

Ammonia has been shown to be toxic to cells (Dang and Visek 1968) and to alter DNA synthesis (Gibson et al 1971). Ammonia concentrations in faecal dialysates increase when dietary intake of protein is increased (Cummings et al 1979b), as would be expected if increased levels of dietary protein result in more entering the colon, the additional protein probably being metabolised to ammonia. The absorptive mechanisms for ammonia from the colon must also be taken into account, but the effect of dietary protein and microbial metabolism on ammonia concentration suggest it may be a potential promoter of carcinogenesis in the human large intestine.

Protein and bacterial species

Very few changes in microbial species occur when protein in the diet is altered. Hentges et al (1977) found counts of bacteroides and an unidentified clostridium significantly higher and *Bifidobacterium adolescentis* significantly lower on a high beef diet compared to a meatless one, but no other differences were found and these workers concluded that protein has little detectable effect on bacterial profiles in man.

Carbohydrate

Of all dietary constituents, carbohydrate, in its variety of forms and sources, has the major influence over the intestinal microflora. Through anaerobic fermentation by the microflora, it provides carbon and energy sources for continued bacterial maintenance and growth.

In the absence of dietary carbohydrate intake, the colonic microflora uses endogenous sources for maintenance, largely the glycoproteins of mucus and sloughed epithelial cells. The endogenous carbohydrate supply to the colon has been examined using intubation studies in healthy individuals (Stephen et al 1983b). Samples taken from the terminal ileum were analysed for total hexosamine, the main constituents of which are glucosamine and galactosamine derived from mucus. During fasting, 70.4 mg/h hexosamine on average passed into the colon, equivalent to 1.69 g/day. Hexosamine constitutes about 40% of the sugar in human mucus (Forstner 1978), and taking into account other sources of hexosamine, it was estimated that 3–4 g/day of endogenous carbohydrate entered the colon from the upper gastro-intestinal tract. There was no effect of meals on the amount of hexosamine passing; indeed, ileal flow increased dramatically after meals and hexosamine concentration fell simultaneously. Hence the suggestion that food causes an increase in mucus secretion (Florey 1955) was not confirmed in this experiment. This study did not take into account any mucus and other sources of carbohydrate within the colon itself however, and these may be substantial.

Carbohydrate in the diet

The major source of carbohydrate from the diet which reaches the intestinal microflora is generally assumed to be in the form of the complex polysaccharides which constitute dietary fibre. The average dietary intake of fibre for individuals on a typical Western diet is about 15–20 g/day, made up of non-starch polysaccharides, which can be further subdivided to cellulose and the non-cellulosic polysaccharides, hexoses, pentoses and uronic acids (Bingham et al 1981). These compounds cannot be broken down by mammalian enzymes, but the intestinal flora can degrade many of them, producing short chain fatty acids, gases and energy in the form of ATP. One mol of hexose produces 3.6–5.6 mol of ATP, one-tenth of that which could be produced if oxygen was present (Owens and Isaacson 1977). The energy produced is used for bacterial cell maintenance and growth, and therefore, the more carbohydrate that is provided, the greater the microbial growth and hence microbial cell mass.

Using the gravimetric procedure described, the dry weight of bacteria excreted each day has been found to be 14.5–15.0 g for healthy volunteers on a typical Western diet (Stephen and Cummings 1980c). When a degradable fibre material, like cabbage, was added to the diet at a dose of 18.4 g/day, faecal bacterial mass increased from 14.5 g/day to 19.3 g/day. Ninety-two per cent of the cabbage was fermented, leaving only 1.6 g of the original 18.4 g to be excreted in the stool. When 16 g wheat bran was given to the same volunteers, faecal bacterial mass increased from 15.0 g/day to 17.3 g/day, but only 27.5% of the bran fibre was fermented, leaving 11.6 g to be excreted in the stool (Stephen and Cummings 1980a) (Figure 5.2).

This study demonstrates how the chemical and physical nature of the carbohydrate affects the extent of its fermentation by the colonic microflora, and what a marked effect this has on faecal bulk. Both the cabbage and bran increased stool weight: cabbage from 88 g/day to 142 g/day and bran from 96 g/day to 197 g/day (Stephen and Cummings 1980a). The greater increase with bran is due to the fibre remaining, which holds water and bulks the stool, in combination with the increased mass of bacteria present, the largest component of stool weight.

It is clear that much of the work relating dietary fibre intake to disease incidence has taken no account of different types of fibre in the diet. Many of the sources of dietary fibre in Africa and other areas of the Third World are

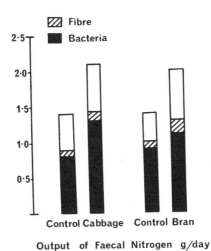

Output of Faecal Nitrogen g/day

Figure 5.2. Changes in daily faecal excretion of total nitrogen and nitrogen in bacteria and fibre (measured as neutral detergent fibre), for individuals during a control period with a dietary fibre intake of 22 g/day and when diet was supplemented with cabbage fibre (18.4 g dietary fibre per day) or bran (16.0 g dietary fibre per day). Number of individuals in each group = 6.

fermentable fibre materials, like plantains, beans or cereals which are not as lignified and resistant to fermentation as wheat. The effects of these materials on the microflora of the large intestine are likely to be similar to those of cabbage and will produce a greater mass of bacteria in the colon than is usually the case in the West. Moreover, African diets contain another carbohydrate source which until recently has been little considered in relation to the colonic microflora, namely starch.

Estimates of the amount of carbohydrate required show that the intake of fibre alone is insufficient to produce the weight of bacteria now known to be excreted on a Western diet. The results of the studies measuring hexosamine indicate that mucus provides only a small contribution to the overall microbial carbohydrate supply and does not fill the 'gap' between carbohydrate required and carbohydrate accounted for. Recent studies, using breath hydrogen tests as an estimate of malabsorption in the small intestine, have shown that even in healthy individuals, some 10–15% of starch from particular foods, including bread and potatoes, is not absorbed in the small intestine and passes into the colon where it is fermented (Anderson et al 1981). In an attempt to obtain more direct estimates of starch malabsorption in normal individuals, intubation studies have been carried out where test meals, containing different amounts of starch, were given to volunteers and samples were aspirated from the terminal ileum during the passage of the meals (Stephen et al 1983b). From measurements of starch concentration and ileal flow, the proportion of the starch in the meals which was not absorbed in the small intestine was calculated (Table 5.3). On average, 9% of meal A, containing 20 g of starch passed into the large intestine (range 2.3–20.1%) and for meal B, containing 61 g starch, 6% on average (range 2.2–10.4%) was not absorbed. The daily intake of starch in the United Kingdom is around 300 g (Bingham et al 1981) and if 7–8% of this escapes absorption in the small

Table 5.3. Passage of unabsorbed starch from two test meals through the ileum of seven healthy subjects.

Subject	Starch		Starch	
	mg	%	mg	%
	Meal A		Meal B	
1	781.8	3.9	2787.3	4.6
2	2632.2	13.2	6352.0	10.4
3	617.2	3.1	1332.4	2.2
4	4023.3	20.1	6253.4	10.3
5	3873.8	19.4	2402.3	3.9
6	452.7	2.3	2775.2	4.6
7	651.6	3.3	3578.8	5.9
Mean	1861.8	9.3	3639.5	6.0
SEM	607.1		732.3	

Meal A contains 20 g of starch, meal B contains 61 g starch.

intestine, it represents a substantial source of substrate for the colonic microflora and may provide much of the carbohydrate required to support the known daily excretion of bacteria. In countries with carbohydrate intakes much greater than in the West, starch may contribute to the large faecal weights, at present solely attributed to large intakes of dietary fibre.

Short chain fatty acids

Anaerobic carbohydrate breakdown results in the formation of short chain fatty acids, the major components of which are acetate, propionate and butyrate, produced in the proportions 60:25:15 (Cummings 1981). These acids are now known to be absorbed from the human large bowel (McNeil et al 1978; Ruppin et al 1980), as they are in other species (Argenzio and Southworth 1974; Remesy and Demigne 1976; Marty and Vernay 1984). In order to produce 15 g of bacteria (dry weight) per day, 60–70 g of carbohydrate must be fermented, and this will yield about 600 mmol of short chain fatty acids (Cummings 1981). Only about 7 mmol/day is recovered in the stools however (Cummings et al 1976), and therefore a vast absorption, hitherto largely ignored is continually proceeding in the human large intestine.

Short chain fatty acids are known to have many metabolic effects in mammals, ranging from inhibition or stimulation of various enzymes of the pathways of glucose and fatty acid metabolism by acetate and propionate (Chan and Freedland 1972; Williamson et al 1981; Snoswell et al 1982) to sparing of free fatty acids from skeletal muscle by acetate (Lundquist et al 1973) and preferential utilisation as an energy source by the colonic mucosal cells by butyrate (Roediger 1980). The integration of short chain fatty acids arising from the gastro-intestinal tract into human biochemical pathways has been given very little serious consideration in the past, and it is clear that this is an area in which animal biochemists are far ahead in their thinking. The possibility that addition of degradable fibre to the diet will result in biochemical changes in the liver or peripheral tissues secondary to short chain fatty acid absorption, must be considered and investigated in detail.

Dietary fibre and effects of other nutrients

The presence of fibre in the diet, whether of a degradable type or not, has implications for the effects of other dietary components on the intestinal microflora. Much work has been done, for example, to examine the effect of fibre on those microbial activities which are affected by increased dietary fat (Table 5.4). In human studies, little or no change has been found in the activity of β-glucuronidase (Drasar et al 1976; Goldin et al 1978; Ross and Leklem 1981), although animal experiments have shown both a decrease in activity with different fibre types (Shiau and Chang 1983) and an increase with pectin (Bauer et al 1979). Some of these contradictions may be explained by differences in the digestibility of different fibre types and the preference of the microflora for a particular substrate, whether it be a degradable fibre or a glucuronide.

Reports on the effect of dietary fibre on bile acid metabolism are contradictory, several studies showing no change in bile acid excretion

Table 5.4. Fibre and bacterial activity.

Forman et al (1968)	+ 15 g metamucil	No change β-glucuronidase
Walters et al (1975)	+ 39 g bran	No change total FBA
Cummings et al (1976)	+ 28 g wheat fibre	Total FBA ↑ [FBA] ↓
Drasar et al (1976)	+ 36 g wheat fibre	No change β-glucuronidase
Kay and Truswell (1977a)	+ 15 g pectin	Total FBA ↑
Kay and Truswell (1977b)	+ 54 g bran	No change total FBA [FBA] ↓
Goldin et (1978)	+ 30 g bran	No change β-glucuronidase
Cummings et al (1979b)	+ 31 g wheat fibre	Total FBA ↑ [FBA] ↓
Kirby et al (1981)	+ 100 g oat bran	[FBA] ↑
Ross and Leklem (1981)	+ 15 g pectin	β-Glucuronidase ↑ (NS) No change 7α-dehydroxylase No change total FBA

FBA = faecal bile acids; NS = not significant.

(Walters et al 1975; Kay and Truswell 1977b), whereas others have demonstrated increases in total bile acid concentration (Cummings et al 1976, 1979b). These studies have all been conducted with wheat fibre. In studies where degradable fibre has been fed, increases in faecal bile acid output have been shown, as is the case when feeding a natural food diet typical of rural Guatemala (Kretsch et al 1979).

The mechanism whereby dietary fibre may increase faecal output of bile acids is generally thought to be related to a capacity to bind acids thus carrying them into the large intestine. Alternatively, dietary fibre may, through a reduction in transit time, reduce the absorption of secondary bile acids, as indicated by recent studies of the effect of transit on the colonic absorption of deoxycholic acid (Marcus and Heaton 1984).

Diet and transit time

It is well accepted that increased intake of dietary fibre reduces intestinal transit time, particularly when the source of fibre is relatively indigestible, like bran or cellulose. Physiological changes brought about by fibre may themselves affect the intestinal microflora. For a group of individuals maintained on identical diets, it has been found that the weight of bacteria excreted each day varies with transit time (Stephen 1980). Moreover, when transit is altered using drugs which affect colonic motility, daily output of bacteria increases with more rapid transit, and is reduced when transit is slowed, in spite of dietary intake remaining constant (Stephen and Cummings 1980b). With a faster turnover rate, the resident population within the colon decreases in size, less of the available carbohydrate energy supply is therefore needed for bacterial cell maintenance, allowing more to be used for growth.

Hence faecal bacterial mass increases and larger stools are produced. Any dietary component which alters transit time will therefore affect the colonic microflora through the change in turnover rate, regardless of any other effects which the nutrient may have. Furthermore, several endogenous components are said to affect colonic motility and some of these, such as deoxycholic acid (Schiff 1979; Flynn et al 1982) or short chain fatty acids (Yokohura et al 1977) are present as a result of microbial action. Hence numerous events occur within the microbial milieu which are modified by, and in turn, may themselves modify, colonic motility.

Bacteria are very susceptible to changes in the rate of turnover of their environment. Not only does a faster rate allow greater growth, but individual cell size increases, as does their content of nitrogen (Herbert 1961) and carbohydrate, often in the form of intracellular glycogen (Cheng et al 1973). Faster turnover rates can also result in different metabolic products, with an increase in the proportion of acetate (Harrison et al 1975). Hence changes in food intake and intestinal motility can lead to marked changes in the microbial population and its activities.

Fibre and bacterial types

Several investigations have been made of the effect of dietary fibre on faecal bacterial species, with few positive results. Drasar and Jenkins (1976) fed bananas and plantain to healthy individuals, but found no changes in microbial species, nor did they find any when bran was added to metabolic diets (Drasar et al 1976). Fuchs et al (1976) found slight increases in streptococci and clostridia and decreases in lactobacilli and eubacteria when bran was fed, but none of these results was significant.

Fibre and nitrogen metabolism

The fermentation of carbohydrate substrate by the intestinal microflora has marked effects on nitrogen metabolism within the colon. Faecal nitrogen excretion varies between 0.6 g/day when subjects are on elemental diets (McCamman et al 1977) to over 4.6 g/day when diets contain large amounts of fibre (Subrahmanyan et al 1955; Calloway and Kretsch 1978). Provided dietary protein is adequate, fibre in the diet brings about an increase in faecal nitrogen, whether the source of fibre is wheat (Cummings et al 1976), oats (Calloway and Kretsch 1978), fruit and vegetables (Kelsay et al 1978), or purified preparations like Isogel (Greenberg 1976) or pectin (Cummings et al 1979c). Several suggestions have been put forward for the mechanism by which fibre increases faecal nitrogen, namely that the extra nitrogen is in the fibre itself (Saunders and Betschart 1980), that the increased bulk impairs the absorption of protein from digestive juices (Bender et al 1979), or that protein degradation is impaired by an effect of fibre on the proteolytic enzymes trypsin and chymotrypsin (Scheeman 1978). However, the finding that degradation of fibre by the intestinal microflora leads to increased faecal bacterial mass suggested that the increase in faecal nitrogen when fibre is fed arises from nitrogen contained within the bacterial organisms themselves. This has been found to be the case (Stephen and Cummings 1980d) (Figure

5.2) and confirms similar findings in the rat (Mason and Palmer 1973) and the pig (Mason et al 1976).

Any condition which encourages bacterial growth should therefore result in increased excretion of faecal nitrogen. Hence, accelerated transit time which produced a greater bacterial mass, also resulted in larger outputs of nitrogen in stools (Stephen 1980).

The source of nitrogen for increased bacterial growth is, as outlined earlier, largely ammonia, from either urea or non-urea sources and a greater utilisation of ammonia implies lower concentrations within the colonic lumen. Fibre has been shown to reduce ammonia concentrations in faecal dialysate (Cummings et al 1981) and faster transit has the same effect (Stephen 1980). The incorporation of ammonia into bacterial mass has been studied using ^{15}N as a marker, and when degradable substrate is provided in the form of the disaccharide lactulose, incorporation was greatly increased, reducing the amount available to be absorbed (Stephen et al 1983b). Hence, if ammonia is toxic or carcinogenic, then to reduce the risk of carcinogenesis, increased microbial growth is a highly desirable aim.

CONCLUSIONS

Of the three methods used to investigate the effect of food on the intestinal microflora, bacterial profiles seem the least informative. Nothing conclusive can be said about diet and the microflora from the numerous studies described using this approach. Enzyme activities and products have been useful, particularly in relation to bile acid metabolism, where evidence from different types of study supports the hypothesis that bile acids are involved in cancer of the colon.

The gravimetric approach has also been useful in assessing those factors which determine faecal output and the amount of carbohydrate required for maintenance of the microflora. This has led to ideas of new sources of carbohydrate which, until recently, had been concentrated on dietary fibre.

In the absence of energy, quite different reactions and activities of the microflora occur, and it is likely that under these circumstances the microflora degrades compounds, which, in the presence of carbohydrate, it would leave alone. All the evidence so far available indicates that to reduce the likelihood of undesirable reactions and the development of intestinal disease, the colonic microflora must be given an adequate energy supply, and this must be in the form of fermentable carbohydrate.

REFERENCES

Anderson I H, Levine A S & Levitt M D (1981) Incomplete absorption of the carbohydrate in all purpose wheat flour. *New England Journal of Medicine* **304**: 891–892.
Antonis A & Bersohn I (1962) The influence of diet on faecal lipids in South African White and Bantu Prisoners. *American Journal of Clinical Nutrition* **11**: 142–155.
Argenzio R A & Southworth M (1974) Sites of organic acid production and absorption in the gastrointestinal tract of the pig. *American Journal of Physiology* **228**: 454–460.

Armstrong B & Doll R (1975) Environmental factors and cancer incidence and mortality in different countries with special reference to dietary practices. *International Journal of Cancer* 15: 617–631.

Attebury H R, Sutter V L & Finegold S M (1972) Effect of a partially chemically defined diet on normal human faecal flora. *American Journal of Clinical Nutrition* 25: 1391–1398.

Banwell J G, Branch W & Cummings J H (1981) The microbial mass in the human large intestine. *Gastroenterology* 80, 1104.

Bauer, H G, Asp N, Oster R, Dahlquist A & Fredlund P (1979) Effect of dietary fiber on the induction of colorectal tumours and fecal β-glucuronidase activity in the rat. *Cancer Research* 39: 3752–3756.

Bender A E, Mohammadiha H & Almas K (1979) Digestibility of legumes and available lysine content. *Qualitas Plantarum* 29: 219–226.

Bingham S A, Williams D R R, Cole T J & James W P T (1979) Dietary fibre and regional large-bowel cancer mortality in Britain. *British Journal of Cancer* 40: 456–463.

Bingham S A, McNeil N I & Cummings J H (1981) The diet of individuals: a study of a randomly-chosen cross section of British adults in a Cambridgeshire village. *British Journal of Nutrition* 45: 23–35.

Bornside G H & Cohn I Jr (1975) Stability of normal human fecal flora during a chemically defined, low residue liquid diet. *Annals of Surgery* 181: 58–60.

Bown R L, Gibson J A, Fenton J C B, et al (1975) Ammonia and urea transport by the excluded human colon. *Clinical Science and Molecular Medicine* 48: 279–287.

Calloway D H & Kretsch M J (1978) Protein and energy utilization in men given a rural Guatemalan diet and egg formulas with and without added oat bran. *American Journal of Clinical Nutrition* 31: 1118–1126.

Chan T M & Freedland R A (1972) The effect of propionate on the metabolism of pyruvate and lactate in the perfused rat liver. *Biochemical Journal* 127: 539–543.

Cheng K-J, Hironaka R, Roberts D W A & Costerton J W (1973) Cytoplasmic glycogen inclusions in cells of anaerobic gram-negative rumen bacteria. *Canadian Journal of Microbiology* 19: 1501–1506.

Costerton J W, Ingram J M & Cheng K-J (1974) Structure and function of the cell envelope of gram-negative bacteria. *Bacteriology Reviews* 38: 87–110.

Crowther J S, Drasar B S, Goddard P, Hill M J & Johnson K (1973) The effect of a chemically defined diet on the faecal flora and faecal steroid concentration. *Gut* 14: 790–793.

Cummings J H (1981) Short chain fatty acids in the human colon. *Gut* 22: 763–779.

Cummings J H, Hill M J, Jenkins D J A, Pearson J R & Wiggins H S (1976) Changes in faecal composition and colonic function due to cereal fiber. *American Journal of Clinical Nutrition* 29: 1468–1473.

Cummings J H, Southgate D A T, Branch W, Houston H, Jenkins D J A & James W P T (1978a) Colonic response to dietary fibre from carrot, cabbage, apple, bran and gua gum. *Lancet* 1: 5–8.

Cummings J H, Wiggins H S, Jenkins D J A et al (1978b) Influence of diets high and low in animal fat on bowel habit, gastrointestinal transit time, fecal microflora, bile acid and fat excretion. *Journal of Clinical Investigation* 61: 953–963.

Cummings J H, Hill M J, Jivraj T, et al (1979a) The effect of meat protein and dietary fibre on colonic function and metabolism. I. Changes in bowel habit, bile acid excretion and calcium absorption. *American Journal of Clinical Nutrition* 32: 2086–2093.

Cummings J H, Hill M J, Bone E S, Branch W J & Jenkins D J A (1979b) The effect of meat protein and dietary fibre on colonic function and metabolism. II. Bacterial metabolism in feces and urine. *American Journal of Clinical Nutrition* 32: 2094–2101.

Cummings J H, Southgate D A T, Branch W J & Wiggins H S (1979c) The digestion of pectin in the human gut and its effect on calcium absorption and large bowel function. *British Journal of Nutrition* 41: 477–485.

Cummings J H, Stephen A M & Branch W J (1981) Implications of dietary fibre breakdown in the human colon. In *Branbury Report 7: Gastrointestinal Cancer: Endogenous Factors*. Cold Spring Harbour Laboratory.

Czerkawski J W (1976) Chemical composition of microbial matter in the rumen. *Journal of the Science of Food and Agriculture* 27: 621–632.

Dang H C & Visek W J (1968) Some characteristics of blood in normal and immune rabbits after urease injection. *American Journal of Physiology* 215: 502–505.

Debongnie J C & Phillips S F (1978) Capacity of the human colon to absorb fluid. *Gastroenterology* 74: 698–703.

Drasar B S & Jenkins D J A (1976) Bacteria, diet and large bowel cancer. *American Journal of Clinical Nutrition* 29: 1410–1416.

Drasar B S, Jenkins D J A & Cummings J H (1976) The influence of a diet rich in wheat fibre on the human faecal flora. *Journal of Medical Microbiology* 9: 423–431.

Finegold S M & Sutter V L (1978) Fecal flora in different populations, with special references to diet. *American Journal of Clinical Nutrition* **31**: S116–S122.

Fletcher M & Floodgate G D (1973) An electron-microscope demonstration of an acidic polysaccharide involved in the adhesion of a marine bacterium to solid surfaces. *Journal of General Microbiology* **74**: 325–334.

Florey H (1955) Mucin and the protection of the body. *Proceedings of the Royal Society of London B* **143**: 147–158.

Flynn M, Hammond P, Darby C & Taylor I (1982) Effect of bile acids on human colonic motor function in vitro. *Digestion* **23**: 211–216.

Forman D T, Garvin J E, Forestner J E & Taylor C B (1968) Increased excretion of fecal bile acids by an oral hydrophilic colloid. *Proceedings of the Society for Experimental Biology and Medicine* **127**: 1060.

Forstner J F (1978) Intestinal mucins in health and disease. *Digestion* **17**: 134–263.

Fuchs H-M, Dorfman S & Floch M H (1976) The effect of dietary fibre supplementation in man. II Alteration in fecal physiology and bacterial flora. *American Journal of Clinical Nutrition* **29**: 1443–1447.

Galbraith H & Miller T B (1973) Physiochemical effects of long chain fatty acids on bacterial cells and their protoplasts. *Journal of Applied Bacteriology* **36**: 647–658.

Gibson J A (1977) Studies of urea and ammonia metabolism. MD thesis, University of Cambridge.

Gibson G E, Zimber A, Krook L & Visek W J (1971) Nucleic acids and brain and intestinal lesions in ammonia intoxicated mice. *Federation Proceedings* **30**: 578.

Glatzel H (1963) Auswirkungen langristigen Fettreicher und Fettarmer Ernahrung auf Lipidstoffwechsel, Kohlenhydrattoleranz, Grundumsatz und Darmflora. *Nutritiv Dieta* **5**: 192–212.

Goerg K J, Specht W, Nell G, Rummel W & Schulz L (1982) Effect of deoxycholate on the perfused rat colon. *Digestion* **25**: 145–154.

Goldin B, Dwyer J, Gorbach S L, Gordon W & Swenson L (1978) Influence of diet and age on faecal bacterial enzymes. *American Journal of Clinical Nutrition* **31**: 5136–5140.

Greenberg C (1976) Studies on the fibre in human diets and its effect on the absorption of other nutrients. PhD thesis, University of Cambridge.

Gustafsson B E (1983) Introduction to the ecology of the intestinal microflora and its general characteristics. In Hallgren B (ed) *Nutrition and the Intestinal Flora*, pp 11–16. Stockholm: Almqvist & Wiksell International.

Haenel H & Bendig J (1975) Intestinal flora in health and disease. *Progress in Food and Nutrition Science* **1**: 21–64.

Harrison D G, Beever D E, Thomson D J & Osbourn D F (1975) Manipulation of rumen fermentation in sheep by increasing the rate of flow of water from the rumen. *Journal of Agricultural Science* **83**: 93–101.

Hayakawa S (1973) Microbial transformations of bile acids. In Paoletti R & Kritchevsky D P (eds) *Advances in Lipid Research*, p 143. New York: Academic Press.

Hentges D J, Maier B R, Burton G C, Flynn M N & Tsutakawa R K (1977) Effects of a high beef diet on the faecal bacterial flora of humans. *Cancer Research* **37**: 568–571.

Herbert D (1961) The chemical composition of microorganisms as a function of their environment. *11th Symposium of the Society of General Microbiology* p 391. London: Cambridge University Press.

Hill M J & Aries V C (1971) Fecal steroid composition and its relationship to cancer of the large bowel. *Journal of Pathology* **104**: 129–139.

Jensen O M, MacLennan R & Wahrendorf J (1982) Diet, bowel function, fecal characteristics, and large bowel cancer in Denmark and Finland. *Nutrition and Cancer* **4**: 5–19.

Kay R M & Truswell A S (1977a) Effect of citrus pectin on blood lipids and fecal steroid excretion in man. *American Journal of Clinical Nutrition* **30**: 171–175.

Kay R M & Truswell A S (1977b) The effect of wheat fibre on plasma lipids and faecal steroid excretion in man. *British Journal of Nutrition* **7**: 227–235.

Kelsay J L, Behall K M & Prather E S (1978) Effect of fiber from fruits and vegetables of human subjects. I Bowel transit time, number of defecations, fecal weight, urinary excretions of energy and nitrogen and apparent digestibilities of energy, nitrogen and fat. *American Journal of Clinical Nutrition* **31**: 1149–1153.

Kies C & Fox H M (1976) Orally administered liquid formula and elemental diets as a sole source of nutrition for normal human adults. *Federation Proceedings* **35**: 261.

Kirby R W, Anderson J W, Sieling B, et al (1981) Oat bran selectively lowers serum low density lipoprotein cholesterol concentrations: studies in hypercholesterolemic men. *American Journal of Clinical Nutrition* **34**: 824–829.

Kramer P, Kearney M M & Ingelfinger F J (1962) The effect of specific foods and water loading on the ileal excreta of ileostomised human subjects. *Gastroenterology* **42**: 535–546.

Kretsch M J, Crawford D L & Calloway D H (1979) Some aspects of bile acid and urobilinogen excretion and fecal elimination in men given a rural Guatemalan diet and egg formulas with and without added oat bran. *American Journal of Clinical Nutrition* **32**: 1492–1496.

Lewis G T & Partin H C (1954) Fecal fat on an essentially fat free diet. *Journal of Laboratory and Clinical Medicine* **44**: 91–93.

Lundquist F, Sestoft L, Damgaard S E, Clausen J P & Trap-Jensen J (1973) Utilization of acetate in the human forearm during exercise after ethanol ingestion. *Journal of Clinical Investigation* **53**: 3231–3235.

Luria S E (1960) The bacterial protoplasm: composition and organization. In Gunsalus I C & Stanier R Y (eds) *The Bacteria*, pp 1–34. New York: Academic Press.

McCamman S, Beyer P L & Rhodes J B (1977) A comparison of three defined formula diets in normal volunteers. *American Journal of Clinical Nutrition* **30**: 1655–1660.

McNeil N I, Cummings J H & James W P T (1978) Short chain fatty acid absorption by the human large intestine. *Gut* **19**: 819–822.

Maczulak A E, Dehority B A & Palmquist D L (1981) Effects of long chain fatty acids on growth of rumen bacteria. *Applied and Environmental Microbiology* **42**: 856–862.

Mallett A K, Bearne C A & Rowland I R (1983) Metabolic activity and enzyme induction in rat fecal microflora maintained in continuous culture. *Applied and Environmental Microbiology* **46**: 591–595.

Mallett A K, Rowland I R & Wise A (1984) Dietary fat and cecal microbial activity in the rat. *Nutrition and Cancer* **6**: 86–91.

Marcus S N & Heaton K W (1984) Intestinal transit rate, deoxycholic bile acid and the cholesterol saturation of bile. *Gut* **25**: A1141.

Marty J & Vernay M (1984) Absorption and metabolism of the volatile fatty acids in the hindgut of the rabbit. *British Journal of Nutrition* **51**: 265–277.

Mason V C, Just A & Bach-Andersen S (1976) Bacterial activity in the hindgut of pigs. Its influence on the apparent digestibility of nitrogen and amino acids. *Zeitschrift fur Tierphysiologie, Tierenahrung und Futtermittelkunde* **36**: 310–324.

Mason V C & Palmer R (1973) The influence of bacterial activity in the alimentary canal of rats on faecal nitrogen excretion. *Acta Agriculturae Scandinavica* **23**: 141–150.

Mastromarino A, Reddy B S & Wynder E L (1976) Metabolic epidemiology of colon cancer: enzymatic activity of fecal flora. *American Journal of Clinical Nutrition* **29**: 1455–1460.

Moore W E C & Holdema L V (1975) Discussion of current bacteriological investigations of the relationships between intestinal flora, diet and colon cancer. *Cancer Research* **35**: 3418–3420.

Moore W E C, Cato E P & Holdeman L V (1978) Some current concepts in intestinal bacteriology. *American Journal of Clinical Nutrition* **31**: 533–542.

Nasset E S (1965) Role of the digestive system in protein metabolism. *Federation Proceedings* **24**: 953–958.

Owens F N & Isaacson H R (1977) Ruminal microbial yields: factors influencing synthesis and bypass. *Federation Proceedings* **36**: 198.

Patterson H, Irvin R, Costerton J W & Cheng K J (1975) Ultrastructure and adhesion properties of *Ruminoccocus albus*. *Journal of Bacteriology* **122**: 278–287.

Pilgrim A F, Gray F V, Weller R A & Belling C B (1970) Synthesis of microbial protein from ammonia in the sheep's rumen and the proportion of dietary nitrogen converted into microbial nitrogen. *British Journal of Nutrition* **24**: 589–598.

Reddy B S & Wynder E L (1973) Large bowel carcinogenesis: fecal constituents of populations with diverse incidence rates of colon cancer *Journal of the National Cancer Institute* **50**: 1437–1442.

Reddy B S, Weisburger J H & Wynder E L (1975) Effects of high risk and low risk diets for colon carcinogenesis on fecal microflora and steroids in man. *Journal of Nutrition* **105**: 878–884.

Reddy B S, Narisawa T, Weisburger J H & Wynder E L (1976) Promoting effect of sodium deoxycholate on colon adenocarcinoma in germfree rats. *Journal of the National Cancer Institute* **56**: 441–442.

Reddy B S, Mangat S, Weisburger J H & Wynder E L (1977) Effect of high risk diets for colon carcinogenesis in intestinal mucosal and bacterial beta-glucoronidase activity in F344 rats. *Cancer Research* **37**: 3533–3536.

Redinger R N, Hermann A N & Small D M (1973) Effect of diet and fasting on biliary lipid secretion and relative composition and bile salt metabolism in the rhesus monkey. *Gastroenterology* **64**: 610–621.

Remesy C & Demigne C (1976) Partition and absorption of volatile fatty acids in the alimentary canal o
the rat. *Annales de Recherches Veterinaires* **1**: 39–55.

Roediger W E W (1980) Role of anaerobic bacteria in the metabolic welfare of the colonic mucosa ir
man. *Gut* **21**: 793–798.

Ross J K & Leklem J E (1981) The effect of dietary citrus pectin on the excretion of human fecal neutra
and acid steroids and the activity of 7-alpha-dehydroxylase and beta-glucuronidase. *Americar
Journal of Clinical Nutrition* **34**: 2068–2077.

Ruppin H, Bar-meir S, Soergel K H, Wood C M & Schmitt M G (1980) Absorption of short chain fatty
acids by the colon. *Gastroenterology* **78**: 1500–1507.

Salter D N, Daneshvar K & Smith R H (1978) The origin of nitrogen incorporated into compounds ir
the rumen bacteria of steers given protein and urea-containing diets. *British Journal of Nutrition* **41**
197–209.

Salyers A A (1983) Metabolic activities of the intestinal bacteria. In Hallgren B (ed) *Nutrition and the
Intestinal Flora* pp 35–44. Stockholm: Almqvist & Wiksell International.

Saunders D R, Hedges J R, Sillery J E, Matsumura K & Rubin C E (1975) Morphological and functiona
effects of bile salts on rat colon. *Gastroenterology* **68**: 1236–1245.

Saunders R M & Betschart A A (1980) The significance of protein as a component of dietary fibre
American Journal of Clinical Nutrition **33**: 960–961.

Scheeman B A (1978) Effect of plant fibre on lipase, trypsin and chymotrypsin activity. *Journal of Fooc
Science* **43**: 634.

Schiff S (1979) Effect of deoxycholic acid on colonic motility in the rabbit. *Gastroenterology* **76**: 1307

Shands J W (1966) Localisation of somatic antigen on gram-negative bacteria using ferritin antibody
conjugates. *Annals of the New York Academy of Sciences* **136**: 292–298.

Shiau S Y & Chang G W (1983) Effects of dietary fiber on fecal mucinase and beta-glucuronidase
activity in rats. *Journal of Nutrition* **113**: 138–144.

Smith R H & McAllan A B (1974) Some factors influencing the chemical composition of mixed rumer
bacteria. *British Journal of Nutrition* **31**: 27–34.

Snoswell A M, Trimble R P, Fishlock R C, Storer G B & Topping D L (1982) Metabolic effects o
acetate in perfused rat liver. Studies on ketogenesis, glucose output, lactate uptake and lipogenesis
Biochimica et Biophysica Acta **716**: 290–297.

Stemmermann G N, Nomina A M Y & Heilbrun L K (1984) Dietary fat and the risk of colorecta
cancer. *Cancer Research* **44**: 4633–4637.

Stephen A M (1980) Dietary fibre and human colonic function. PhD thesis, University of Cambridge.

Stephen A M & Cummings J H (1980a) Mechansim of action of dietary fibre in the human colon. *Nature
284: 283–284.

Stephen A M & Cummings J H (1980b) Effect of changing transit time on faecal bacterial mass in man
Gut **21**: A905.

Stephen A M & Cummings J H (1980c) The microbial contribution to human faecal mass. *Journal o
Medical Microbiology* **13**: 45–56.

Stephen A M & Cummings J H (1980d) The effect of dietary fibre on faecal nitrogen excretion in man
Proceedings of the Nutrition Society **38**: 141A.

Stephen A M, Haddad A C & Phillips S F (1983a) The effect of lactulose and dietary fibre on colonic
metabolism of nitrogen. *Gastroenterology* **84**: 1323.

Stephen A M, Haddad A C & Phillips S F (1983b) Passage of carbohydrate into the colon: direc
measurements in humans. *Gastroenterology* **85**: 589–595.

Subrahmanyan V, Narayanarao M, Ramarao G & Swaminathan M (1955) The metabolism of nitrogen
calcium and phosphorus in human adults on a poor vegetarian diet containing ragi (*Eleusine
coracana*) *British Journal of Nutrition* **9**: 350–357.

Takahashi M, Benno Y & Mitsuoka T (1980) Utilization of ammonia nitrogen by intestinal bacteri:
isolated from pigs. *Applied and Environmental Microbiology* **39**: 30–35.

Tremolières J, Bonfils S, Carre L & Sautier C (1961) Une methode d'étude de la digestibilite chez
l'homme, le fecalogramme. *Nutritiv Dieta* **3**: 281–289.

Van Houte J & Gibbons R J (1966) Studies on the cultivatable flora of normal human faeces. *Antonie
van Leewenhoek* **32**: 212–222.

Vince A, Down P F, Murison J, Twigg F J & Wrong O M (1976) Generation of ammonia from non-urea
sources in a faecal incubation system. *Clinical Science and Molecular Medicine* **51**: 313–322.

Walters R L, McLean Baird I, Davies P S, et al (1975) Effects of two types of dietary fibre on faeca
steroid and lipid excretion. *British Medical Journal* **4**: 536–538.

Webb J P W, James A T & Kellock T D (1963) The influence of diet on the quality of faecal fat ir
patients with and without steatorrhea. *Gut* **4**: 37–41.

Wiggins H S, Howell K E, Kellock T D & Stalder J (1969) The origin of faecal fat. *Gut* **10**: 400–403.

Williamson J R, Martin-Requero A, Corkey B E, Brandt M & Rothman R (1981) Interactions between alpha-ketoisovalerate, propionate and fatty acids on gluconeogenesis and ureogenesis in isolated hepatocytes. *Developmental Biochemistry* **18**: 105–117.

Winitz M, Adams R F, Seedman D A, et al (1970) Studies in metabolic nutrition employing chemically defined diets. *American Journal of Clinical Nutrition* **23**: 546–559.

Wise A, Mallett A K & Rowland I R (1983) Dietary protein and cecal microbial metabolism in the rat. *Nutrition and Cancer* **4**: 267–272.

Wolpert E, Phillips S F & Summerskill W H J (1971) Transport of urea and ammonia production in the human colon. *Lancet* **2**: 1387–1390.

Yokohura T, Yajima T & Hashimoto S (1977) Effect of organic acid on gastrointestinal motility of the rat in vitro. *Life Sciences* **21**: 59–62.

Chapter 6
Diet and Short Chain Fatty Acids in the Gut

John H. Cummings

The principal short chain fatty acids found in the human gut are the C_2 (acetic), C_3 (propionic) and C_4 (butyric) members of the aliphatic monocarboxylic acid series, which include the more familiar C_8 (caprylic), C_{10} (capric) and C_{12} (lauric) medium chain fatty acids used in the dietary management of certain malabsorptive states, and C_{14} (myristic), C_{16} (palmitic) and C_{18} (stearic) long chain fatty acids which, together with oleic acid ($C_{18:1}$), are the major ones in food and in faecal fat. The short chain fatty acids (SCFA) are sometimes referred to as volatile fatty acids (VFA) because they are volatile in aqueous solutions at acid pH. It was this property that led to their identification in faeces more than 100 years ago (Brieger 1878). However the term VFA has never been clearly defined and it is probably better to call these acids SCFA, or better still by their individual names, since the borderline between short and medium chain fatty acids has never been defined either.

Table 6.1 summarises some of the chemical properties of the major SCFA found in the human gut and lists other fatty acids occasionally reported to be present. They are all low molecular weight substances with substantial or complete water solubility. Their pK's (dissociation constant) are on average around 4.8, so that at the pH of the small and large intestine they will be ionised and therefore present as fatty acid anions.

SPECIES DISTRIBUTION OF SHORT CHAIN FATTY ACIDS

Short chain fatty acids are found in the gut of many, if not all, mammalian species. Their presence is always associated with a significant anaerobic microbial population. They are produced largely as a result of the breakdown of carbohydrate in the gut by the flora, a process conventionally referred to as fermentation. This reaction can be summarised by the equation

$$58\ (C_6H_{12}O_6) \rightarrow 62\ CH_3COOH + 22\ CH_3CH_2COOH + 16\ CH_3(CH_2)_2COOH + 60.5\ CO_2 + 33.5\ CH_4 + 27\ H_2O$$

which has been derived from extensive studies on the rumen (Wolin 1960; Hungate 1966). From Table 6.2 it will be evident that the major areas of fermentation in the gut are the rumen and/or the caecum/large intestine. Total short chain fatty acid levels in the rumen are around 100 mmol/l. The rumen is a part of the fore-stomach of plant-eating species which has become

Table 6.1. Predominant short chain fatty acids in the human colon.

Common name	Proper name	Formula	Molecular weight	pK
Acetic acid	Acetic acid (ethanoic acid)	CH_3COOH	60	4.75
Propionic acid	Propanoic acid	CH_3CH_2COOH	74	4.87
Butyric acid	Butanoic acid	$CH_3(CH_2)_2COOH$	88	4.81

Other short chain fatty acids and related substances which may be found in the human gut:

Formic acid	Formic acid (methanoic acid)	$HCOOH$	46	3.75
Lactic acid	2-Hydroxy-propanoic acid	$CH_3CH(OH)COOH$	90	3.08
Isobutyric acid	2-Methyl-propanoic acid	$(CH_3)_2CHCOOH$	88	4.84
Valeric acid	Pentanoic acid	$CH_3(CH_2)_3COOH$	102	4.82
Isovaleric acid	3-Methyl-butanoic acid	$(CH_3)_2CHCH_2COOH$	102	4.77
Caproic acid	Hexanoic acid	$CH_3(CH_2)_4COOH$	116	4.83

specially adapted to allow the microbial breakdown of plant cell-wall polysaccharides or 'fibre' which constitute a major part of the diet. All dietary carbohydrates entering the rumen are converted to short chain fatty acids which are then absorbed and provide the major source of energy for ruminant metabolism. The rumen is an area of slow transit; large particulate matter spends around two days there, being returned to the mouth for regrinding from time to time (chewing the cud) in order to facilitate its breakdown by the bacteria.

Measurable amounts of SCFA are found in the true stomach, although these are rarely greater than 25 mmol/l and often much less. In species such as the pig, the high levels reflect the division of the stomach. A proximal or cranial half is lined by a stratified squamous epithelium and cardiac mucosa and contains a significant microflora including anaerobic lactobacilli; a distal or caudal part of the stomach is lined by proper gastric and pyloric mucosa and is acid secreting. Gastric acid secretion is the primary factor limiting growth of microbial species in this area. In the small bowel, short chain fatty acid levels are low, usually less than 10 mmol/l. Transit rate through the small

Table 6.2. Total short chain fatty acid* concentrations (mmol/l) in the gut of various mammalian species.

Species	Rumen	Stomach	Small intestine	Caecum	Colon		Reference
					Proximal	Distal	
Cow	59–120	12–20	6–12	34–46	17–49		Elsden et al (1946) Kern et al (1974)
Sheep	141	6	12	102	89	75	Elsden et al (1946)
Giraffe	106	17	11	69	64	45	Clemens and Maloiy (1983)
Buffalo	83	6	13	37	19	15	Clemens and Maloiy (1983)
Oryx	183	29	43	91	74	55	Clemens and Maloiy (1983)
Pony	—	10–40	0–5	60–100	75–120	35–70	Argenzio et al (1974)
Pig	—	5–60	0–40	104–200	103–240	86–200	Argenzio and Southworth (1974) Elsden et al (1946)
Dog	—	10–40	0–5	60–100	75–120	35–70	Banta et al (1979)
Baboon	—	16–21	24–37	172	173–192	101–139	Clemens and Maloiy (1981)
Bush Baby	—	20–22	23–34	156	122–139	142–157	Clemens and Maloiy (1981)
Rabbit	—	4	5	62	39		Elsden et al (1946)
Rat	—	12–57	1–10	103–190	78–106		Remesy and Demigne (1976) Elsden et al (1946)
Man	—	?	0–4	?	?	?	Newton et al (1972) Chernov et al (1972)

*Predominantly the sum of acetate, propionate and butyrate although readers should consult the original papers since the methods of measurement varied considerably particularly in earlier studies. Some data recalculated from original papers, or read from graphs.

bowel is probably too rapid to allow the development of significant flora. Two attempts to measure short chain fatty acids in the human small bowel have been made and levels of less than 4 mmol/l were reported, although they increased in the stagnant loop syndrome (Chernov et al 1972; Newton et al 1972).

In the large intestine, short chain fatty acid levels are substantial in all mammalian species examined, reaching up to 200 mmol/l or more in some cases. In such circumstances the osmolarity of colonic contents must be considerably in excess of that in plasma (approximately 280–300 mosmol/kg). The caecum and colon, with their slow turnover and neutral pH, favour fermentation in non-ruminant species such as the horse, rabbit and some primates. In these animals the large intestine is, like the rumen, a major source of energy for the host through the absorption of short chain fatty acids.

Short chain fatty acids are in fact the predominant anion in the colon of many species and from Table 6.3 it will be seen that acetate is the principal one, occurring at a concentration greater than the sum of propionate + butyrate. The relative proportions of the three principal SCFA show a remarkable similarity, the molar ratios of acetate : propionate : butyrate always being approximately 60 : 25 : 15, despite the wide variety of sampling techniques used, and of the diets of the various animals. An exception to this observation is the lower termite where acetate accounts for 94–98% of hind-gut SCFA. This is probably due to the unusual diet of the termite which consists almost entirely of wood cellulose and hemicellulose, most of the acetate being produced by flagellate protozoa which are essential for the degradation of wood polysaccharides in these creatures. No information is at present available on SCFA levels in the human colon, but total concentration in faeces varies between 60 and 170 mmol/l, depending on the method of obtaining faecal fluid for analysis.

In all species, small amounts of other SCFA such as isobutyrate, valerate and isovalerate are usually present. These are partly the products of the fermentation of branched chain amino acids (leucine, isoleucine and valine) and may appear in significant quantities only when carbohydrate fermentation is limited (Russell and Jeraci 1984) or altered by diet in some way (Thomsen et al 1984).

EFFECT OF DIET

The study of diet and its effects on short chain fatty acid generation in the animal gut is relatively easy, since access can be gained to different sites in the gut with reasonable ease. A number of reports give data which show that SCFA levels and production rates are related to diet, particularly the supply of energy-yielding substrates such as carbohydrate. In man, however, until recently the only material readily available for analysis was faeces and hence much of the work relating diet to short chain fatty acid metabolism has been based on its effect on SCFA excretion. Perhaps not surprisingly therefore, dietary change has much less apparent effect on SCFA concentration or molar ratios than might be anticipated. In Table 6.4 are shown SCFA values from a dictary study involving four healthy adult males. During the first

Table 6.3. Acetate, propionate and butyrate concentrations (mmol/l) in the large intestine and faeces of various non-ruminant mammals*.

Species	Site	Acetate	Propionate	Butyrate	Reference
Horse	Caecum	53	12	8	Elsden et al (1946)
Pig	Caecum	118	68	25	Argenzio and Southworth (1974)
Greater glider (*Petauroides volans*)	Caecum	23	8	6	Rubsamen et al (1983)
Rat	Caecum	101	57	32	Remesy and Demigne (1976)
	Colon	70	29	7	
	Faeces	75	27	16	
Termite (*Reticulitermes flavipes*)	Hind-gut	81	3	2	Odelson and Breznak (1983)
Man	Faecal dialysate	46	17	15	Rubinstein et al (1969)
		39	19	14	Bjork et al (1976)
		41	12	13	Cummings et al (1979)
		55	18	10	Vernia et al (1984)
	Faecal water	93	46	24	Bjork et al (1976)
	Faeces	48	11	5	Zijlstra et al (1977)

*See footnote to Table 6.2.

Table 6.4. Short chain fatty acids and ammonia in faecal dialysate during dietary change (mean ± SEM).

Diet	Total SCFA (mmol/l)	Molar ratio (%) acetate: propionate: butyrate					Ammonia (mmol/l)
Low protein	65.7 ± 4.6	63	:	18	:	19	14.8 ± 1.3
High protein	57.7 ± 4.7	55	:	23	:	22	30.4 ± 1.1
High protein + wheat fibre	66.1 ± 4.2	60	:	19	:	21	28.2 ± 1.1

Data from Cummings et al (1979).

period they ate a controlled diet which included 63 g/day protein and 23 g/day dietary fibre; they then changed to an equicaloric diet with 136 g/day protein and 22 g/day dietary fibre; finally they were placed on a further equicaloric diet with 164 g/day protein and 53 g/day fibre. Faecal SCFA and NH_4 concentrations were measured using the dialysis bag technique of Wrong et al (1965). SCFA concentrations and molar ratios were unchanged, despite the large alterations in fibre and protein intake. By contrast, ammonia concentration increased as protein intake increased, although it was unchanged by the addition of fibre. In a larger study of 19 subjects on a constant protein intake but consuming varying amounts of dietary fibre (Figure 6.1), again no change was seen in faecal short chain fatty acid concentrations with diet, but ammonia and SCFA levels were related, indicating some common factor in their metabolism in the gut.

In another study (Rubinstein et al 1969), when five healthy subjects changed from an ad lib diet to one containing only carbohydrate (soluble carbohydrate + methylcellulose 40 g/day), SCFA concentrations in faecal dialysate fell from 85 to 46 mmol/l but there was little difference in the molar ratios 59 : 22 : 19 (ad lib diet) to 58 : 17 : 13 (carbohydrate only diet). Two of these subjects then lived for four days on only methylcellulose and water: SCFA concentration fell to 23 mmol/l, but molar ratios were again unchanged. When a similar group of subjects were given antibiotics (neomycin, bacitracin, colistin and gramicidin) in addition to their normal diet, acetate, propionate and butyrate all fell to very low levels whilst succinate increased from 4 to 40 mmol/l.

Faecal short chain fatty acids are therefore not a particularly sensitive guide to colonic SCFA metabolism in man. It is most likely that diet influences their production and absorption but unless changes are extreme, or antibiotics are given, faecal concentrations and molar ratios remain relatively

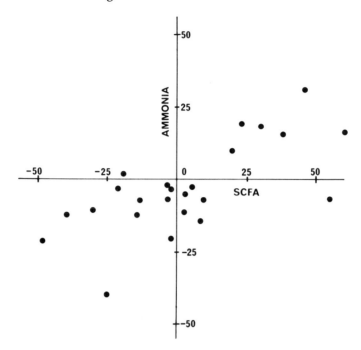

Figure 6.1. Change in mean faecal dialysate ammonia and total SCFA concentration in 19 healthy volunteers when going from a control diet to one supplemented with 15–20 g of dietary fibre from either bran, cabbage, carrot, apple or guar gum, $r = 0.69$, $P < 0.001$. From Cummings and Branch (1985), with kind permission of the publisher, Alan R. Liss.

constant. From this, one might predict that faecal output of SCFA is closely related to total stool weight. This is in fact the case. Figure 6.2 shows average daily stool weight (or faecal water output) and faecal SCFA output from three separate studies of diet and gastro-intestinal function. Study A is a controlled diet study of six healthy volunteers taking a standard UK diet for three weeks and then the same diet with the addition of about 30 g dietary fibre from wheat; this was added by exchanging white bread for wholemeal bread, cornflakes for All-Bran, and giving a bran biscuit and raw bran. The dietary changes led to a three-fold increase in stool output and three-fold increase in short chain fatty acid output (Cummings et al 1976). SCFA concentrations were unchanged. In study B the subjects were given varying doses of the non-absorbable carbohydrates mannitol, lactulose or raffinose as a single dose and faeces collected over the ensuing 48 h. Stool weight increased three-fold and short chain fatty acid excretion two-fold (Saunders and Wiggins 1981). Perhaps more significant in this context is the study of Grove et al (1929: Study C), in which four healthy subjects were given magnesium sulphate. Stool weight increased substantially as did SCFA output, an observation confirmed by Saunders and Wiggins in their paper. Other work has been reported in which the effect on stool and SCFA output of bran pentosan (Olmsted et al 1935), a variety of vegetable and cereal foods

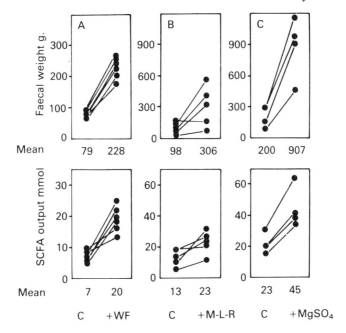

Figure 6.2. Mean daily stool weight (g/day) and total SCFA output (mmol/day). C = control diet. Study A: *The effect of wheat bran (WF)*. Six healthy subjects first ate a control diet, typical of that eaten in the UK, and then the same diet with 36 g of dietary fibre from wheat added. Study B: *The effect of non-absorbable sugars*. Four healthy volunteers eating either an ad lib diet, or after a single test dose containing approximately 150 mmol of either mannitol (M), lactulose (L) or raffinose (R). Values are the mean of two days of faecal collection. Data from Saunders and Wiggins (1981). Study C: *The effect of catharsis*. Four healthy medical students were studied whilst eating controlled high carbohydrate diets for seven days and were then given about 30 g of magnesium sulphate for 2–7 days. Data from Grove et al (1929).

(Williams and Olmsted, 1936a, 1936b), cellulose and pectin (Spiller et al 1980) and cellulose, xylan, corn bran or pectin (Fleming and Rodriguez 1983) have been observed. In general SCFA output rises in conjunction with faecal output, even in subjects with diarrhoea (Cummings et al 1973). Only limited information can be gained, therefore, from the study of faecal SCFA, since no specific patterns of SCFA excretion in human stools have emerged which relate to events occurring within the large intestine. The role of SCFA in the colon would be much clearer if production rates were known.

SHORT CHAIN FATTY ACID PRODUCTION RATES

Knowledge of the amounts of SCFA produced in the hind-gut would facilitate a much clearer understanding of colonic function and of the significance of fermentation. Measuring production rates has proved to be exceedingly difficult however, and accurate data are few, even in ruminant physiology. In animals where fermentation occurs mainly in the fore-gut, SCFA production and metabolism has been assessed by two methods. The first uses concentration differences between portal, hepatic and arterial blood together with estimates or assumptions about blood flow to calculate net clearance. The second general approach is the use of isotope dilution methods to measure turnover (Bergman 1975). The problem with these studies is that each fatty acid is metabolised differently and at a number of sites in the body, for example in colonic epithelium, liver and muscle. Moreover, the picture is further complicated by endogenous production of acetate. This type of study has not been attempted in man, and the prospects of being able to obtain blood from the relevant sites in a person eating a reasonably normal diet at the time of study are not good.

An alternative approach (Cummings 1981) is to measure the supply of substrate for fermentation and from this, using fermentation balance equations derived for the ruminant, calculate theoretical production rates. Substrates available for fermentation in the human colon will include dietary carbohydrate which escapes digestion in the small intestine, and endogenous carbohydrate from both the small and large bowel. The principal dietary carbohydrates which pass into the large bowel are the cell wall polysaccharides of plants (non-starch polysaccharides, NSP). Much work remains to be done in conclusively demonstrating that the small intestine is not a major site of breakdown of NSP in the human gut. However preliminary studies have shown that NSP, taken as part of a normal diet, can be substantially recovered in ileostomy effluent (Holloway et al 1978; Sandberg et al 1981, 1983; Englyst and Cummings 1985). The amount available for fermentation in the colon will therefore depend largely on dietary intakes. These vary between 15 to 30 g/day in the UK, Scandinavia and Japan (Bingham et al 1979, 1984; Englyst et al 1982; Minowa et al 1983) to probably in excess of 100 g/day in parts of Africa (Bingham and Cummings 1980).

Starch may also escape breakdown in the small bowel, although at the moment it is not at all clear how much and for what reason this failure of digestion occurs. Anderson et al (1981), using breath hydrogen excretion as a marker of fermentation in man, have suggested that 10–20% of the carbohydrate in white flour is malabsorbed. Using a very different approach but with the same aim, Stephen et al (1983) measured the amount of starch reaching the terminal ileum in seven healthy volunteers; samples were collected by means of a multilumen tube, passed by mouth and positioned close to the ileo-caecal valve. Between 6 and 9% of the carbohydrate in a liquidised meal of banana, rice and other vegetables reached the ileum (see Chapter 4). Englyst and Cummings (1985), in a study of cereal starches, found a maximum of 4% not absorbed, and in a preliminary report of similar studies Chapman et al (1984) found only 2.4% malabsorbed from mixed diets. If one concludes from these studies that 5–10% of dietary starch is available for fermentation in subjects living on Western style diets, then this would add another 15–20 g to that available from NSP. In addition to this, small amounts (5 g/day) of soluble carbohydrate may also pass into the colon (Bond et al 1980; McNeil et al 1982). The only other source of carbohydrate available to the colonic microflora will be that derived from intestinal mucus. Although mucus degrading bacteria are present in the colon (Salyers et al 1977; Hoskins and Boulding 1981), the amounts degraded can only be surmised at present. An overall figure for total carbohydrate entering the large intestine in those living on Western style diets may be something between 40 and 50 g/day.

If the amount of carbohydrate fermented is known, then some idea of SCFA production can be obtained using equations derived from rumen metabolism (Hungate 1966) or proposed for man (Miller and Wolin 1979). From these equations it can be predicted that

$$10 \text{ g hexose fermented} \rightarrow 100 \text{ mmol SCFA} + 850 \text{ ml } CH_4 + 1200 \text{ ml } CO_2$$

Thus 40–50 g of carbohydrate will theoretically yield 400–500 mmol SCFA which, given the molar ratios in Table 6.3, would include 240–300 mmol acetate and 80–100 mmol of both propionate and butyrate. However, a number of assumptions have to be made in doing these calculations, not all of which may be appropriate. For example, it is believed that a close parallel between rumen and hind-gut fermentation exists, although in man there is apparently much less methane (CH_4) produced in the hind-gut than there is in the rumen and the hind-gut also contains few, if any, protozoa. Furthermore, the carbon/nitrogen ratio of available substrate is likely to be different in the rumen and hind-gut. It is also supposed that carbohydrate breakdown in the colon is entirely an anaerobic process. Whilst the great majority of the colonic flora are anaerobic (99.9%) some aerobes are present and could exert an important effect on SCFA production. Finally the overall efficiency of fermentation in the large bowel is unknown (see Chapter 5).

What other substrates have the potential to be fermented and produce SCFA in the colon? Long chain fatty acids are not fermented, but proteolysis is known to occur in the large intestine and many species of the microflora can break down amino acids (Hespell and Smith 1983). In man, ileostomy effluent contains 2–3 g/day of nitrogen, most of which must be protein (equivalent to 12–18 g/protein) since ileal effluent contains little urea or ammonia (Gibson 1977; McNeil et al 1982). Faecal nitrogen, which is usually less than ileostomy nitrogen (1–2 g/day), is present largely in microbial cells (Stephen and Cummings 1979). Protein is therefore available for fermentation in the colon and during passage through this organ some protein nitrogen is probably incorporated into microbial nitrogen. Only 7% of total faecal nitrogen comes from urea diffusion into the gut (Wrong et al 1982). It is likely that after deamination, the carbon skeletons of amino acids are fermented by the microflora and used as an energy source, whilst nitrogen is available for microbial protein synthesis. The carbon skeletons will yield acetate and propionate, together with the branched-chain fatty acids isobutyrate, iso-valerate and 2-methylbutyrate. The relative contribution of proteolytic fermentation in man is unknown and may well be influenced by the concomitant availability of carbohydrate for fermentation.

ABSORPTION

There can be little doubt that short chain fatty acids are absorbed from the human colon. If this was not so, man would be unique in the animal kingdom. All mammalian species studied absorb these acids, including the rat (Remesy and Demigne 1976; Umesaki et al 1979), pig (Argenzio and Southworth, 1974; Argenzio and Whipp 1979), horse (Argenzio et al 1974) and goat (Argenzio et al 1975). Absorption of all three SCFA from the human colon has been shown (Dawson et al 1964; McNeil et al 1978; Ruppin et al 1980). McNeil (1980) measured SCFA absorption in the human rectum, descending and transverse colon and showed that absorption rates are comparable with those observed in animals: i.e. human 6.1 – 12.6 μmol/sq.cm/h; cf. horse 8 μmol/sq.cm/h (Argenzio et al 1977), pig 8–10 μmol/sq.cm/h (Argenzio and Southworth, 1974) and from the cow's rumen 10.5 μmol/sq.cm/h (Stevens and Stettler 1966a,b). Net movement out of the colonic lumen of SCFA is more rapid than net sodium transport (Argenzio 1975; McNeil et al 1978).

The exact mechanism whereby these acids are absorbed still requires further study in all species, but a number of general characteristics emerge from published reports. Transport from the lumen is invariably associated with the appearance of bicarbonate ions, with the stimulation of sodium absorption (except in the horse: Argenzio et al 1977) and is independent of bulk water flow (Argenzio and Whipp 1979; Argenzio et al 1975). In man, important unanswered questions are whether they are absorbed primarily as acids or in the ionised form, whether there is a specific membrane carrier for SCFA, how SCFA transport affects that of other ions and, more particularly, the influence of mucosal SCFA metabolism on their transport.

MUCOSAL METABOLISM

Unlike the electrolytes sodium, potassium, chloride and bicarbonate, short chain fatty acids are potential substrates for energy metabolism in the colonic mucosa. In the ruminant, butyrate is almost entirely metabolised in the epithelium, whilst about 50% of propionate and some acetate are also utilised (Bergman 1975). In isolated colonocytes of the guinea-pig, it has been shown, using ^{14}C-labelled substrate, that all three acids are metabolised in the order butyrate > propionate > acetate (Wirthensohn 1981). Using colonocyte isolated from the rat, Roediger (1982) has shown that SCFA are substantially metabolised and suppress glucose oxidation. Studies of carbon dioxide production using mixtures of SCFA indicate that activation of fatty acids is in the order butyrate > acetate > propionate, as in the rumen (Ash and Baird 1973).

The main products of short chain fatty acid metabolism in the colonic epithelium are ketone bodies (acetoacetate, β-hydroxybutyrate), CO_2 and water. In the intact rat, Remesy and Demigne (1976) observed that about 12% of butyrate is transformed to ketone bodies in the caecal wall, as evidenced by studies of arterio-venous differences, the caecal artery (A) concentration for acetoacetic acid being 0.070 ± 0.005 mmol and caecal vein (V) 0.107 ± 0.005 mmol and for β-hydroxybutyrate (A) 0.083 ± 0.006 mmol and (V) 0.133 ± 0.007 mmol. Significantly, no evidence of ketogenesis was found in the colons of these rats, a finding similar to that of Henning and Hird for the rabbit (1972a,b) and in contrast to the considerable ketogenesis found in vitro.

In isolated human colonocytes, Roediger has shown (1980) that butyrate is actively metabolised to both CO_2 and ketone bodies. In comparison with metabolism by cells from proximal and distal colon, acetoacetate production was significantly diminished in the distal colon. Butyrate metabolism accounted for about 80% of oxygen consumption by colonocytes in both regions, but glucose utilisation was suppressed by butyrate to a larger degree in proximal than in the distal colonocytes. This, together with diminished ketone body production by the distal colon, suggests a greater dependence on butyrate as a fuel in the distal bowel.

The net effect of SCFA metabolism on colonic absorption is unknown. Since the three SCFA are metabolised at different rates in the cell, yet have similar stimulatory effects on sodium absorption, their intraceullular fate may not be important in ion transport (von Engelhardt and Rechkemmer 1983). Regional differences in metabolism may be significant however and in the guinea-pig regional differences in SCFA absorption occur (Rechkemmer and von Engelhardt 1981); Such differences have not been shown for man (McNeil and Cummings 1979).

DIARRHOEA

It has been suggested that changes in human stool output are due to the effect of short chain fatty acids generated in the colon. In man, these acids were once thought of as poorly absorbed anions, causing fluid retention in the colon by an osmotic effect. This view has been strengthened by the finding that, in children with diarrhoea due to carbohydrate malabsorption, stool output correlates with SCFA output (Torres-Pinedo et al 1966; Weijers et al 1961) and similarly in adults with diarrhoea due to malabsorption (Bustos-Fernandez et al 1971), lactose intolerance (McMichael et al 1965) and catharsis with magnesium sulphate (Grove et al 1929) (Figure 6.2). In some circumstances, short chain fatty acids may even induce fluid secretion in the colon (Bustos-Fernandez et al 1976). Other evidence for the laxative role of SCFA comes from a series of studies of the effect of dietary fibre on stool composition in man by Williams and Olmsted (1936a,b). They showed that stool weight correlated with SCFA output, and concluded that breakdown of dietary fibre produced short chain fatty acids which, being unabsorbed, increased faecal weight.

However, it is now clear that short chain fatty acids are absorbed from the colon and that the increase in faecal weight with dietary fibre is due to physical effects of undigested fibre and bacterial mass (Stephen and Cummings 1980). As faecal SCFA levels remain more or less constant despite dietary changes, any factor increasing stool weight will increase output of these acids, even laxatives. The change in stool output in diarrhoea caused by carbohydrate malabsorption is now thought to be partly due to the osmotic effect of malabsorbed sugars (Launiala 1968, 1969; Christopher and Bayless 1971; Saunders and Wiggins 1981). Furthermore, Argenzio (1978) has pointed out that SCFA production from glucose results in only a small increase in the theoretical osmotic pressure, as carbon dioxide is absorbed and bicarbonate reacts with short chain fatty acids as follows

$$\text{NaHCO}_3 + \text{CH}_3\text{COOH} \rightarrow \text{CH}_3\text{COONa} + \text{CO}_2 + \text{H}_2\text{O}$$

He also points out that these acids are the most rapidly absorbed ions in the colon and that their likely contribution to an increase in osmotic pressure will be small. In addition, acetate stimulates absorption of sodium and water from the colon at pH 6.4 and it is more likely that absorption from the colon is impaired in the absence of SCFA (Crump et al 1980).

The case against these acids being involved in diarrhoea is strong. However, where short chain fatty acids are rapidly generated, the colonic buffering system may not be able to deal with production of acid and pH will fall. This may impair absorption of salt and water by the colonic mucosa (Rousseau and Sladen 1971) and, in addition, promote lactate formation (a less well-absorbed anion) by the bacteria. Lactate may be important in the diarrhoea of childhood malabsorption, since significant quantities of it are found in the stools of these children. In general, however, it is difficult to implicate short chain fatty acids directly in either the control of faecal output or the genesis of diarrhoea in man.

FATE OF SHORT CHAIN FATTY ACIDS

Once across the colonic mucosa, short chain fatty acids enter the portal vein and are transported to the liver. All three SCFA are present in portal blood (Dankert et al 1981), but only acetate reaches peripheral tissues. Pomare et al (1985) have measured acetate in the venous blood of healthy subjects, following an overnight fast and then ingestion of various amounts of fermentable carbohydrate. Fasting venous blood acetate was 53.8 ± 4.4 μmol/l; the level rose to 181.3 ± 23.9 μmol/l 2.5 h after 20 g of lactulose and to 95.8 ± 11.7 μmol/l about 7 h after a similar amount of pectin. Thus short chain fatty acids produced in the colon may reach every tissue in the body and potentially may have wide-ranging effects on metabolism. The fact that they are largely the product of the breakdown of dietary polysaccharides provides a further mechanism whereby diet influences physiology and metabolism outside the confines of the gastro-intestinal tract.

REFERENCES

Anderson I H, Levine A S & Levitt M D (1981) Incomplete absorption of the carbohydrate in all-purpose wheat flour. *New England Journal of Medicine* **304**: 891–892.

Argenzio R A (1978) Physiology of diarrhoea — large intestine. *Journal of American Veterinary Association* **173**: 667–672.

Argenzio R A & Southworth M (1974) Sites of organic acid production and absorption in gastrointestinal tract of the pig. *American Journal of Physiology* **228**: 454–460.

Argenzio R A & Whipp S C (1979) Interrelationship of sodium, chloride, bicarbonate and acetate transport by the colon of the pig. *Journal of Physiology* **295**: 315–381.

Argenzio R A, Southworth M & Stevens C E (1974) Sites of organic acid production and absorption in the equine gastrointestinal tract. *American Journal of Physiology* **226**: 1043–1050.

Argenzio R A, Miller M & von Engelhardt W (1975) Effect of volatile fatty acids on water and ion absorption from the goat colon. *American Journal of Physiology* **229**: 997–1002.

Argenzio R A, Southworth M, Lowe J E & Stevens C E (1977) Interrelationship of Na, HCO₃ and volatile fatty acid transport by equine large intestine. *American Journal of Physiology* **233**: E469–E478.

Ash R & Baird G D (1973) Activation of volatile fatty acids in bovine liver and rumen epithelium. *Biochemical Journal* **136**: 311–319.

Banta C A, Clemens E T, Krinsky M M & Sheffy B E (1979) Sites of organic acid production and patterns of digesta movement in the gastrointestinal tract of dogs. *Journal of Nutrition* **109**: 1592–1600.

Bergman E N (1975) Production and utilization of metabolites by the alimentary tract as measured in portal and hepatic blood. In McDonald I M & Warner A C I (eds) *Digestion and Metabolism in the Ruminant* pp 292–305. Australia: University of New England Publishing Unit.

Bingham S & Cummings J H (1980) Sources and intakes of dietary fibre in man. In Spiller G A & Kay R M (eds) *Medical Aspects of Dietary Fibre* pp 261–284 New York: Plenum.

Bingham S, Cummings J H & McNeil I (1979). Intakes and sources of dietary fibre in the British population. *American Journal of Clinical Nutrition* **32**: 1313–1319.

Bingham S A, Englyst H N, Williams D R R & Cummings J H (1985) Dietary fibre consumption in Britain: new estimates and their relation to large bowel cancer mortality. *British Medical Journal* (in press).

Bjork J T, Soergel K H & Wood C M (1976) The composition of 'free' stool water. *Gastroenterology* **70**: A6/864.

Bond J H, Currier B E, Buchwald H & Levitt M D (1980) Colonic conservation of malabsorbed carbohydrate. *Gastroenterology* **78**: 444–447.

Brieger L (1878) Ueber die fluchtigen Bestandtheile der menschlichen Excremente. *Journal für praktische Chemie.* **17**: 124–138.

Bustos-Fernandez L B, Gonzalez E, Marzi A & Paolo M I L (1971) Faecal acidorrhoea. *New England Journal of Medicine* **284**: 295–298.

Bustos-Fernandez L B, Gonzalez E, Paolo, M I. L, Celemer D & de Furuya K O (1976) Organic anions induce colonic secretion. *American Journal of Digestive Diseases* **21**: 329–332.

Chapman R W, Sillery J & Saunders D R (1984) Physiological starch malabsorption: direct quantitation in ileostomates and effect of small bowel transit time. *Gut* **25**: A1158–A1159.

Chernov A J, Joe W F & Gompertz D (1972) Intrajejunal VFAs in the stagnant loop syndrome. *Gut* **13**: 103–106.

Christopher N L & Bayless T M (1971) Role of the small bowel and colon in lactose induced diarrhoea. *Gastroenterology* **60**: 845–852.

Clemens E T & Maloiy G M O (1981) Colonic electrolyte flux and gut composition as seen in four species of sub-human primates. *Comparative Biochemistry and Physiology* **69A**: 543–549.

Clemens E T & Maloiy G M O (1983) Digestive physiology of East African wild ruminants. *Comparative Biochemistry and Physiology* **76A**: 319–330.

Crump M H, Argenzio R A & Whipp S C (1980) Effects of acetate on absorption of solute and water from the pig colon. *American Journal of Veterinary Research* **41**: 1565–1568.

Cummings J H (1981) Short chain fatty acids in the human colon. *Gut* **22**: 763–779.

Cummings J H & Branch W J (1985) Fermentation and the production of short chain fatty acids in the human large intestine. In Vahouny G V & Kritchevsky D (eds) *Basic and Clinical Aspects of Dietary Fibre*, in press. New York: Alan R. Liss.

Cummings J H, James W P T & Wiggins H S (1973) Role of the colon in ileal-resection diarrhoea. *Lancet* **1**: 344–347.

Cummings J H, Hill M J, Jenkins D J A, Pearson J R & Wiggins H S (1976) Changes in faecal composition and colonic function due to cereal fibre. *American Journal of Clinical Nutrition* **29**: 1468–1473.

Cummings J H, Hill M J, Bone E S, Branch W J & Jenkins D J A (1979) The effect of meat protein and dietary fibre on colonic function and metabolism. II. Bacterial metabolites in faeces and urine. *American Journal of Clinical Nutrition* **32**: 2094–2101.

Dankert J, Zijlstra J B & Wolthers B G (1981) Volatile fatty acids in human peripheral and portal blood: quantitative determination by vacuum distillation and gas chromatography. *Clinica et Chimica Acta* **110**: 301–307.

Dawson A M, Holdsworth C D & Webb J (1964) Absorption of short chain fatty acids in man. *Proceedings of the Society for Experimental Biology and Medicine* **177**: 97–100.

Elsden S R, Hitchcock M W S, Marshall R A & Phillipson A T (1946) Volatile acid in the digestion of ruminants and other animals. *Journal of Experimental Biology* **22**: 191–202.

Englyst H N & Cummings J H (1985) Digestion and absorption of the polysaccharides of some cereal foods in the human small intestine. *American Journal of Clinical Nutrition* (in press).

Englyst H N, Bingham S A, Wiggins H S et al (1982) Non-starch polysaccharide consumption in four Scandinavian populations. *Nutrition and Cancer* **4**: 50–60.

Fleming S E & Rodriguez M A (1983) Influence of dietary fibre in faecal excretion of volatile fatty acids by human adults. *Journal of Nutrition* **113**: 1613–1626.

Gibson J A (1977) Studies of urea and ammonia metabolism. MD thesis, University of Cambridge.

Grove E W, Olmsted W H & Koenig K (1929) The effect of diet and catharsis on the lower volatile fatty acids in the stools of normal men. *Journal of Biological Chemistry* **85**: 127–136.

Henning S J & Hird F J (1972a) Transport of acetate and butyrate in the hind-gut of rabbits. *Biochemical Journal* **130**: 791–796.

Henning S J & Hird F J R (1972b) Ketogenesis from butyrate and acetate by the caecum and the colon of rabbits. *Biochemical Journal* **130**: 785–790.

Hespell R B & Smith C J (1983). Utilization of nitrogen sources by gastrointestinal tract bacteria. In Hentges D J (ed) *Human Intestinal Microflora in Health and Disease*, pp 167–188. New York Academic Press.

Holloway W D, Tasman-Jones C & Lee S P (1978) Digestion of certain fractions of dietary fiber in humans. *American Journal of Clinical Nutrition* **31**: 927–930.

Hoskins L C & Boulding E T (1981) Mucin degradation in human colon ecosystems: evidence for the existence and role of bacterial subpopulations producing glycosidases as extra-cellular enzymes *Journal of Clinical Investigation* **67**: 163–172.

Hungate R E (1966) *The Rumen and Its Microbes*. New York: Academic Press.

Kern D L, Slyter L L, Leffel E C, Weaver J M & Oltjen R R (1974) Ponies vs. steers: microbial and chemical characteristics of intestinal ingestion. *Journal of Animal Science* **38**: 559–564.

Launiala K (1968) The mechanisms of diarrhoea in congenital disaccharide malabsorption. *Acta Paediatrica Scandinavica* **57**: 425–432.

Launiala K (1969) The effect of malabsorbed sucrose or mannitol-induced accelerated transit on absorption in the human small intestine. *Scandinavian Journal of Gastroenterology* **4**: 25–32.

McMichael H B, Webb J & Dawson A M (1965) Lactose deficiency in adults. *Lancet* **1**: 717–720.

McNeil N I (1980) Short chain fatty acid absorption in the human large intestine. M D thesis, University of Cambridge.

McNeil N I & Cummings J H (1979) Evidence for regional variation in large intestinal function. *Gut* **20** A439.

McNeil N I, Cummings J H & James W P T (1978) Short chain fatty acid absorption by the human large intestine. *Gut* **19**: 819–822.

McNeil N I, Bingham S, Cole T J, Grant A M & Cummings J H (1982) Diet and health of people with an ileostomy. 2 Ileostomy function and nutritional state. *British Journal of Nutrition* **47**: 407–415.

Miller T L & Wolin M J (1979) Fermentation by saccharolytic intestinal bacteria. *American Journal of Clinical Nutrition* **32**: 164–172.

Minowa M, Bingham S & Cummings J H (1983) Dietary fibre intake in Japan. *Human Nutrition Applied Nutrition* **37A**: 113–119.

Newton C R, Bennett A N, Billings J A & Milton-Thompson G J (1972) Ileal short chain fatty acid concentrations after a chemically defined meal. *Archives de Maladies de l'appareil Digestif et de la Nutrition* **61**: 37C.

Odelson D A & Breznak J A (1983) Volatile fatty acid production by the hindgut microbiota of xylophagous termites. *Applied and Environmetal Microbiology* **45**: 1602–1613.

Olmsted W H, Curtis G & Timm O K (1935) Stool volatile fatty acids. IV. The influence of feeding bran pentosan and fibre to man. *Journal of Biological Chemistry* **108**: 645–652.

Pomare E W, Branch W J & Cummings J H (1985) Carbohydrate fermentation in the human colon and its relation to acetate concentrations in venous blood. *Journal of Clinical Investigation* (in press)

Rechkemmer G & von Engelhardt W (1981) Absorptive processes in different colonic segments of the guinea-pig and the effects of short chain fatty acids. In Kasper H & Goebell H (eds) *Colon and Nutrition*, pp 61–67. Lancaster: MTP Press.

Remesy C & Demigne C (1976) Partition and absorption of volatile fatty acids in the alimentary canal of the rat. *Annales de Recherches Veterinaires* **7**: 39–55.

Roediger W E W (1980) Role of anaerobic bacteria in the metabolic welfare of the colonic mucosa in man. *Gut* **21**: 793–798.

Roediger W E W (1982) Utilization of nutrients by isolated epithelial cells of the rat colon. *Gastroenterology* **83**: 424–429.

Rousseau B & Sladen G C (1971) Effect of luminal pH on the absorption of water, sodium and chloride by the rat intestine in vivo. *Biochimica et Biophysica Acta* **233**: 591–593.

Rubinstein R, Howard A V & Wrong O M (1969) In vivo dialysis of faeces as a method of stool analysis IV. The organic anion component. *Clinical Science* **37**: 549–564.

Rubsamen K, Hume I D, Foley W J & Rubsamen U (1983) Regional differences in electrolyte, short chain fatty acid and water absorption in the hindgut of two species of arboreal marsupials. *Pflügers Archiv. European Journal of Physiology* **399**: 68–73.

Ruppin H, Bar-Meir S, Soergel K H, Wood C M & Schmitt M G (1980) Absorption of short chain fatty acids by the colon. *Gastroenterology* **78**: 1500–1507.

Russell J B & Jeraci J L (1984) Effect of carbon monoxide on fermentation of fibre, starch, and amino acids by mixed rumen microorganisms in vitro. *Applied and Environmental Microbiology* **48**: 211–217.

Salyers A A, Vercellotti J R, West S E H & Wilkins T D (1977) Fermentation of mucin and plant polysaccharides by strains of Bacteroides from the human colon. *Applied and Environmental Microbiology* **33**: 319–322.

Sandberg A-S, Andersson H, Hallgren B, Hasselblad K, Isaksson B & Hulten L (1981) Experimental model for in vivo determination of dietary fibre and its effect on the absorption of nutrients in the small intestine. *British Journal of Nutrition* **45**: 283–294.

Sandberg A-S, Ahderinne R, Andersson H, Hallgren B & Hulten L (1983) The effect of citrus pectin on the absorption of nutrients in the small intestine. *Human Nutrition: Clinical Nutrition* **37C**: 171–183.

Saunders D R & Wiggins H S (1981) Conservation of mannitol, lactulose and raffinose by the human colon. *American Journal of Physiology* **24**: G397–G402.

Spiller G A, Chernoff M C, Hill R A, Gates J E, Nassar J J & Shipley E A (1980) Effect of purified cellulose, pectin, and a low-residue diet on faecal volatile fatty acids, transit time and faecal weight in humans. *American Journal of Clinical Nutrition* **33**: 754–759.

Stephen A M & Cummings J H (1979) The influence of dietary fibre on faecal nitrogen excretion in man. *Proceedings of the Nutrition Society* **38**: 141A.

Stephen A M & Cummings J H (1980) Mechanism of action of dietary fibre in the human colon. *Nature, London* **284**: 283–284.

Stephen A M, Haddad A C & Phillips S F (1983) Passage of carbohydrate into the colon. Direct measurement in humans. *Gastroenterology* **85**: 589–595.

Stevens C E & Stettler B K (1966a) Factors affecting the transport of volatile fatty acids across rumen epithelium. *American Journal of Physiology* **210**: 365–372.

Stevens C E & Stettler B K (1966b) Transport of fatty acid mixtures across rumen epithelium. *American Journal of Physiology* **211**: 264–271.

Thomsen L L, Roberton A M, Wong J, Lee S P & Tasman-Jones C (1984) Intra-caecal short chain fatty acids are altered by dietary pectin in the rat. *Digestion* **29**: 129–137.

Torres-Pinedo R, Lavastida M, Rivera C L, Rodriguez H & Ortiz A (1966) Studies on infant diarrhoea. I. A comparison of the effects of milk feeding and intravenous therapy upon the composition and volume of the stool and urine. *Journal of Clinical Investigation* **45**: 469–480.

Umesaki Y, Yajima T, Yokokura T & Mutai M (1979) Effect of organic acid absorption on bicarbonate transport in rat colon. *Pflugers Archiv. European Journal of Physiology* **379**: 43–47.

Vernia P, Breuer R I, Gnaedinger A, Latella G & Santoro M L (1984) Composition of faecal water. Comparison of 'in vitro' dialysis with ultrafiltration. *Gastroenterology* **86**: 1557–1561.

von Engelhardt W & Rechkemmer G (1983). The physiological effects of short chain fatty acids in the hind gut. In Wallace G & Bell L (eds) *Fibre in Human and Animal Nutrition*, pp 149–155. Wellington, New Zealand: Royal Society of New Zealand.

Weijers H A, van de Kamer J H, Dicke W K & Ijsseling J (1961) Diarrhoea caused by deficiency of sugar splitting enzymes. *Acta Pediatrica (Stockholm)* **50**: 55–71.

Williams R D & Olmsted W H (1936a) The effect of cellulose, hemicellulose and lignin on the weight of stool. A contribution to the study of laxation in man. *Journal of Nutrition* **11**: 433–449.

Williams R D & Olmsted W H (1936b) The manner in which food controls the bulk of faeces. *Annals of Internal Medicine* **10**: 717–727.

Wirthensohn K (1981) Der Stoffwechsel kurzkettiger Fettsauren im Colonepithel des Meerschweinchens und seine Bedeutung fur die Natriumresorption. Thesis, University of Hohenheim.

Wolin M J (1960) A theoretical rumen fermentation balance. *Journal of Dairy Science* **40**: 1452–1459.

Wrong O, Metcalfe-Gibson A, Morrison B I, Ng S T & Howard V (1965) In vivo dialysis of faeces as a method of stool analysis. 1. Technique and results in normal subjects. *Clinical Science* **28**: 357–375.

Wrong O M, Vince A J & Waterlow J C (1982) The origins and bacterial metabolism of faecal ammonia. In Kasper H & Goebell H (eds) *Colon and Cancer*, p 133. Lancaster: MTP Press.

Zijlstra J B, Beukema J, Wolthers B G, Byrne B M, Groen A & Donkert L (1977) Pretreatment methods prior to gas chromatographic analysis of volatile fatty acids from faecal samples. *Clinica et Chimica Acta* **78**: 243–250.

Chapter 7
Immunological Responses to Food

Glenis K. Scadding and Jonathan Brostoff

As well as its functions of digestion, absorption and elimination, the gut also acts as a barrier between the internal and external environment. Mucosal integrity, gastric acid, mucus, bacterial flora, and peristaltic movement play a part; so do several immunological mechanisms (Tables 7.1, 7.2).

The common mucosal associated lymphoid tissue (MALT) is present at all epithelial surfaces that are in contact with the external environment, is largely independent of the systemic immune response and is governed by antigenic stimuli at epithelial surfaces. A failure or abnormality in one of these mechanisms can result in symptoms such as anaphylaxis, rhinitis and skin rashes, classified as food allergy.

Peyers' patches

Peyers' patches are covered with an epithelium which includes a unique cell type, the membranous or microfold (M) cell. This appears to provide preferential and controlled antigen uptake: M cells take up carbon particles

Table 7.1. Non-immunological gastro-intestinal barriers.

Intact epithelium	— Decreased turnover, e.g. methotrexate, alcohol, uraemia, ischaemia: associated with diarrhoea, malabsorption and the passage of toxins and bacteria into the circulation.
Normal gut flora	— Maintained by peristalsis: imbalance from blind loop, antibiotics, malabsorption.
Gastric acid	— Decrease is associated with increased gastro-intestinal infections and with increased circulating antibovine serum antibodies (Kraft et al 1967).
Lysozyme	— Leads to bacterial lysis with/without IgA and complement (Adinolfi et al 1966).
Bile salts	— Decreased proliferation of some micro-organisms (Dixon et al 1960).
Glycoproteins	— Prevent attachment of bacteria, viruses, parasites to epithelium. Interact with allergens and toxins to decrease epithelial penetration. Synthesis is increased during immunological reactions (Miller et al 1979; Lake et al 1980).

Table 7.2. Gut-associated lymphoid tissues (GALT).

Immunoglobulins
   IgA ⎫
   IgM ⎭ in secretions

   IgA in bile

Cells
   Solitary lymphoid follicles and Peyers' patches
      B cells (in follicles)
      T cells (in deep cortex, mainly OKT4+)

   Diffuse lymphoid tissues
      Intra-epithelial lymphocytes (T cells, mainly OKT8+)
      Lamina propria T lymphocytes (mainly OKT4+)
         Plasma cells (mainly IgA producing)

      Macrophages

      Mast cells ⟨ mucosal mast cell / connective tissue mast cell

      Eosinophils
   Mesenteric lymph nodes
   Reticulo-endothelial cells of liver

---

and horseradish peroxidase from the intestinal lumen by pinocytosis and transport such particles through the epithelium in vesicles for release into the space occupied by migrating lymphoid cells (Bockman and Cooper 1973; Owen 1977). It is possible that this route is also utilised by certain invading micro-organisms such as reoviruses and *Salmonella typhi* (Kumagai 1922; Owen 1983).

Studies in a rabbit with two Thiery-Vella loops, one loop containing Peyers' patches, the other not, showed that it was necessary to expose the Peyers' patch containing loop to antigen to obtain a secretory response in both loops (Cebra et al 1977). Thus, the Peyers' patch immunoblasts appear to play a primary role in the induction of the secretory immune response. Once primed, these cells pass along afferent lymphatics to the mesenteric nodes where they are 'processed' and become lymphoblasts. These then migrate via the thoracic duct to the systemic circulation where they mature (Parrott 1976). The lymphocytes then migrate through the spleen and other organs, eventually 'homing' to the lamina propria and to extra-intestinal sites of IgA antibody production. The mechanism of 'homing' is not understood: antigen does not appear to be necessary since IgA lymphoblasts migrate to tissues which have never been exposed to antigen (Moore and Hall 1972; Parrott and Ferguson 1974). This continuous traffic of lymphocytes from the nodular lymphoid tissues of the gut, via lymph and blood back to the mucosa of small bowel and colon, allows for widespread distribution of antibody-producing cells and T blasts and the capacity for specific immune reactions to antigen is spread throughout the length of the gut.

In summary, priming results in antigen-specific IgA plasmablasts in gut lamina propria and after a second challenge includes:

(i)   antigen-stimulated expansion and differentiation of specific B cells;
(ii) generation of specific helper T cells required for maturation of plasma-blasts and subsequent synthesis and secretion of IgA antibodies;
(iii) in vivo redistribution of antigen-specific B and T cells.

Plasma cells, the main humoral effector cells in the mucosa, are derived from the B immunoblasts that have followed this traffic route; the T immunoblasts are later found as intra-epithelial lymphocytes. The function of these latter cells is unknown, but the majority are OKT8 positive and Ia negative (in contrast to the majority of lamina propria T cells which are OKT8 negative) (Selby et al 1983). They are capable of modulating Ia expression by intestinal epithelial cells (Cerf-Bentussan 1984) and may show mitogen-induced cytotoxicity (Chiba et al 1981). They could be important: (i) in processing intraluminal antigens possibly by suppression/cytotoxicity (Selby et al 1981) and are in an environment which is suited to such reactions being HLA ABC positive, with weak DR (Ia) antigens; (ii) in food tolerance; (iii) in the control of bacterial and viral infection; and (iv) in parasite defence. In the gut, T helper cells are mainly directed towards aiding IgA production, while T suppressors inhibit IgG and IgM production. In contrast, there are in Peyers' patches Ia positive veiled cells, similar to Langerhans cells in skin, which could enhance humoral immunity to antigen encountered there.

Secretory immunity

IgA containing cells greatly outnumber cells producing IgG and IgM in the lamina propria (Crabbé and Heremans 1966). Less than 1% of cells contain IgE (Brandtzaeg 1981) and IgD containing cells are also very sparse. In germ-free animals, the lamina propria is practically devoid of antibody-producing cells, but following exposure to a normal environment the numbers of mucosal lymphocytes and plasma cells increase over a few weeks to reach normal levels. Similarly, in neonates there is no IgA or IgM in exocrine secretions (Ogra et al 1972), but the levels gradually increase with exposure to bacterial and food antigens. The IgA producing cell system is probably mature by 1–2 months (Haneberg and Aarskog 1975). IgM is probably important in infants as judged by *E. coli* oral vaccination (Girard and de Kalbermatten 1979), but in the adult IgA is the major immunoglobulin in intestinal juice, reaching levels of 28 mg per 100 ml in jejunal secretions (Bull et al 1971).

In external secretions, IgA is found as an 11 S dimer, secretory IgA, which consists of two monomers of 7 S IgA, jointed by a covalently linked peptide, the J chain of which is also secreted by the plasma cell. To this is added, by the epithelial cell, a glycopeptide secretory component which is involved in the transport of IgA across the epithelium (Brandtzaeg 1978; Brown 1978) and also protects it from digestion by the proteolytic enzymes bathing the mucosal surface (Tomasi 1970). Among the other immunoglobulin classes, only IgM binds secretory piece and is transported across the epithelium as secretory immunoglobulin (Brandtzaeg 1973).

The function of gut-associated immunoglobulin lies probably in immune exclusion at mucosal surfaces. This is important in the defence against micro-organisms: secretory IgA prevents bacterial adherence to mucosal surfaces and plays a part in the resistance to viruses such as poliomyelitis; IgE appears in secretions during parasitic infections and may be a factor in worm expulsion. Immune exclusion is also important in the control of antigen absorption. In rats locally immunised with horseradish peroxidase or bovine serum albumin, the amount of absorbed antigens is decreased.

Oral tolerance

Immunological tolerance, a state of unresponsiveness to a particular antigen, can be induced by oral feeding of that antigen (Chase 1946). Since Besredka (1919) showed that oral immunisation of rabbits with killed salmonellae provided protection against a fatal live dose, irrespective of the titres of serum antibody, the concept of a local secretory immune system has grown in importance.

The mechanism by which a state of specific immunological non-responsiveness occurs is not understood and several factors have been implicated: serum factors (Andre et al 1975), immunoglobulin (Kagnoff 1978), B lymphocytes (Asherson et al 1977) and T lymphocytes (Richman et al 1978; Ngan and Kind 1978; McDonald, 1983). It is possible that digestion of antigen generates tolerogenic fragments, whereas whole antigen acts through the macrophage-T helper B-cell route and induces a humoral response. Animal experiments suggest that the sequence of the response to fed antigen is: (i) initial gastro-intestinal contact with new antigen; (ii) secretory antibody response, IgA in plasma cells and in gut lumen; (iii) little or no serum IgG or IgM production and no evidence of immune cell reactions; (iv) tolerance to that antigen then occurs; and (v) little or no production of IgE in the gut or elsewhere (Royal College of Physicians Report on Food Allergy 1983) (Figure 7.1).

ABNORMAL IMMUNOLOGICAL RESPONSES TO FOOD

The concept of food allergy has gained in popularity recently. Allergy is defined as an untoward immunological reaction, but it must be emphasised that many instances of reactions to foods do not involve the immune system and are therefore not allergic in nature. The main categories of food reactions are listed in Table 7.3.

This chapter will deal exclusively with reactions involving the immune system; many of the other mechanisms are described elsewhere in this book.

Type I reactions to foods

In Type I reactions, mast cells sensitised with antibody are made to degranulate and release mediators when the coating antibodies are cross-linked by the relevant antigen. The occurrence of Type I reactions to food antigens is undisputed. Such reactions include anaphylaxis, urticaria and

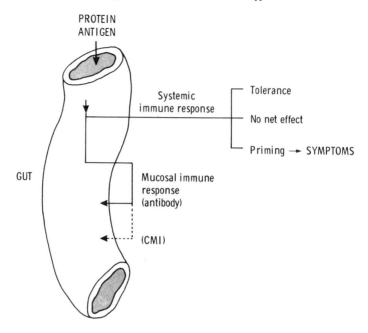

Figure 7.1. Food antigen in the gut can elicit a local mucosal immune response, involving antibody, mainly IgA, and possibly cell-mediated immunity (CMI). The systemic immune system often remains uninvolved, unless intestinal permeability is increased.

angio-oedema, rhinorrhoea, asthma, diarrhoea and vomiting. Symptoms usually occur within a few minutes of food ingestion and are often associated with a positive skin prick test and a positive radio-allergosorbent test (RAST; see p. 104) to the relevant food, and elevated serum IgE levels. They are probably IgE mediated. Reactions have been transferred to normal individuals as a Prausnitz–Kustner reaction at the site of injection of serum from allergic individuals (Wilson and Waltzer 1935). Such reactions are commoner in children (7–12% of all infants are allergic to cow's milk protein; Bahna and Heiner 1978) and there is a tendency for the allergy to disappear with age.

Delayed reactions to foods

These are more controversial. Atopic asthma and eczema in young children are sometimes associated with food allergy, particularly to milk and eggs, and elimination diets are often successful (Rowe and Rowe 1951; Atherton et al 1978). In adults, late responses occurring hours or days after ingestion of specific food have been described. These can affect the gut, but may also involve a variety of other organs such as lungs (Brostoff et al 1979), brain (Monro et al 1980), nose (Shiada et al 1979) and joints (Parke and Hughes 1981). The evidence for these reactions being food related depends on their

Table 7.3. Reactions to food.

A. Non-immunological

Psychological	— food aversion
Contamination	— chemical, e.g. preservatives
	microbiological — toxins
	— parasites
Idiosyncrasy	— enzyme disorders — lactase deficiency
	— glucose-6-phosphate dehydrogenase
	— phenylketonuria
	— pharmacological effect — caffeine
	— tyramine
	direct histamine release, e.g. strawberries, shellfish
	prostaglandin metabolism — salicylates

Irritation of gastro-intestinal tract, especially if diseased
Fermentation   — unabsorbed residues by bowel flora

B. Immunological

— immediate Type I allergy — local
— systemic (anaphylaxis)

— delayed ⟨ local / systemic ⟩ ? Type III

— enteropathy ⟨ gluten / cows' milk ⟩ ? Types III & IV

---

disappearance when food is withdrawn and their reappearance on challenge with the relevant food or foods.

Involvement of some immunological mechanism must be demonstrated before these reactions can be described as food allergic.

MECHANISMS

Gut permeability

In order for food allergy to occur, food antigens must be absorbed through the gastro-intestinal tract. Despite the immunological and non-immunological gut barriers, some macromolecules are transported intact across the mucosa. This occurs most in premature and newborn infants (Gruskay and Cooke 1955; Rothberg 1969). The uptake and transport of gamma-globulin markedly decreases when the epithelial cells of the small intestine mature in the neonate (Bamford 1966; Rodewald 1970) and it had been assumed that macromolecular absorption ceases entirely at this time. However, reports have appeared suggesting that small, nutritionally insignificant amounts of antigenically intact macromolecules may be transmitted across the mature mammalian gut (Dack and Petran 1934; Wilson and Waltzer 1935; Danforth and Moore 1959; Bernstein and Ovary 1968; Korenblat et al 1968). Studies with horseradish peroxidase, which can be detected histochemically by light and electron microscopy, have confirmed this (Clarke and Hardy 1971; Cornell et al 1971).

Absorption appears to be related to protein concentration; there must be sufficient to escape intraluminal proteolysis and subsequent lysosomal digestive capacity, to permit intact molecules to be transported out of the cell and into the circulation. At physiological or low levels, luminal antigens are directed via the M cells to the MALT. Obviously increased gut permeability, or decreased levels of secretory IgA could result in more macromolecules entering the systemic circulation with subsequent sensitisation (Cunningham-Rundles et al 1978). Increased permeability to polyethylene glycol (PEG) has been described in children with eczema (Jackson et al, 1981) although gut histology is normal (Perkkio 1980) (see Chapter 3). Gut irradiation with ^{60}Co resulted in the development of egg allergy in an atopic patient (Ciprandi et al 1984), presumably as a result of increased intestinal permeability. Bacterial or viral gut infections may precipitate food allergy in this way.

Immune complexes

The formation of immune complexes in the small intestine and the specialised uptake of large molecules as complexes is a physiological event (WHO 1977). These complexes usually contain IgG or IgA and appear transiently in the serum following a meal. They are normally removed by the liver and transported into the bile (Jackson et al 1978; Orlans et al 1978; Stokes et al 1980).

In contrast, food allergic individuals form immune complexes containing allergens and specific IgG and IgA in concentrations greater than those in the blood of normal subjects (André et al 1975; Paganelli et al 1979). Circulating immune complexes containing IgE and IgG have been demonstrated in the blood of food allergic patients and the appearance of these correlated with symptoms. Brostoff et al (1982) postulate that a primary mucosal IgE-mediated hypersensitivity is the gate-keeper, via mast cell degranulation and mediator release, for increased permeability of the gut mucosa. Antigen absorption is thus increased, with the formation of immune complexes and the occurrence of symptoms resulting from a form of serum sickness (Figure 7.2). Genetic factors controlling mast cells, complement components (Turner et al 1978) and neutrophil activity (Soothill 1976) could be relevant in determining which individuals are food allergic. It is possible that other immunoglobulins may be involved, especially in delayed reactions, for example IgG4 (Gwynn et al 1982) and IgD (Miller 1982) in the reaction to tartrazine and other colouring agents.

Mediators

Whether or not immunological mechanisms are implicated, the sequence of events which follows a food challenge in a sensitised or food-intolerant person involves the release of a number of mediators. There is evidence of histamine

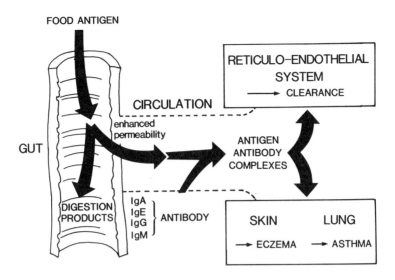

Figure 7.2. Enhanced intestinal permeability results in food antigen–antibody immune complex formation. These may exceed the clearing capacity of the reticuloendothelial system and result in disease at various sites.

release (May 1976), prostaglandin release and of benefit from cyclooxygenase inhibitors such as aspirin (Buisseret et al 1978). Recently, raised levels of 5-hydroxyindoleacetic acid after food challenge have been reported in the serum of patients with rheumatoid arthritis, whose symptoms increase following challenge with certain foodstuffs (Little et al 1983). A rise in prostaglandin E_2 has been reported in patients with diarrhoea resulting from irritable bowel syndrome (Alun Jones et al 1982). In this study, double-blind challenges with selected foodstuffs demonstrated intolerance in six out of six patients. However, the serum IgE was not raised and no immunological abnormality was found (see Chapter 14). It has been suggested (Wright and Burton 1982) that some atopic subjects have abnormal prostaglandin synthesis pathways because of a deficiency of enzymes for converting linoleic to gamma-linolenic acid. In such a case, milk, which contains linoleic acid and arachidonic acid, might stimulate the synthesis of thromboxane and other metabolites. The resting plasma $PGF_{2\alpha}$ levels in ten aspirin sensitive urticaria patients were significantly higher than ten normal subjects in a recent study, and the $PGF_{2\alpha}/PGE$ ratio in aspirin sensitive urticaria patients was significantly higher than that in normal subjects.

FOOD ALLERGY AS A CAUSE OF GUT DISEASE

Immediate hypersensitivity

This can occur in both children and adults and can present with any of the following symptoms: diarrhoea and vomiting, nausea, pain, distension and flatus. There is usually a positive skin prick test and RAST to the relevant antigen, although the skin prick test may remain positive in a child who has outgrown his gastro-intestinal sensitivity.

Eosinophilic gastro-enteritis

This syndrome comprises inflammation of the stomach and intestine, characterised by a peripheral blood eosinophilia and a localised or diffuse eosinophilic infiltration of the intestine. The symptoms vary according to the layer of gut wall involved; mucosal involvement giving nausea, vomiting, diarrhoea and pain with anaemia and hypoproteinaemia. Muscle layer involvement results in intestinal obstruction, and serosal inflammation, which is rare, gives eosinophilic ascites. The patients are frequently atopic and the symptoms may be relieved by exclusion diets (Scudamore et al 1982). Skin prick tests to the relevant antigen can be negative.

Cows' milk-sensitive enteropathy

This has been shown to be a cause of gastro-intestinal bleeding, protein-losing enteropathy, colitis and subtotal villous atrophy in young children (see Chapter 12).

Gluten-sensitive enteropathy (see Chapter 13).

This syndrome, first described by Samuel Gee in 1888, involves an intolerance to the gliadin fraction of gluten which results in severe intestinal epithelial damage and malabsorption. Several observations suggest an immunological basis. The proportion of atopic people suffering from coeliac disease is significantly higher than the proportion in the normal population; 75% of coeliacs possess HLA B8, DR3 and 1 in 50 has secretory IgA deficiency. Half of them have other auto-antibodies, including those to reticulin (Hodgson et al 1976). Those with gliadin antibodies were all of Gm allotype G2m(n). Many show decreased complement function (Doe et al 1974) and poor cell-mediated immunity (Scott and Lowsowsky 1976). IgE levels are usually normal and no IgE against wheat fractions has been demonstrated. It is possible that Type III (immune complexes) and Type IV (delayed hypersensitivity) immune mechanisms are involved. Recently sequence homology between gliadin and an adenovirus type XII protein has been described (Kagnoff 1984). There is evidence of prior infection with this adenovirus in 38% of patients with coeliac disease and 7% of controls, as assessed by neutralising antibody to a different viral protein.

Ulcerative colitis

Histologically there is an increase in mast cells in the lamina propria (Juhlin 1963), which also have a high histamine content. There are increased numbers of plasma cells producing IgA, IgM and IgG (Söltoft et al 1973) but IgE plasma cells were reported as increased in only one of several studies (Heatley et al 1975a), and serum IgE is usually normal. Immune complexes do occur, but levels are not related to disease activity.

The aetiology is unknown. Intravenous feeding or an elemental diet rarely gives relief from symptoms, while there are sometimes exacerbations following certain foods, especially milk. Disodium cromoglycate was of benefit in only one series of ulcerative proctitis (Mani et al 1976), and is generally considered to be of little value in this condition.

Crohn's disease

This topic is reviewed in Chapter 15.

Oral and pharyngeal pruritus

This condition is noted by some atopic patients after the ingestion of certain foods. Antigenic cross-reactivity suggests that a carbohydrate side chain may be involved (Aalberse et al 1981).

Hypersensitve furrowed mouth

This syndrome of non-congenital fissuring of the lips, tongue, buccal mucosa and pharynx is associated with positive skin prick and RAST tests to specific foods, and with increased levels of salivary IgE. The skin window technique shows an influx of eosinophils. These all suggest an allergic response to food antigens.

Irritable bowel syndrome (see Chapter 14)

A recent survey of 2000 patients referred to a gastro-intestinal out-patient clinic (Theodossi 1983) showed that 880 were categorised as having non-organic disorders. The largest subgroup of these (449) had altered bowel habit with abdominal pain. The author admitted that it was possible that these patients could be reclassified as having food intolerance. Since the symptoms are similar to those noted in immediate hypersensitivity, it would seem logical to search for possible food allergens in these patients.

Our recent studies (Scadding et al unpublished data) have shown no increase in IgE containing immune complexes after feeding suspect foods to patients with irritable bowel syndrome; this contrasts with the findings of 90% positive in food responsive arthralgia and suggests that if there is an immunological abnormality in irritable bowel syndrome the reaction is localised within the gut wall.

DIAGNOSIS

Skin tests, RAST and serum IgE levels are helpful in Type I hypersensitivity, but they are usually unhelpful in patients with delayed reactions to foods except in confirming that a patient is atopic with multiple sensitivities. The lack of evidence of IgE-mediated abnormalities on skin tests or serum studies does not necessarily exclude a local IgE response within the gastro-intestinal tract. Patients with haemorrhagic proctitis have an increased number of IgE containing plasma cells in their rectal mucosae (Rosenkrans et al 1980; Heatley et al 1975a) and patients with food sensitivity may have intense eosinophilic gastroenteritis without other evidence of a response to specific foods (Klein et al 1970).

IgE

Attempts to show an IgE-mediated immunological mechanism can be performed by skin testing or by the RAST test, which was devised by Wide et al (1967). In this procedure allergens are covalently bound to solid phase supports, reacted with the test serum, which may contain IgE antibody, and any solid phase allergen–IgE antibody complex is detected by radiolabelled anti-IgE. It is important to ensure that certain technical details are correct. First, all relevent allergens must be coupled to the solid phase support material; sensitivity of the test can be improved by utilising purified food extracts, but the relevance of RAST assays using enzymatic digests and breakdown products of food cannot be evaluated with our present knowledge (Schwartz et al 1980). Second, the assay should contain negative control serum samples to reflect non-specific IgE binding. There should also be a positive control serum to confirm that relevant allergens have been coupled to the solid phase support. The assay must be performed in a technically correct fashion, all reagents should be used in the proper quantity and stored in a manner designed to preserve their activity. Different laboratories use different scoring methods and criteria for positivity of RAST results. A positive RAST does not necessarily indicate clinical sensitivity to that allergen: false positive results to cereal grain occur in patients with inhalant allergies. A negative RAST does not exclude clinical sensitivity. In a study of 127 children with a reasonably positive clinical history of food intolerance to at least one food, in which the symptoms were produced consistently on ingestion of this food, only 59% of patients showed at least one positive RAST (Hoffman and Haddad 1974).

RAST inhibition can also be used in food allergy (Gillespie et al 1976). It provides a tool to confirm the specificity of IgE antibody.

Other tests

Many tests (sublingual and intracutaneous challenge, cytotoxicity, pulse rate, examination of hair, dowsing) have been claimed to be diagnostic of food allergy but there is as yet no definite scientific evidence for any of them.

Exclusion diets

The main means of diagnosis is time consuming and difficult and involves putting patients on elimination diets to see if symptoms remit and subsequent challenge with suspected foodstuffs and placebo, preferably double-blind (May and Bock 1978). On the first few days of allergen elimination the patient's symptoms may actually worsen, and it may be necessary to warn patients about this. The elimination diets should only be used for a short time since they may not be nutritionally adequate and patients who have had a reaction to food, such as anaphylaxis, should not be challenged with this food again.

Reappearance of symptoms on food challenge on more than one occasion suggests that that particular food is involved, but does not prove an allergic mechanism.

Histamine release

The basophil or leucocyte histamine release assay is a specific and reproducible test. It can either be performed using cells in the patient's blood, or by passively sensitising chopped lung tissue from monkey or human or peripheral blood basophils with patient's serum. This test is technically demanding and is mainly used in a research setting (McLaughlan et al 1983).

TREATMENT OF FOOD ALLERGY

Avoidance of specific food allergens is the treatment of choice in food allergy. It is safe, effective and easy except if multiple foodstuffs are involved or if the patient suffers from anaphylaxis to a minute quantity. Even then, avoidance can be managed with dietetic help about hidden allergens. It may be necessary to avoid airborne food allergen when the patient is extremely sensitive. Each patient should receive professional dietary advice, to ensure, first, that the antigen is really eliminated and second, that the long-term diet is nutritionally adequate. Each patient should be instructed in reading the labels on foodstuffs.

Allergy to a food may decrease over months to years, especially in children under three. Therefore it is advisable to attempt reintroduction of the food at intervals of a few months.

Breast-fed children can react to foodstuffs contained in breast milk and it may be necessary for the mother herself to avoid certain foodstuffs, especially milk, eggs, wheat, nuts, citrus fruits, shellfish and fish. Patients who are allergic to peanuts and soya can usually tolerate peanut oil and soya oil, excepting those who are very sensitive.

When the offending food items cannot be identified or are multiple, a rotation diet may prove helpful; certain food groups are eaten on one day and then not eaten again until three or four days later. In this way, the intestine never receives a build-up of one particular food-group antigen. A typical rotation diet is shown in Table 7.4.

Pharmacological treatment

This is intended to be in addition to the basic treatmet by avoidance or rotation diet. It is a useful adjunct in patients with multiple food allergies or for those with additional unrecognised allergies and for patients who are eating out and cannot be certain of avoiding a particular food.

Antihistamines (anti-H1 receptors). Antihistamines are useful in the treatment of urticaria/angio-oedema and also in conjunctivitis/rhinitis. Their value in gastro-intestinal allergy has never been demonstrated.

Table 7.4. Rotation diet.

Day	Meat, fish, etc.	Vegetables	Fruits	Beverages	Grains, flour	Nuts	Oils, fats	Sweetener
1	Beef Lamb Cheese	Parsley family: carrot, celery, parsnip, parsley Fungi: mushroom	Rose family: strawberry raspberry Apple family: apple, pear	Milk Tea Apple juice	Oats	Brazil Cashew	Beef dripping Butter	Beet sugar (Silver Spoon)
2	Fish Shellfish	Sunflower family: lettuce, chicory, endive, artichoke (Jerusalem) Potato family: tomato, potato, peppers	Citrus family: orange, lemon grapefruit, lime Avocado Rhubarb	Orange juice Grapefuit juice Camomile tea	Buckwheat Sunflower seeds Tapioca	Filbert Hazel	Olive Sunflower oil Safflower oil	100% Maple syrup Maple sugar
3	Poultry Eggs	Mustard family: cabbage, broccoli, cauliflower, turnip Gourd family: marrow, cucumber, courgette	Banana Melon Pineapple Gooseberry family: gooseberry, currant	Pineapple juice Mint tea	Wheat Corn(maize) Rice Sago	Walnut	Corn oil	Cane sugar Molasses
4	Pork Rabbit	Legume family: pea, bean, lentil, soya, chickpea Sweet potato Lily family: onion, garlic, chive, leek, asparagus	Grape family: grape, raisin Plum family: cherry, peach, apricot Palm family: coconut, date	Grape juice Rosehip tea	Lentil Chickpea Soya	Peanut Almond	Peanut oil Soya oil Pork lard	

Disodium cromoglycate (DSCG). This substance is thought to inhibit the release of mast cell mediators. Side-effects are rare, and it is poorly absorbed by the gastro-intestinal tract, making it suitable for local therapy. Trials in children have shown that some 75% of food sensitive children respond to DSCG, and that some of them can continue to tolerate food to which they have been allergic after the DSCG is stopped (Freier and Berger 1973; Dannaeus et al 1977; Molkhou and Waquet 1981; Buscinco et al 1983). In adults, DSCG protected against food-induced asthma, but not against salicylate-induced asthma, if given orally, not by inhalation (Dahl 1981). In another study (Harries et al 1978) one week's therapy with DSCG failed to give any protection against food induced asthma and urticaria with the exception of one patient in whom the symptoms involved the gastro-intestinal tract.

Oral DSCG does not always help symptomatic food allergic subjects. However, if the offending food is removed from the diet and symptoms are relieved, the patient who was previously unresponsive may be protected from a subsequent food challenge by pretreatment with DSCG. This change in responsiveness may be related to the two populations of mast cells in the gut (Table 7.5), the connective tissue mast cell being DSCG responsive while the mucosal mast cell is not (Befus et al 1982; Pearce et al 1982). Following antigen challenge in the gut, there is a local recruitment of mucosal, but not connective tissue, mast cells (Pearce et al 1982). In this situation, the total mast cell population will be unresponsive to DSCG. If the antigen is removed there will be a reduction in the mucosal mast cell population and a relative increase in the proportion of connective mast cells, thus restoring the gut to a state of DSCG responsiveness. This hypothesis, which fits the clinical observations, will need to be tested formally.

Corticosteroids. These cause a dramatic improvement in milk-induced allergic gastro-enteropathy and are also useful in eosinophilic gastro-enteritis.

Table 7.5. Morphological heterogeneity of rat mast cells.

	Connective tissue mast cells	Mucosal mast cells
Site	Skin, submucosa, serosal surfaces	Mucosa
Size	Large	Smaller
Granules	Many	Few
T-cell-dependent	No	Yes
Proteoglycan	Heparin	Chondroitin sulphate
Fixation with formalin	Stable	Labile
Staining properties	Safranin positive	Alcian blue positive
Protease	RMCP I	RMCP II

Intravenous corticosteroid is also used in severe hypersensitivity responses such as anaphylaxis.

Poorly absorbed corticosteroids taken by mouth also seem to be effective in some cases of atopic eczema (Heddle et al 1984). This is presumably due to the reduction in gut permeability in these patients, secondarily decreasing antigen and perhaps immune complex absorption.

Adrenergic agents. Adrenaline is useful in anaphylaxis and largyngeal oedema, a dose of 0.01 mg/kg of a 1 : 1000 dilution being given subcutaneously. This can be repeated at 15–20 minute intervals. A kit, known as Anakit, is available from Hollister Stier Laboratories. This contains a syringe loaded with adrenaline for use by those patients who suffer from anaphylaxis in response to food. Orally inhaled isoprenaline (Medihaler Iso) is useful early in the onset of angio-oedema of the tongue and larynx. However, it is not useful where there is complete obstruction, and the absorption is variable, so this should not be relied upon totally.

Prostaglandin inhibitors. Prostaglandins are associated with the mediation of abnormal increases in intestinal motility and secretions. Prostaglandin E_2 and $F_{2\alpha}$ can give nausea and vomiting, colic, distention and diarrhoea (Barr and Naismith 1972). Prostaglandin inhibitors decrease diarrhoea in ulcerative colitis. Buisseret et al (1978) used prostaglandin synthetase inhibitors and showed them to be helpful in three out of six patients.

Immunotherapy. Classical desensitisation, although useful in airborne allergens, has not been convincingly demonstrated to have a role in food allergy. Provocation/neutralisation techniques have been variously reported as being successful or unsuccessful, and at the moment the American Academy of Allergy and Immunology regards the case as not proven (1983). Two more recent reports (Rea et al 1984; McGovern et al 1984) support the use of such methods in food allergy following double-blind evaluation. Our own studies demonstrate that certain patients derive benefit from these techniques.

REFERENCES

Aalberse R C, Koshte V & Clements J G J (1981) IgE antibodies that cross react with vegetable foods, pollen and hymenoptera venom. *Journal of Allergy and Clinical Immunology* 68: 356–364.
Adinolfi M, Glynn A A, Lindsay M & Milne C M (1966) Serological properties of IgA antibodies to *E.coli* present in human colostrum. *Immunology* 10: 517–526.
Alun Jones V, McLaughlan P, Shorthouse M, Workman E & Hunter J O (1982) Food intolerance: a major factor in the pathogenesis of irritable bowel syndrome. *Lancet* 2: 1115–1117.
American Academy of Allergy and Immunology (1983) Adverse reactions to foods. *NIH Publication* No. 842442.
Andre C J F, Heremans J F, Vaerman J P & Cambiaso L L (1975) A mechanism for the induction of immunological tolerance by antigen feeding: antigen–antibody complexes. *Journal of Experimental Medicine* 142: 1509.
Asherson G L, Zembala M, Perera M A C C, Mayhew B & Thomas W R (1977) Production of immunity and unresponsiveness in the mouse by feeding contact sensitising agents and the role of

suppressor cells in the Peyers' patches, mesenteric lymph nodes and other lymphoid tissues. *Cellular Immunology* **33**: 145–155.

Atherton D J, Sewell M, Soothill J F, Wells R S & Chilvers C E D (1978) A double-blind crossover trial of an antigen avoidance diet in atopic eczema. *Lancet* **1**: 401–403.

Bahna S L & Heiner D C (1978) Cow's milk allergy. *Advances in Paediatrics* **25**: 1–37.

Bamford D R (1966) Studies in vitro of passage of serum proteins across the intestinal wall of young rats. *Proceedings of the Royal Society of London Series B* **166**: 30–47.

Barr W & Naismith W C (1972) Oral prostaglandins in the induction of labour. *British Medical Journal* **2**: 188–191.

Befus A D & Bienenstock J (1982) Factors involved in symbiosis and resistance at the mucosa–parasite interface. *Progress in Allergy* **31**: 76–177.

Befus A D, Pearce F L, Gauldie, J, Horsewood P & Bienenstock J (1982) Mucosal mast cells. Isolation and functional characteristics of rat intestinal mast cells. *Journal of Immunology* **128**: 2475–2480.

Bernstein I D & Ovary Z (1968) Absorption of antigens from the gastrointestinal tract. *International Archives of Allergy and Applied Immunology* **33**: 521–529.

Besredka A (1919) De la vaccination contre les etats typhoides par le voie buccale. *Annales de l'Institute Pasteur* **33**: 882.

Bockman D E & Cooper M D (1973) Pinocytosis by epithelium associated with lymphoid follicles in the bursa of Fabricius, appendix and Peyers' patches. *American Journal of Anatomy* **136**: 455–577.

Brandtzaeg P (1973) Structure, synthesis and transfer of mucosal immunoglobulins. *Annual Review of Immunology* **1246**: 417.

Brandtzaeg P (1978) Polymeric IgA is complexed with secretory component (SC) on the surface of human intestinal epithelial cells. *Scandinavian Journal of Immunology* **8**: 39–52.

Brandtzaeg P (1981) The humoral immune systems of the gastrointestinal tract. *Monographs in Allergy* **17**: 195–221.

Brostoff J, Carini C, Wraith D G & Johns P (1979) Production of IgE complexes by allergen challenge in atopic patients and the effect of sodium cromoglycate. *Lancet* **2**: 1268–1270.

Brostoff J, Carini C & Wraith D G (1982) Food allergy. An IgE immune complex disorder. In *Skandia International Symposium on Theoretical and Clinical Aspects of Allergic Diseases*, pp 104–122. Stockholm: Almqvist & Wiksell International.

Brown W R (1978) Relationships between immunoglobulins and the intestinal epithelium. *Gastroenterology* **75**: 129–138.

Buisseret P D, Youlten L J F, Heinzelmann D I & Lessof M H (1978) Prostaglandin synthesis inhibitors in prophylaxis of food intolerance. *Lancet* **1**: 906–908.

Bull D M, Bienenstock J & Tomasi T B (Jr) (1971) Studies on human intestinal immunoglobulin A. *Gastroenterology* **60**: 370–380.

Businco L, Cantani A, Benincori N, et al (1983) Effectiveness of oral sodium cromoglycate (SCG) in preventing food allergy in children. *Annals of Allergy* **51**: 47–50.

Cebra J J, Kamat R, Gearhart P J, Robertson S M & Tseng J (1977) The secretory IgA system of the gut. In *Immunology of the Gut. Ciba Foundation Symposium* **46**: 5–28.

Cerf-Bensussan Quaroni A, Kurnick J T & Bhan A K (1984) Intraepithelial lymphocytes modulate Ia expression by intestinal epithelial cells. *Journal of Immunology* **132**: 1244–1252.

Chase M W (1946) Inhibition of experimental blood allergy by prior feeding of sensitised agents. *Proceedings of the Society of Experimental Biology and Medicine* **61**: 257–259.

Chiba M, Bartnik W, Remine S G, Thayer W R & Shorter R G (1981) Human colonic intraepithelial and lamina propria lymphocytes: cytotoxicity in vitro and the potential effects of the isolation method on their functional properties, *Gut* **22**: 177–186.

Ciprandi G, Dirienzo W, Canonica G W & Fudenberg H H (1984) ^{60}Co therapy as an 'allergic breakthrough' in a case of food allergy. *New England Journal of Medicine* **311**: 861.

Clarke R M & Hardy R N (1971) Factors influencing the uptake of ^{125}I polyvinyl pyrrolidine by the intestine of the young rat. *Journal of Physiology (Lond)* **212**: 801–807.

Cornell R, Walker W A & Isselbacher K J (1971) Intestinal absorption of horseradish peroxidase. A cytochemical study. *Laboratory Investigation* **25**: 42–48.

Crabbé P A & Heremans J F (1966) The distribution of immunoglobulin containing cells among the human gastrointestinal tract. *Gastroenterology* **51**: 305–309.

Cunningham-Rundles C, Brandeis W E, Good R A & Day N K (1978) Milk precipitins, circulating immune complexes and IgA deficiency. *Proceedings of the National Academy of Sciences (USA)* **75**: 3387–3389.

Dack G M & Petran E (1934) Bacterial activity in different levels of intestine and in isolated segments of small and large bowel in monkeys and in dogs. *Journal of Infectious Diseases* **54**: 204–207.

Dahl R (1981) Oral and inhaled sodium cromoglycate in challenge tests with food allergens o acetylsalicylic acid. *Allergy* **36**: 161–165.

Danforth E & Moore R D (1959) Intestinal absorption of insulin in the rat. *Endocrinology* **65**: 118–126.

Dannaeus A, Foucard T & Johansson S G O (1977) The effect of orally administered sodium cromoglycate on symptoms of food allergy. *Clinical Allergy* **7**: 109–115.

Dixon J M (1960) Fate of bacteria in the small intestine. *Journal of Pathology and Bacteriology* **79** 131–140.

Doe W F, Henry K & Booth C C (1974) Complement in coeliac disease. In Hekkens W Th J M & Pena S (eds) *Coeliac Disease. Proceedings of the 2nd International Coeliac Symposium*, pp 189–196 Leiden: Stefert Kroese.

Freier S & Berger H (1973) Disodium cromoglycate in gastrointestinal protein intolerance. *Lancet* **1** 913–915.

Gee S (1888) On the coeliac affectation. *St. Bartholomew's Hospital Reports* **24**: 17–20.

Gillespie D N, Nakajima S & Gleich G J (1976) Detection of allergy to nuts by the radioallergosorben test. *Journal of Allergy and Clinical Immunology* **57**: 307–309.

Girard J P & de Kalbermatten A (1970) Antibody activity in human duodenal fluid. *European Journal of Clinical Investigation* **1**: 185–195.

Gruskay F L & Cooke R E (1955) The gastrointestinal absorption of unaltered protein in normal infant and in infants recovering from diarrhoea. *Pediatrics* **16**: 763–768.

Gwynn C M, Ingram J, Almousaur T & Stanworth D R (1982) Bronchial provocation tests in atopi patients with allergen-specific IgG4 antibodies. *Lancet* **1**: 254–256.

Haneberg B & Aarskog D (1975) Human fecal immunoglobulin in healthy infants and children and i some with disease affecting the gastrointestinal tract or immune system. *Clincal and Experimenta Immunology* **22**: 210–222.

Harries G, O'Brien I M, Burge P S & Pepys J (1978) Defects of orally administered sodium cromoglycate in asthma and urticaria due to foods. *Clinical Allergy* **8**: 423–427.

Heatley R V, Rhodes J, Calcraft B J, et al (1975a) Immunoglobulin E in rectal mucosa of patients wit proctitis. *Lancet* 1010–1012.

Heatley R V, Calcraft B J, Rhodes J, Owen E & Evans B K (1975b) Disodium cromoglycate in the treatment of chronic proctitis. *Gut* **16**: 559–563.

Heddle R J, Soothill J F, Bulpitt C J & Atherton D J (1984) Combined oral and nasal beclomethason diproprionate in children with atopic eczema: a randomised controlled trial. *British Medical Journa* **289**: 651–654.

Hodgson H J, Davies R J & Gent A E (1976) Atopic disorders and adult coeliac disease. *Lancet* **1** 115–7.

Hoffman D R & Haddad Z H (1974) Diagnosis of IgE-mediated reactions to food antigens b radioimmunoassay. *Journal of Allergy and Clinical Immunology* **54**: 165–173.

Jackson G D F, Lemaitre-Coelho I, Vaerman J P, Bazine H & Beckers A (1978) Rapid disappearanc from serum of intravenously injected rat myeloma IgA and its secretion into bile. *European Journa of Immunology* **8**: 122–126.

Jackson P G, Baker R W, Lessof M H, Ferret J & MacDonald D M (1981) Intestinal permeability i patients with eczema and food allergy. *Lancet* **1**: 1285–1286.

Juhlin L (1963) Basophil leucocytes in ulcerative colitis. *Acta Medica Scandinavica* **173**: 351–359.

Kagnoff M F (1978) A mechanism for suppression of IgM humoral antibody responses after antige feeding. *Clinical Research* **26**: 321A.

Kagnoff M F, Austin R K, Hubert J J, Bernardin J E & Kasarda D D (1984) Possible role for a huma adenovirus in the pathogenesis of celiac disease. *Journal of Experimental Medicine* **160**: 1544–1557.

Klein N C, Hargrove R L, Sleisenger M H & Jeffries G H (1970) Eosinophilic gastroenteritis. *Medicin (Baltimore)* **49**: 299–319.

Korenblat R E, Rothberg R M & Minden P (1968) Immune response of human adults after oral an parenteral exposure to bovine serum albumin. *Journal of Allergy* **41**: 226–235.

Kraft S C, Rothberg R M, Knauer C M, et al (1967) Gastric acid output and circulating anti-bovin serum antibodies in adults. *Clinical and Experimental Immunology* **2**: 321–330.

Kumagai K (1922) Uber den resorptions Vergang der Corpuscularen. *Kekkaku-Zassi* **4**: 429–431.

Lake A M, Bloch K J, Sinclair K J & Walker W A (1980) Anaphylactic release of intestinal goblet cel mucus. *Immunology* **39**: 173–178.

Little C H, Stewart A G & Fennessy M R (1983) Platelet serotonin release in rheumatoid arthritis: study in food-intolerant patients. *Lancet* **2**: 297–299.

Mani V, Lloyd G, Green F H Y, Fox H & Turnberg L A (1976) Treatment of ulcerative colitis with ora disodium cromoglycate. A double-blind controlled trial. *Lancet* **1**: 439–441.

May C D (1976) Objective clinical and laboratory studies of immediate hypersensitivity reactions to foods in asthmatic children. *Journal of Allergy and Clinical Immunology* **58**: 500–515.

May C D & Bock S A (1978) Adverse reactions to food due to hypersensitivity. In Middleton E (Jr), Reed L E & Elli E F (eds) *Allergy, Principles and Practice*, Vol. 2, pp 1159–1171. St Louis: C V Mosby.

McDonald T T (1983) Immunosuppression caused by antigen feeding. III. Suppressor T cells mask Peyer's patch B cell priming to orally administered antigen. *European Journal of Immunology* **12**: 767–773.

McGovern J J, Rapp D J, Gardner R W, et al (1984) Double blind studies support reliability of provocative-neutralisation test. *Acta Oto-Laryngologica* (in press).

McLaughlan P & Coombs R R (1983) Latent anaphylactic sensitivity of infants to cows' milk proteins. Histamine release from blood basophils. *Clinical Allergy* **13**: 1–9.

Miller K (1982) Sensitivity to tartrazine. *British Medical Journal* **285**: 1597–1598.

Miller H R P, Nawa Y & Parish C R (1979) Intestinal goblet cell differentiation in *Nippostrongylus*-infected rats after transfer of fractionated thoracic duct lymphocytes. *International Archives of Allergy and Applied Immunology* **59**: 281–285.

Molkhou P & Waquet J-C (1981) Food allergy and atopic dermatitis in children: treatment with oral sodium cromoglycate. *Annals of Allergy* **47**: 173–175.

Monro J, Carini C, Brostoff J & Zilkha K (1980) Food allergy in migraine. *Lancet* **2**: 1–4.

Moore A R & Hall J (1972) Evidence for primary association between immunoblasts and small gut. *Nature, London* **239**: 161–162.

Ngan J & Kind L S (1978) Suppressor T cells for IgE and IgG in Peyers' patches of mice made tolerant by the oral administration of ovalbumin. *Journal of Immunology* **120**: 861–865.

Orlans E, Peppard J, Reynolds J & Halls J (1978) Rapid active transport of immunoglobulin A from blood to bile. *Journal of Experimental Medicine* **147**: 588–592.

Ogra S S, Ogra P L, Lippes J & Tomasi T B (1972) Immunohistologic localisation of immunoglobulin, secretory component and lactoferrin in the developing human fetus. *Proceedings of the Society of Experimental Biology and Medicine* **139**: 570–574.

Owen R L (1977) Sequential uptake of horseradish peroxidase by lymphoid follicle epithelium of Peyers' patches in the normal unobstructed mouse intestine: an ultrastructural study. *Gastroenterology* **72**: 440–451.

Owen R L (1983) And now pathophysiology of M cells — good news and bad news from Peyers' patches. *Gastroenterology* **85**: 470–472.

Paganelli R, Levinsky R J, Brostoff J & Wraith D G (1979) Immune complexes containing food proteins in normal and atopic subjects after oral challenge and the effect of sodium cromoglycate on antigen absorption. *Lancet* **1**: 1270–1272.

Parke A L & Hughes G R V (1981) Rheumatoid arthritis and food: a case study. *British Medical Journal* **282**: 2027–2078.

Parrott D M V (1976) The gut as a lymphoid organ. *Clinics in Gastroenterology* **5**: 211–228.

Parrott D M V & Ferguson A (1974) Selective migration of lymphocytes within the mouse small intestine. *Immunology* **26**: 571–588.

Pearce F L, Befus A D, Gauldie J & Bienenstock J (1982) Mucosa mast cells. II. Effects of anti-allergic compounds on histamine secretion by isolated intestinal mast cells. *Journal of Immunology* **128**: 2481–86.

Perkkio M (1980) Immunohistochemical study of intestinal biopsies from children with atopic eczema due to food allergy. *Allergy* **35**: 573–581.

Rea W J, Podell, R N, Willliams M L, et al (1984) Intracutaneous neutralization of food sensitivity: a double blind evaluation. *Archives of Otolaryngology* **110**: 248–253.

Richman L K, Chiller J M, Brown W R, Hanson D G & Vaz W M (1978) Enterically induced immunological tolerances. I. Induction of suppressor T lymphocytes by intragastric administration of soluble proteins. *Journal of Immunology* **121**: 2429–2434.

Rodewald R D (1970) Selective antibody transport in the proximal small intestine of the neonatal rat. *Journal of Cell Biology* **45**: 635–640.

Rosenkrans P C M, Meijer C J L M, Wal A M van der & Lindeman D (1980) Allergic proctitis, a clinical pathological entity *Gut* **21**: 1017–1023.

Rothberg R M (1969) Immunoglobulin and specific antibody synthesis during the first weeks of life of premature infants. *Journal of Pediatrics* **75**: 391–399.

Rowe A & Rowe A H (1951) Atopic dermatitis in infants and children. *Journal of Pediatrics* **39**: 80–86.

Royal College of Physicians Report on Food Allergy (1984) Food intolerance and food aversion. A joint report of the Royal College of Physicians and the British Nutrition Foundation. *Journal of the*

Royal College of Physicians of London **18**: 1–41.

Schwartz H R, Nerurkar L S, Spies J R, Scanlon R T & Bellanti J A (1980) Milk hypersensitivity: RAS studies using new antigens generated by pepsin hydrolysis of β-lactoglobulin. *Annals of Allergy* **45** 242–245.

Scott B B & Losowsky M S (1976) Depressed cell-mediated immunity in coeliac disease. *Gut* **17** 900–905.

Scudamore H H, Phillips S F, Swedlund H A & Gleich G J (1982) Food allergy manifested b eosinophilia, raised IgE levels and protein losing enteropathy: the syndrome of allergic gastroenter opathy. *Journal of Allergy and Clinical Immunology* **70**: 129–138.

Selby W S, Janossy G, Goldstein G & Jewell D P (1981) T lymphocyte subsets in normal huma intestinal mucosa — the distribution and relationship to MHC derived antigens. *Clinical an Experimental Immunology* **44**: 453–458.

Selby W S, Janossy G, Bofill M & Jewell D P (1983) Lymphocyte subpopulations in the human smal intestine. The findings in normal mucosa and in the mucosa of patients with adult coeliac disease *Clinical and Experimental Immunology* **52**: 219–228.

Shiada H, Mishima T, Yamada S, Shiada S & Nakai Y (1979) Nasal smears in the diagnosis of foo allergy. In Pepys J & Edwards A M (eds) *Mast Cell*, p 422. London: Pitman.

Söltoft J, Binder V & Gudmand-Hoyer E (1973) Intestinal immunoglobulins in ulcerative colitis *Scandinavian Journal of Gastroenterology* **8**: 293–300.

Soothill J F (1976) Some intrinsic and extrinsic factors predisposing to allergy. *Proceedings of the Roya Society of Medicine* **69**: 439–442.

Stokes C R, Swarbrick E T & Soothill J F (1980) Immune eliminations and enhanced antibod responses: functions of circulating IgA. *Immunology* **40**: 455–458.

Theodossi A (1983) Organic or functional? Analysis of 2000 gastroenterology outpatients. *Gastroenter ology in Practice* **1**: 36–38.

Tomasi T B (Jr) (1970) Structure and function of mucosal antibodies. *Annual Review of Medicine* **21** 281.

Turner M W, Mowbray J F, Harvey B A M, et al (1978) Defective yeast opsonisation and C2 deficienc in atopic patients. *Clinical and Experimental Immunology* **34**: 253–259.

Wide L, Bennich H & Johansson S G O (1967) Diagnosis of allergy by an in vitro test for allerge antibodies. *Lancet* **2**: 1105–1107.

Wilson S J & Waltzer M (1935) Absorption of undigested proteins in human beings. IV. Absorption o unaltered egg protein in infants and children. *American Journal of Diseases of Children* **50**: 49–57

World Health Organization (1977) *The Role of Immune Complexes in Disease.* Report of a WH(Scientific Group. OMS Publication no. 2204.

Wright S & Burton J L (1982) Oral evening primose-seed oil improves atopic eczema. *Lancet* **2** 1120–1122.

Chapter 8
The Scope for Pseudo-Allergic Responses to Food

D. R. Stanworth

With the impact of the application of immunology to the study of allergic reactions it has become apparent in recent years that not all immediate responses with clinical symptomology characteristic of Type I allergy (asthma, hay fever, urticaria) are mediated by anaphylactic antibodies. There is growing evidence, for instance, that certain individuals respond in a so-called pseudo-allergic manner following exposure to pharmaceutical agents, such as radiographic contrast media, some antibiotics, and intravenous anaesthetics.

In this article, the possibility will be considered that the adverse reactions exhibited by some people in response to foods, or food additives, can be attributed to a similar non-antibody mediated mechanism. In other words, the scope for pseudo-allergy to foods will be explored in the light of present knowledge of the immunopathology underlying such responses to other forms of 'allergenic' agent.

MOLECULAR BASIS OF IgE ANTIBODY-MEDIATED HYPERSENSITIVITY REACTIONS

Before considering the probable mechansims of peseudo-allergic reactions, it is important to outline the role attributed to IgE antibodies in classical, immediate type, hypersensitivity responses.

Our passive skin sensitisation inhibition studies in humans and monkeys, using cleavage fragments of human myeloma IgE (Stanworth et al 1968; Stanworth 1973), were the first to demonstrate that anaphylactic antibodies bind strongly to Fc receptors on mast cells, where they can persist for long periods (i.e. up to several weeks). In later studies, the fate of radio-labelled whole human myeloma IgE administered intravenously to baboons was followed by autoradiographic and histochemical examination of tissue sections taken from various organs at autopsy (McLaughlan 1973). This form of systemic passive sensitisation of sub-human primates resulted in the IgE being localised mainly in the skin together with the respiratory, gastrointestinal and female genital tracts. It might be assumed that IgE antibodies which are actively synthesised in atopic individuals (in the reticulo-endothelial system) will end up in similar locations. It could be significant, therefore, that we found the passively administered radio-labelled human IgE to be localised mainly in the lamina propria of the gut of the recipient baboons, and only occasionally associated with tissue mast cells in that region.

It is the subsequent presentation of specific antigen (allergen) to such IgE antibody-sensitised mast cells which sets in train a complex series of biochemical events culminating in the energy and calcium-ion dependent, non-lytic, release of histamine and other mediators of immediate-type hypersensitvity responses (Figure 8.1). This response is, of course, manifested by the characteristic weal and flare reaction which occurs within minutes of pricking specific allergen into the skin of a hay fever sufferer, whilst in vitro, similar allergen challenge of the patient's basophils results in their rapid and explosive degranulation.

One of our research interests has been the definition of the molecular events underlying this antibody mediated process of exocytosis. Although some investigators (notably in the USA) claim that the immunological triggering stimulus responsible for initiating mediator release merely involves

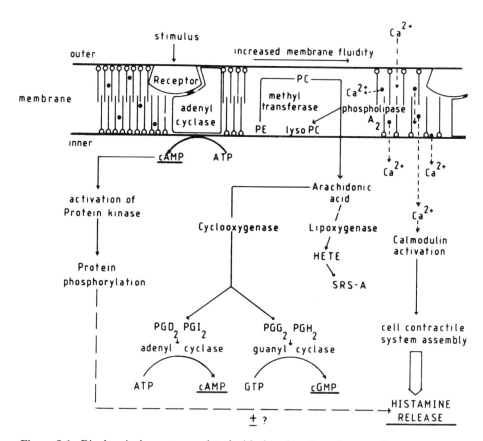

Figure 8.1. Biochemical events associated with the triggering of mast cells culminating in the release of mediators of immediate-type allergic reactions. Courtesy of D. S. Burt.

the cross-linking of Fc receptors on the mast cell plasma membrane indirectly, through the bridging by allergen of IgE antibody bound to those receptors, we have always contended that the latter process results in the antibody molecules becoming altered in conformation and providing a direct triggering signal to the target mast cells (Figure 8.2). Such a mechanism offers an explanation for some forms of pseudo-allergic reaction, notably those resulting from administration of certain polypeptides, such as the synthetic ACTH-(1–24)-peptide (adrenocorticotrophic homone: Synacthen) and the antibiotic polymyxin B (Stanworth 1984a).

Studies over a number of years, employing synthetic peptides representative of human ϵ-chain sequences, have enabled us to delineate the precise part of the IgE antibody Fc region (within the $C_\epsilon 4$ domain) which appears to be responsible for providing the direct triggering signal to the mast cell in response to allergen challenge (Stanworth 1984b; Stanworth et al 1984).

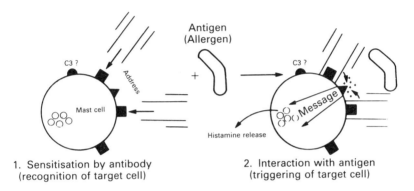

Figure 8.2. Suggested manner in which antigen (allergen) challenge initiates a conformational change in mast cell bound IgE antibody molecules with the transmission of a direct triggering signal by an effector site located within their Fc regions.

Recent collaborative model membrane studies (Dufton et al 1984) suggest that a sequence of around 10 amino acid residues (Figure 8.3) represents that part of the ϵ-chain which penetrates mast cell plasma membranes via the C-terminal hydrophobic region. The cationic N-terminal region then causes the aggregation of those protein components within the membrane which provide the primary stimulus for initiating mediator release.

It is interesting to note that substance P, an undecapeptide released from primary afferent neurones, which is thought to act indirectly on neighbouring mast cells to release histamine, shows remarkably similar structural features to our histamine releasing synthetic ϵ-chain peptide (Figure 8.3). It seems that basic peptide ligands, other than those comprising the supposed IgE antibody Fc effector site, are capable of eliciting non-cytolytic mediator release from mast cells. Recent detailed structure–activity studies on the histamine releas-

COMPARISON OF PRIMARY STRUCTURES

HUMAN ε·DECAPEPTIDE	Lys.Thr.Lys.	Gly.Ser.Gly.	Phe.Phe.Val.Phe.	NH₂
SUBSTANCE P.	Arg.Pro.Lys.	Pro.Gln.Gln.	Phe.Phe.Gly.Leu.	Met NH₂

Figure 8.3. Primary structures of (top) the region within the IgE antibody molecule which supposedly provides the mast cell triggering signal, (bottom) substance P, a neuropeptide with mast cell triggering ability.

ing capacity of a range of synthetic ε-chain analogues have indicated that the essential structural requirement for this effect is a cationic 'head' separated by a suitable number of 'inert' amino acid residues from a hydrophobic 'tail' (Stanworth et al 1984). Thus, unlike the situation which is found in hormone agonist receptor interactions, there appears to be no absolute amino acid specificity requirement for mast cell triggering.

PSEUDO-ALLERGIC REACTIONS TO PHARMACEUTICAL AGENTS

It is becoming apparent that pseudo-allergic reactions to pharmaceutical agents, which fortunately only occur in a relatively small number of sensitive individuals, can result from non-antibody dependent mechanisms. Nevertheless the outcome of these various non-immunological processes is very similar to that produced by IgE antibody–allergen interactions on the mast cell (or basophil) plasma membrane.

Adverse reactions to basic polypeptides

The mechanism of immunological triggering of mast cells, outlined in the previous section, offers an explanation as to how certain pharmaceutical compounds, usually basic peptides like substance P, might by-pass the IgE antibody–allergen induced mediator release process, but lead to similar effects (Stanworth 1980a). Thus, studies undertaken in our laboratory on sera from a group of patients who had had severe and apparently anaphylactic reactions to the administration of Synacthen, failed to reveal any evidence of the formation of anaphylactic antibodies directed against this synthetic polypeptide hormone (which possesses the same primary structure as the first 24 amino acid residues of human ACTH). In contrast, we have been able to demonstrate consistently that such polypeptides are capable of eliciting the non-cytolytic release of histamine from normal rat mast cells in vitro, at relatively low doses (10^{-6} M), effecting a release of the order of 50% of the total available histamine (Jasani et al 1973). Hence, it seems reasonable to suppose that such polypeptides act directly on the mast cell plasma membrane, in a similar manner to that ascribed to the synthetic ε-chain peptides (as discussed above). A similar mechanism may explain reactions to amino-glycosides and basic polypeptide antibiotics such as polymixin B, colistin and bacitracin.

Interestingly, the whole 39 amino acid residue native ACTH molecule is much less effective than the synthetic (1–24) peptide in causing histamine release from mast cells. This can be attributed to the preponderance of acid amino acid residues in the 25–39 region of the native ACTH. Our structure activity studies on ACTH analogues and melittin cleavage fragments (Jasani et al 1973) revealed that the presence nearby of acidic residues can inhibit the activity of basic amino acid residues, such as lysine and arginine. Such structural effects need to be borne in mind when considering the potential of food protein digests to produce pseudo-allergic reactions by this type of mechanism.

Other apparently pseudo-allergic reactions occur to different types of pharmaceutical compounds, such as radiographic contrast media. Evidence put forward to suggest that these are also caused by a direct triggering action on mast cells is much less convincing.

Indirect mast cell triggering via the products of alternative complement pathway activation

It seems likely that other pseudo-allergic reactions may be mediated by the anaphylatoxic complement sub-components C3a and C5a formed as a result of activation of the alternative complement pathway. It is probable, for instance, that adverse reactions to radiographic contrast media (RCM) and the solvent Cremophor E. L. (a surfactant produced by epoxylation of castor oil, and used in the formulation of intravenous anaesthetics) arise in this manner (Stanworth 1984a). The experimental evidence in support of this conclusion is only indirect, however, and it seems that RCM (tri-iodinated benzoic acid derivatives) injected intravenously in relatively large amounts interact with the complement system in a manner which differs from the typical alternative complement pathway activation (produced by agents such as zymosan particles). Studies aimed at delineating the structural basis of the histamine releasing activities of the basic anaphylatoxic C3a and C5a components (which have 77 amino acid residues) have pointed to a key role for the C-terminal arginyl residues (Stanworth 1980a,b). Cleavage of these by carboxypeptidases results in a dramatic reduction in mast cell triggering activity. For this reason, it seems unlikely that such complement sub-components could play a significant role in the mediation of pseudo-allergic reactions attributable to food products.

PSEUDO-ALLERGIC RESPONSES TO FOODS

There would appear to be few, if any, documented cases of food allergy which can be convincingly attributed to non-antibody mediated responses although, as is becoming increasingly recognised, immunologically based reactions to foods sometimes involve anaphylactic antibodies of the IgG4 (rather than IgE) class.

Thus all one can do at this stage is to speculate about the scope for such reactions, in the light of current knowledge of the likely basis of pseudo-allergic responses to pharmaceutical agents. In doing this, it is important to recognise that the normal individual might react immunologically to certain foods in a different manner to patients suffering from a food sensitive enteropathy. Coeliac disease is, of course, a well studied example of the latter, although this is not to imply that the pathological basis of gluten sensitivity is necessarily an allergic one (using this term in its narrow, immunological, sense).

It would seem unlikely, on first consideration, that the multi-step degradation process to which food polypeptides are normally submitted, as a result of the progressive action of a range of endo- and exopeptidases in the gut, would lead to the survival of a short chain peptide with the requisite structural credentials (outlined on p. 115) for the triggering of mediator release from gut mucosal mast cells. On the other hand, pharmacologically active peptides from foods are produced in the gut (see Chapter 9); moreover, it is conceivable that a defect in peptide hydrolysing capacity, such has been postulated in coeliac disease (see Chapter 13), might impair peptide breakdown. It is interesting to note, therefore, that histological and ultrastructural findings have led to the suggestion (Kingston et al 1979) that the damage induced within the mucosa of the small intestine of children intolerant to cow's milk or gluten, as a result of 'antigen' challenge, involves degranulation of mast cells triggered by IgE 'not necessarily produced by local immunocytes'. But no direct evidence is provided in support of the conclusion that the mast cell degranulation observed in jejunal biopsies taken after dietary challenge is indeed mediated by IgE anaphylactic antibody, rather than the manifestation of a pseudo-allergic reaction.

In the latter connection, it is difficult to establish from the available literature whether any gluten fraction or sub-fractions, which are toxic to coeliac patients, have the structural characteristics necessary for direct mast cell triggering activity (as demonstrated in our peptide studies outlined on p. 115). Total amino acid composition determinations have revealed toxic α-, β- and γ-gliadin fractions to contain a greater proportion of basic amino acids than the less toxic ω-gliadin (Jos et al 1978) (see also Chapter 9) but, as our work has already indicated (Jasani et al 1973), a cluster of basic amino acid residues in the absence of neighbouring acid residues is the predominant structural requirement for histamine releasing activity.

There is, however, another mechanism whereby gluten fractions could evoke pseudo-allergic reactions in patients with coeliac disease, which is entirely consistent with the alternative 'lectin hypothesis' of the aetiology of this condition. It has been established for some time that agents capable of cross-linking IgE in the same way as specific allergens likewise cause the non-cytolytic release of histamine and other mediators from isolated mast cells. These include anti-IgE antibody and the lectin concanavalin A, which has been shown to cross-link mast cell bound IgE antibody molecules by binding to mannose residues within their carbohydrate moieties. It seems to be of particular significance, therefore, that a toxic gluten fraction has been shown to possess lectin-like properties, and to be capable of forming a complex with high mannose type proteins. Its activity is calcium ion-dependent and inhibited by mannan (Kuttgen et al 1982). Thus, it has been suggested that gluten binds to oligomannose residues within glycoconjugates of the intestinal tract of coeliac patients, which are exposed owing to a genetically determined enzyme deficiency expressed in such patients. Substantiation of these speculations would add further support to the idea that pseudo-allergic reactions play a prominent role in the pathogenesis of gluten-sensitive enteropathy.

CONCLUSION

The considerable strides which have been made in recent years in the understanding of the molecular basis of allergic reactions mediated by IgE antibodies have been reviewed briefly. As a result of this progress, it is suggested that it is possible to begin to explain the mechanism of certain forms of pseudo-allergic reaction; notably those to polypeptide hormones and antibiotics.

It is possible that pseudo-allergic reactions to certain food products could also fall within this category. Perhaps in certain individuals, under specific clinical conditions, peptides with the requisite structural features for direct mast cell triggering survive the normal intestinal proteolytic cleavage procedures. It is also possible that certain food products, or additives, initiate the formation of anaphylatoxic components as a result of activation of the alternative complement pathway. But no documented cases of pseudo-allergic reactions to food products attributable to this type of mechanism are known; it is conceivable that anaphylatoxins formed in the gut would be subject to rapid deactivation by carboxypeptidases before they were able to trigger local mast cells.

However, the role of histamine in some clinical reactions to food has been stressed by Moneret-Vautrin (1983). Prostaglandin release after food challenge has also been documented (Alun Jones et al 1982). In both these studies no evidence of IgE antibodies was obtained, and the mechanism of release of mediators is not understood.

In contrast, as discussed in the previous section, it might be expected that food products with lectin-like properties (such as gluten fractions in coeliac patients) would be capable of effecting mediator release from intestinal mast cells by cross-linking bound IgE molecules. This proposal deserves further experimental investigation.

Even if adverse reactivity to certain foods experienced by some individuals turns out to be attributable to one of the mechanisms discussed here, it will still be necessary to explain — as with pseudo-allergic reactions to pharmaceutical agents — why such responses are not more widespread. Further studies of this aspect of the problem may lead ultimately to a means of anticipating the possibility of such adverse reactions occurring in susceptible individuals.

REFERENCES

Alun Jones V, McLaughlan P, Shorthouse M, Workman E. & Hunter J O (1982) Food intolerance: a major factor in the pathogenesis of irritable bowel syndrome. *Lancet* 2: 1115–1117.

Dufton M J, Cherry R J, Coleman J W & Stanworth D R (1984) The capacity of basic peptides to trigge exocytosis from mast cells correlates with their capacity to immobilize band 3 proteins erthyrocyte membranes. *Biochemical Journal* **223**: 67–71.

Jasani B, Mackler B, Kreil G & Stanworth D R (1973) Studies on the mast cell triggering action certain histamine liberators. *International Archives of Allergy and Applied Immunology* **45**: 74–8

Jos J, Charbonnier L, Mougenot J F, Mosse J & Wrey J (1978) Isolation and characterisation of t toxic fraction of wheat gliadin in coeliac disease. In McNicholl B, McCarthy C F & Fottrell P (eds) *Perspectives in Coeliac Disease* pp 75–89. Lancaster: MTP Press.

Kingston D, Pearson J & Shiner M (1979) The mast cell in gastrointestinal allergy. In Pepys J Edwards A M (eds) *The Mast Cell: its Role in Health and Disease* pp 394–405. London: Pitm Medical.

Kuttgen E, Volk B, Kluge F & Gerok W (1982) Gluten, a lectin with oligomannosyl specificity and th causative agent of gluten-sensitive enteropathy. *Biochemical and Biophysiological Researc Communications* **109**: 168–173.

McLaughlan P (1973) *In vitro and in vivo studies with radio-labelled IgE and anti-IgE.* PhD thes University of Birmingham.

Moneret-Vautrin D A (1983) False food allergies: non-specific reactions to foodstuffs. In Lessof M (ed) *Clinical Reactions of Food* pp 135–153. Chichester: John Wiley and Sons.

Stanworth D R (1973) *Immediate Hypersensitivity: the Molecular Basis of the Allergic Respon* North-Holland Research Monographs: Frontiers of Biology, vol. 28. Amsterdam: North-Hollan

Stanworth D R (1980a) Oligo-peptide induced release of histamine. In Dukor P et al (ed *Pseudo-Allergic Reactions. 1. Genetic Aspects and Anaphylactoid Reactions*, pp 56–107. Basl Karger.

Stanworth D R (1980b) Contribution of complement receptors to the triggering of mast cells ar basophils. *Proceedings of Symposium on Triggering of Phagocytic Cells*, pp 217–233. Székesferé var, Budapest: Kultura.

Stanworth D R (1984a) Mechanisms of pseudo-allergy. *Proceedings of International Seminar on t Immunological system as a Target for Toxic Damage*, Luxembourg, November 1984 (in press).

Stanworth D R (1984b) The role of non-antigenic receptors in mast cell signalling processes. *Molecul Immunology* **21**: 1183–1190.

Stanworth D R, Humphrey J H, Bennich H & Johansson S G O (1968) Inhibition of Prausnitz–Küstn reaction by proteolytic cleavage fragments of a human myeloma protein of immunoglobulin class *Lancet* **1**: 17–18.

Stanworth D R, Coleman J W & Khan Z (1984) Essential structural requirements for triggering of ma cells by a synthetic peptide comprising a sequence in the $C_\epsilon 4$ domain of human IgE. *Molecul Immunology* **21**: 243–247.

Chapter 9
Production of Pharmacologically Active Peptides from Foods in the Gut

Michael L. G. Gardner

Although the popular view that protein components in the diet may be responsible for dysfunction has begun to attract scientific credence, remarkably little attention has yet been paid to the possibility that partially digested fragments of proteins may modulate or compromise normal physiological functions. Undoubtedly, a major reason stems from the widely held presumption that protein digestion proceeds to completion in the lumen of the gastro-intestinal tract and within the epithelial cells lining it, and this 'fact' appears in many reputable texts. Other reasons, as will be clear from the following account, relate to the fact that it is extremely difficult, if not impossible, to characterise fully all the peptides formed during the normal digestion and assimilation of a protein meal; also, the assignation of pharmacological activities to given peptides is an enormous task. The number of potential activities that might be elicited by such molecules is colossal, and the activities that have been found are inevitably those which have been selected for specific investigation.

Until 1968, it was supposed that only free amino acids were absorbed by the intestinal cells; since then it has become clear that small peptides are actively transported into these cells by specific carrier mechanisms, and that the terminal phases of peptide digestion occur under the action of cytoplasmic peptidases within the mucosal cells (see reviews by Gardner 1981, 1984; Matthews 1975, 1977). The question of the form in which the amino-N arising from dietary protein enters these cells has thus received much more attention than that of the form — not necessarily the same — in which it enters the circulation. However, there is now a substantial body of evidence showing that small amounts of intact peptides can and do enter the circulation (Gardner 1984); also, there are grounds for belief that this amount may be increased in some pathological circumstances, especially ones affecting intestinal permeability or intestinal peptidase activities (see below).

Interest in the biological roles of small peptides has exploded recently, fuelled especially by the discovery of endogenous ligands for opiate receptors in brain. These are now known to be peptides, the endorphins. Many related peptides, for example the enkephalins which are pentapeptides, have been shown to be intensely potent substances, although their physiological and pathophysiological roles are still the subject of much curiosity. Further, at least 32 neuroactive peptides are now known, and many are regarded as putative neurotransmitters or modulators of neurotransmission (Iversen 1983, 1984); it is possible that several hundred such peptides are involved in normal regulatory processes (Snyder 1980). Knowledge that numerous peptides, formerly regarded as peptide hormones, have been identified in neural tissue has led to the concept that peptides play a key role in the integration of the neural and endocrine systems (e.g. Polak and Bloom 1982), and investigation of the neuropharmacological aspects of peptides is currently a major area of research.

Hence, there are many questions to be answered as to whether pharmacologically active peptides can be produced during dietary protein assimilation, and whether they can interfere with, or modulate, physiological regulatory processes, either in the gut itself or in peripheral tissues.

ABSORPTION OF ACTIVE PEPTIDES

Although the subject of absorption of intact peptides and proteins across the gut has been thoroughly reviewed elsewhere (Gardner 1983a,b, 1984), and that of intestinal permeability is covered in Chapter 3, it is appropriate to repeat here some of the evidence that biologically active peptides can exert systemic effects even after oral administration.

Figure 9.1, reproducing data of Amoss et al (1972), shows that oral administration of luteinising hormone releasing hormone (luliberin; LHRH) is effective in promoting release of luteinising hormone in steroid-blocked ovariectomised rats. Similar results were reported independently by Nishi et al (1975) and Humphrey et al (1973). Luliberin is a decapeptide with structure:

pGlu-His-Trp-Ser-Tyr-Gly-Leu-Arg-Pro-GlyNH$_2$

Corresponding experiments in animals and in man have shown that thyrotropin releasing hormone (TRH), a blocked tripeptide pGlu-His-ProNH$_2$, also is active after oral administration. The blocked termini, pyroglutamate (pyrrolidone carboxylate) at the N-terminus and an amidated C-terminus, are a common feature among endogenous peptide hormones; the significance is probably not that they directly confer biological activity or enhance potency but that they reduce the susceptibility of the peptide to enzymic hydrolysis by tissue peptidases. The data of Chang et al (1981) show that C-terminal amidation of the β-casomorphin, Tyr-Pro-Phe-Pro, markedly increases the activity in several assays. Although the intestinal tract of many species including man contains a pyrrolidone carboxylic acid peptidase (Szewczuk and Kwiatkowska 1970; Woodley 1972), the resistance of TRH to degradation within the gut has been demonstrated (Masson et al 1979).

Absorption of hydrolysis-resistant peptides in intact form has already been exploited in several pharmacological trials. For example, Kastin and Barbeau (1972) reported the successful use of oral Pro-Leu-GlyNH$_2$ (melanocyte-stimulating hormone release-inhibitory factor; MIF); Mycroft et al (1982) pointed out that the non-amidated sequence Pro-Leu-Gly occurs in α-gliadin and in bovine α$_{s1}$-casein.

Other data, reviewed by Gardner (1984), show the intestinal absorption of insulin, a synthetic opioid peptide, carnosine, vasopressin and various other

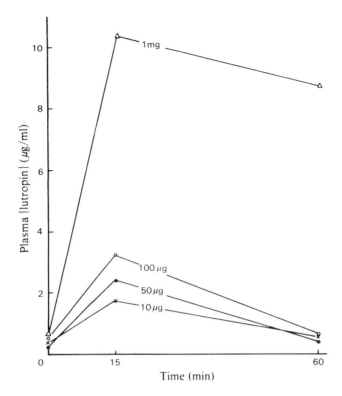

Figure 9.1. Plasma levels of luteinising hormone (LH; luteotrophin; lutropin) in rats after oral administration of the decapeptide luliberin (luteinising hormone releasing hormone; LHRH). These results suggest that physiologically significant amounts of the active peptide (or an active fragment therefrom) reach the systemic circulation after oral administration. Based on data from Amoss et al (1972). Reprinted with permission from Gardner (1983a). Copyright © 1983 The Biochemical Society, London.

pharmacologically active molecules in intact or bioactive form. Hence, any pharmacologically active peptides produced in the gut during digestion may act either locally or systemically, and these actions may be relevant in the pathogenesis of gut disease or of other diseases. The possibility of such peptides reaching receptor sites, either in the gut itself or in peripheral tissues, obviously is enhanced in intestinal dysfunction associated with increased 'permeability' or with decreased digestive protease/peptidase activity (Gardner 1984).

PROTEIN DIGESTION — PEPTIDE PRODUCTION

The normal process of protein digestion is so complex in terms of sequential and parallel processing by a substantial number of enzymes that it is not possible to predict in detail the composition (or number) of the many partially digested materials present in the intestinal lumen. Although the specificities of the major proteases and peptidases are known, these are not absolute. Further, the rates of hydrolysis of individual peptide bonds depend on a vast number of variables including the neighbouring amino acids, degree of denaturation, product accumulation (amino acid and peptide), as well as on the rate at which these bonds are exposed by the co-action of other proteases. So while it is possible to predict most of the peptide fragments produced by, for example, prolonged peptic digestion of a known protein in vitro, it is impossible to predict reliably the composition of those existing in the small intestine after ingestion of that protein.

Protein digestion is initiated in the stomach by pepsin (or, rather, by a group of pepsins with slightly differing specificities), with preferential hydrolysis of peptide bonds at the amino side of aromatic amino acids. In the small intestine, there is simultaneous attack by the pancreatic exopeptidases trypsin (essentially specific for the carbonyl side of the basic amino acids lysine and arginine), chymotrypsin (at a variety of sites, but favouring the carbonyl side of aromatic or hydrophobic amino acids especially leucine, isoleucine and methionine) and elastase (with fairly broad specificity, but preferentially at the carbonyl side of small neutral amino acids). There is simultaneous action from the pancreatic exopeptidases, carboxypeptidases A and B, the former removing neutral amino acids and the latter basic amino acids from the C-terminus, one at a time. Neither removes proline, nor will cleave if proline is the penultimate residue at the C-terminus. Also present in the intestinal lumen are a series of aminopeptidases, mainly originating from sloughed off mucosal cells (see, for example, Adibi and Kim (1981) for discussion of their specificities).

Hence, theoretical attempts to predict the occurrence of pharmacologically active peptides in the course of digestion are likely to be unrealistic. However, it is clear that small peptides greatly predominate over amino acids in the lumen, even as digestion and absorption proceed both with time and with progression down the length of the gut (Figure 9.2).

BIOLOGICAL ACTIVITY AND SPECIFICITY OF PEPTIDES

A dramatic example of the possible pharmacological effects of partial digests of proteins is provided by the old literature on 'peptone shock' (Chittenden et al 1899; see also Matthews and Payne 1976). Intravenous infusion of enzymic digests of proteins in animals was well known to cause a variety of undesirable effects, including inhibition of blood coagulation and hypotension, the latter often being profound and lethal. Unfortunately, these phenomena have never been understood. The original preparations of the digests were generally extremely complex; while they probably were conducted with meticulous care, there must be much uncertainty about the composition of the media infused. Also, adequate control experiments were lacking. Nevertheless, more recent work has confirmed that '... the ability to increase capillary permeability was a property shared by a large number of different peptides' (Spector 1958). Spector reviews the actions of peptides in increasing capillary permeability with special reference to the production of inflammation.

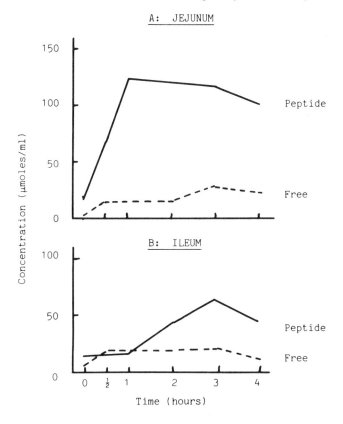

Figure 9.2. Data showing the predominance of small peptides over free amino acids in both jejunal and ileal lumen of human small intestine as digestion proceeds after ingestion of a test meal containing bovine serum albumin (50 g), carbohydrate (120 g) and fat (40 g). The peptides were said to be mainly di-, tri-, and tetra-peptides. Data from Adibi and Kim (1981). Similar results were reported by Chung et al (1979) who noted also that at 2 hours all the proline in the jejunum was in the peptide-bound form.

Clearly, peptides are strong potential candidates, although a specific role in inflammatory bowel disease has not been tested.

It is impossible to provide even a partial catalogue of the pharmacological activities that have been claimed to be elicited by various small peptides. However, the examples given by Edminson et al (1982) and Matthews and Payne (1976) serve to demonstrate the diversity of such activities; this in turn emphasises the futility of supposing that one might screen a known peptide or mixture of peptides, such as the contents of the gastro-intestinal tract, for all possible pharmacological or biological activities. Walsh (1981), in discussing the biological activities of gastro-intestinal hormones, lists no fewer than 25 putative activities attributed to pharmacological doses of cholecystokinin. Little wonder that it is difficult to establish the truly physiological roles of such peptides! It would thus be surprising if very many intermediates in protein digestion were not pharmacologically active in appropriate assay systems. Indeed, it may be true that virtually all peptides are pharmacologically active in some system or another; bioactivity seems more likely to be the 'rule' than the 'exception'.

There is a growing number of reports of association between peptiduria and a number of psychiatric and behavioural disorders, and several urinary peptides have been identified. Also, behavioural responses to injection of various small peptides have been reported. Roles of peptides in autism, schizophrenia, regulation of appetite and of sleep have been suggested. For examples, see De Wied (1977), Trygstad et al (1980) and Edminson et al (1982). While these observations must not be ignored, it should be stressed that: (i) behavioural phenomena are, as yet, seldom explicable in chemical terms; (ii) recording of behavioural parameters generally involves subjective assessment which is always less acceptable to the critic than, for example, chemical quantitation; and (iii) the interpretation of such associations in terms of direct cause and effect is extremely risky. Hence it is not easy to interpret the significance of many of these reports.

It must not be assumed that only medium-sized or large oligopeptides are active; a number of active dipeptides are known. Two interesting examples are carnosine (β-alanyl-histidine) and kyotorphin (tyrosyl-arginine). The former is present in the skeletal muscle of many species and is commonly ingested. It is regarded as a putative neurotransmitter, and deficiency of carnosinase enzyme activity has been reported to be associated with neurological disorder (Perry et al 1967; see also Gardner 1984). Kyotorphin, isolated from bovine brain, is reported to induce analgesia after intracisternal injection in mice. This effect was antagonised by naloxone, and it has been proposed that this dipeptide acts as a met-enkephalin releasing-factor (Takagi et al 1979a,b). We have no idea, however, what is the half-life of such a peptide in the circulation.

In the meantime, it seems appropriate to consider a few activities, especially ones that are currently attracting attention in other fields such as the endorphins and exorphins (see below), but the possibility that unrelated biological activities may be involved in the pathogenesis of gut or systemic disease must not be overlooked.

Although it has been stressed that the structural specificity and spectrum of biological activities of active peptides is unpredictable, it is worth considering whether the amino acid sequences of known active peptides occur frequently or rarely in known proteins. Mycroft et al (1982) point out that the Pro-Leu-Gly sequence (cp. the amide which is MIF) occurs in the sequences of α-gliadin and α_{s1}-casein. A preliminary search through a computer database containing sequences of 2511 proteins (albeit mainly bacterial and viral, rather than dietary, proteins) now shows that active tri-peptide sequences (or closely related ones) occur quite frequently (Table 9.1). Details of all the individual proteins are not given in this table, and this study should be taken only to indicate that the occurrence of particular active sequences in proteins must be regarded as likely rather than rare.

Table 9.1. Summary of results of a search through the computer database of protein structures of Barker et al (1984) for the occurrence of amino acid sequences the same as, or related to, those of several biologically active peptides.

I. Amino acid sequence	II. Related active peptide	III. Proteins in which sequence I is found to occur
Gln-His-Pro	pGlu-His-ProNH$_2$, TRH	Twelve proteins including myoglobin (carp), α-crystallin A chain, various viral and *E. coli* proteins
Gln-His-Trp	pGlu-His-TrpNH$_2$, active N-terminal fragment of LHRH	Nine proteins including bacterial α-amylase, plasminogen, somatostatin II precursor, angiotensinogen precursor
		(The C-terminal tripeptide sequence — probably inactive — occurs in 119 known protein sequences)
Gln-Leu-Tyr	pGlu-Leu-Tyr, active N-terminal fragment of neurotensin	Thirty proteins including fibrinogen, ω-gliadin, papain, keratin
Pro-Leu-Gly	Pro-Leu-GlyNH$_2$, MIF	Fifty-eight proteins including rhodopsin, proglucagon precursor, apolipoprotein A-1 (twice in molecule), angiotensinogen precursor, histocompatibility antigens, α$_{s1}$-casein, keratin, oxytocin

No occurrences were found for the enkephalins Tyr-Gly-Gly-Phe-Met, Try-Gly-Gly-Phe-Leu or for β-casomorphin-4 Tyr-Pro-Phe-Pro

Note that these results are given only to illustrate the occurrence of biologically active sequences in proteins. The contents of the database are, of course, not complete; many dietary proteins are not included.

EXORPHINS, CASOMORPHINS, ETC.

A particularly interesting and provocative series of observations in the present context is that several dietary proteins can, on digestion with pepsin in vitro, give rise to hydrolysis-resistant peptides with biological activity in opioid or opiate-binding assays. This phenomenon has been studied by several independent groups, notably those of Zioudrou and Klee, and Brantl and Teschemacher; the exogenous peptides have been named exorphins (cp. their endogenous counterparts, the endorphins) or, in the case of those arising from digestion of caseins, casomorphins.

The endorphins comprise a family of endogenous peptides, naturally occurring in brain, that bind to morphine receptors. Their discovery in 1975 appeared to answer the puzzle as to what were the normal physiological ligands for opiate receptors, but also initiated a substantial new field of neuropharmacology: the physiological roles of endorphins are certainly not fully understood. Nevertheless, it is believed that they are, at least, involved in the perception of pain, the aetiology of psychotic illness, and in learning, mood and behaviour; possibly also in the regulation of eating, drinking, and blood pressure (see review by Bloom 1983).

Although only a limited number of proteins have yet been examined for 'exorphin' activity, it appears that such active peptides arise during digestion of several dietary proteins including α-casein, β-casein, wheat gluten, maize zein, barley hordein, and bovine serum albumin (Zioudrou et al 1979; Brantl et al 1979). Other peptides active in an adenylate cyclase assay, but whose activities were not reversed by (−)-naloxone and hence cannot be classed as opioid, were obtained in similar digests of soy protein, α-lactalbumin, and a cytochrome (Zioudrou et al 1979).

One of the original stimuli for this work came from the epidemiological observations made by Dohan (1966, 1969; Dohan and Grasberger 1973) implicating gluten and, possibly, bioactive peptides derived therefrom, in the pathogenesis of schizophrenia and suggesting certain features as common to coeliac disease and schizophrenia (see below). These searches for exorphin activity have concentrated mainly on gluten and casein, two proteins that are among those most frequently accused of causing food-related disturbances. A few of the active peptides have been isolated and sequenced (see below), but it should be noted that these have been selected individual ones and the total number of active peptides seems to be very much greater. For example, 'pepsin hydrolysates of gluten are very complex mixtures that contain a number of different fragments with stimulatory or with opiate activities' (Zioudrou et al 1979). In these authors' study, the binding of gluten exorphin to brain receptors was of similar potency to that of morphine, and probably more potent than met-enkephalin. The exorphin derived from α-casein was, however, much less potent. The synthetic peptide, 'morphiceptin', which is the amide of an active fragment from β-casein, was as active as morphine in a guinea pig ileum assay, but less active in a vas deferens assay (Chang et al 1981).

It should be noted that different opioid assays give different relative potencies for different putative ligands; one reason is that there are at least four or five discrete types of opiate receptor (e.g. Cox 1982). It should be noted also that receptor-binding assays or isolated-organ assays (e.g. effect on electrically stimulated vas deferens) do not necessarily reflect the true situation in vivo, where permeability barriers can restrict the access of a ligand to its receptors; also, rapid degradation of the ligand can annul its effects; in other words, biological half-life is as important a factor as pharmacological potency in determining effects in vivo.

Brantl and Teschemacher (1979) also detected material active in the opioid bioassay in baby food, fresh cows' milk and human milk. The amount present in the fresh cows' milk did, however, vary inexplicably. Teschemacher et al (1980) then developed a radio-immunoassay for β-casomorphins; they were originally unable to detect β-casomorphins in plasma of cows or calves after milk ingestion, but they did detect immunoreactive material in some batches of bovine milk (i.e. unhydrolysed) or milk products, and it was suggested that these had been produced by bacterial action. Current work suggests that β-casomorphins are detectable in plasma after milk ingestion (M. Hautefeuille, personal communication); also it appears that bovine and rat plasma contains a peptidase (possibly dipeptidyl-peptidase IV) active against β-casomorphins (Kreil et al 1983).

The same research group fractionated and sequenced the active peptide in commercial casein peptone, apparently a tryptic digest from bovine casein (Henschen et al 1979); this was a heptapeptide, Tyr-Pro-Phe-Pro-Gly-Pro-Ile, corresponding to residues 60–66 of the known sequence of β-casein. It proved to be highly resistant to further proteolysis, even by pronase; carboxypepti-dases (except bacterial carboxypeptidase Y) were also ineffective. The high content of prolyl bonds may be responsible for this stability. These authors' subsequent experiments showed that the related hexa-, penta-, and tetra-peptides derived by removal of the C-terminal amino acids were all active, the pentapeptide Tyr-Pro-Phe-Pro-Gly being the most potent (Brantl et al 1981). The relative specificities of these peptides in several opioid assays led Brantl et al (1981) to the view that they were acting as agonists of the μ-type opiate receptors, the type that appears to predominate in the gut.

Corresponding studies by Loukas et al (1983) on the exorphins derived by Zioudrou et al (1979) from peptic digestion of α-casein showed that they corresponded to the hepta- and hexa-peptide fragments from residues 90–96 and 90–95 respectively; viz. Arg-Tyr-Leu-Gly-Tyr-Leu-Gly and Arg-Tyr-Leu-Gly-Tyr-Leu. Activity was confirmed in synthetic peptides, and it was clear that they were also stable against tryptic digestion although they were partially inactivated by chymotrypsin. The results of Ryle and Auffret (1979) suggest that the Tyr-Leu bond would be a good substrate for pepsin C (gastricsin, pepsin 5); we do not know whether this particular pepsin was present in the preparations used by these workers.

The few studies reported hitherto have failed to resolve whether or not the casomorphins have any functional or physiological (as opposed to ex-perimental) relevance. Petrilli et al (1984) thought that β-casomorphin was unlikely to reach physiologically significant concentrations in the intestinal lumen in vivo. However, Schusdziarra et al (1983a,b) believed that the presence of β-casomorphins in a test meal stimulated insulin release in dogs; naloxone reversibility suggested that this phenomenon involved opiate recep-tors although not necessarily directly. Likewise, Morley et al (1983) reported that ingestion of pepsin-hydrolysed gluten produced a naloxone-reversible increase in plasma somatostatin-like activity in man; a reversible increase in intestinal transit time was also observed.

Experiments in stripped rabbit ileum showed that natural β-casomorphin-4 peptide did not evoke any change in short-circuit current, but that synthetic hydrolysis-resistant analogues did; the response was naloxone-reversible and was elicited by addition of the peptide to either the mucosal or serosal side of the preparation (Hautefeuille et al 1984). The question of whether or not β-casomorphins are detectable in plasma after milk ingestion is clearly an important one needing urgent verification (see above).

These studies have confirmed beyond doubt that potent pharmacological-ly active peptides *can* be produced during enzymic digestion of common dietary proteins. Whether or not they *are* produced during dietary digestion in vivo, whether such peptides are absorbed in intact form or whether they are locally active on the gut, and whether these findings have any pathophysiological significance are currently unresolved (but very interesting) questions.

POSSIBLE SITES OF ACTION OF ACTIVE PEPTIDES

Nothing definite is known of the actual site(s) of actions of peptides produced during food digestion, but it should be reiterated that three general sites need to be considered:

(1) Intestinal — luminal/mucosal: there is no evidence that any peptides may act locally on the gut before absorption across the mucosa. Indeed, it would be surprising if such luminal receptors existed.

(2) Intestinal — sub-mucosal/serosal: Morley has suggested that 'food hormones' have a potential physiological role as exogenous regulators of gastro-intestinal activity (Morley 1982; Morley et al 1983). In view of the known peptide receptors (including opiate receptors) in the sub-mucosa and myenteric plexus of intestine, this site is a plausible one. Furthermore, peptides crossing the mucosa will not have been exposed to the liver peptidases. The work of Hautefeuille et al (1984) suggested this as a more likely site of action of synthetic (blocked) casomorphin analogues than the mucosal side of their intestinal preparation.

(3) Peripheral: Peptides crossing the gut in intact form and escaping hydrolysis by hepatic, renal and other peptidases will have access to receptors in all peripheral tissues including the central nervous system. This latter site has been discussed in detail by Zioudrou and Klee (1979) and Klee and Zioudrou (1980).

COELIAC DISEASE AND SCHIZOPHRENIA

Is there a common factor — gluten peptides?

In the present context, it is appropriate to mention the hypothesis that gluten may be implicated in the pathogenesis of schizophrenia; it has been suggested that pharmacologically active peptides, possibly but not necessarily exorphins, arising from intestinal digestion of gluten, may be an aetiological factor in genetically susceptible subjects (Dohan 1966, 1969, 1978, 1980, 1983; Dohan et al 1984). The proponents of this theory thus believe that schizophrenia (or, at least, some schizophrenias) and coeliac disease share certain common factors, genetic and dietary. Gluten exclusion is of proven value in coeliac disease, even though the fundamental aetiology is still not understood; but the evidence as to whether gluten exclusion is helpful to some schizophrenics is equivocal — perhaps because the exclusion must be prolonged and absolute, or because this factor is relevant only in a sub-set of schizophrenic patients. Ingestion of gluten by some coeliac patients is claimed to evoke psychiatric symptoms, and Dohan (1980) cites, among other examples, an interesting case of such a coeliac patient who was the sister of a schizophrenic.

While the evidence implicating gluten or gluten peptides in psychiatric illness is plausible, much of it relies on subjective (if not anecdotal) case histories rather than controlled trials. The relationship is far from proven and this theory does not receive wide support, although Ross-Smith and Jenner (1980) cautiously accede that, 'the clinical evidence, therefore, seems to go halfway to providing a consistent picture of a relation between gluten and schizophrenia.' However, it must be stressed that if gluten (or, indeed, any other protein) damages the intestinal mucosa, then this is likely to promote the absorption of intact peptides and proteins. Gluten undoubtedly damages the mucosa of coeliac patients, but in large doses it can also induce mucosal changes in apparently healthy subjects, especially relatives of coeliac patients (Doherty and Barry, 1981). At least two independent reports have described peptidaemia or peptiduria in coeliac patients, but although intestinal mucosal peptidase activities are depressed in the untreated disease repeated searches for a 'missing peptidase' have been inconclusive (Peters and Bjarnason 1984). We still do not know whether absorption of intact peptides is a characteristic feature of coeliac disease; if it is, we shall need to know whether it relates not only to peptides derived from gluten digestion, but also to those from other dietary proteins.

These issues assume special relevance in the light of the knowledge discussed above, that digestion of gluten (and casein) can give rise, at least under some circumstances, to active exorphins. Also, it must be stressed that recent experiments on the active principle, toxic to coeliac patients, suggest that a number of distinct entities may be involved and that several of them are small peptides. Not only are whole gluten and gliadin toxic, but symptoms are elicited by peptic + tryptic digests of gliadin (Cornell and Maxwell 1982). Several peptic + tryptic peptides from gliadin were also cytotoxic to mucosa cultures in vitro, another index of pharmacological activity (Jos et al 1983).

CONCLUSIONS

It would be conjectural to conclude that significant amounts of pharmacologically active peptides are definitely produced in the gut from dietary protein either in healthy subjects or in sick patients, or that such peptides have established pathogenic relevance. However, it is clear that:

(1) During digestion, the small intestinal lumen contains large quantities of small peptides, especially di-, tri-, and tetra-peptides, of very diverse composition.
(2) Biologically active peptides are known to be produced by enzymic digestion, albeit in vitro, of typical dietary proteins, and the amino acid sequences of several known biologically active peptides occur in a variety of proteins.
(3) Significant amounts of some intact peptides can and do cross the healthy intestinal mucosa.
(4) Intestinal permeability, also intestinal peptidase activities, can be altered in a number of gastro-intestinal diseases, malnutrition and other ther-

apeutic situations, in such a way as to promote the likelihood of intact peptides (and proteins) being absorbed.

(5) An enormous range of biological/pharmacological activities, including neuroactivity, can be elicited by numerous small peptides including di-peptides, although the structural specificity and nature of activity of such peptides cannot reliably be predicted empirically.

(6) The intestine and the nervous system contain numerous peptide and opioid-receptors, whose physiological functions are currently attracting much attention.

The relevance of these facts calls for further attention, and it would be particularly timely for this to coincide with the current impetus in the study of the key roles of peptides in biology.

Acknowledgements

I am grateful to Professor Andrew Miller for support and continued provision of facilities. I also thank Dr J F Collins, Dr A F W Coulson and Mr A Lyall (Department of Molecular Biology, University of Edinburgh) for the computer searches of the protein sequence database and Professors R B Fisher and D M Matthews with whom I have had many beneficial discussions.

REFERENCES

Adibi S A & Kim Y S (1981) Peptide absorption and hydrolysis. In Johnson L R (ed) *Physiology of the Gastrointestinal Tract*, pp 1073–1095. New York: Raven Press.

Amoss M, Rivier J & Guillermin R (1972) Release of gonadotrophins by oral administration of synthetic LRF or a tripeptide fragment of LRF. *Journal of Clinical Endocrinology and Metabolism* **35** 175–177.

Barker W C, Hunt L T, Orcutt B C et al (1984) Protein Sequence Database from the Atlas of Protein Sequence and Structure, Version 8.1, January 1984, Washington: National Biomedical Research Foundation, Georgetown University Medical Center.

Bloom F E (1983) The endorphins: a growing family of pharmacologically pertinent peptides. *Annual Review of Pharmacology and Toxicology* **23**: 151–170.

Brantl V & Teschemacher H (1979) A material with opioid activity in bovine milk and milk products *Naunyn-Schmeideberg's Archives of Pharmacology* **306**: 301–304.

Brantl V, Teschemacher H, Henschen A & Lottspeich F (1979) Novel opioid peptides derived from casein (β-casomorphins). I. Isolation from bovine casein peptone. *Hoppe-Seyler's Zeitschrift für Physiologische Chemie* **360**: 1211–1216.

Brantl V, Teschemacher H, Blasig J, Henschen A & Lottspeich F (1981) Opioid activities of β-casomorphins. *Life Sciences* **28**: 1903–1909.

Chang K-J, Killian A, Hazum E, Cuatrecas P & Chang J-K (1981) Morphiceptin (NH_2-Tyr-Pro-Phe Pro-$CONH_2$): a potent and specific agonist for morphine (μ) receptors. *Science* **212**: 75–77.

Chittenden R H, Mendel L B & Henderson Y (1899) A chemico-physiological study of certain derivatives of the proteids. *American Journal of Physiology* **2**: 142–181.

Chung Y C, Kim Y S, Shadchehr A et al (1979) Protein digestion and absorption in human small intestine. *Gastroenterology* **76**: 1415–1421.

Cornell H J & Maxwell R J (1982) Amino acid composition of gliadin fractions which may be toxic to individuals with coeliac disease. *Clinica Chimica Acta* **123**: 311–319.

Cox B M (1982) Endogenous opioid peptides: a guide to structures and terminology. *Life Sciences* **31** 1645–1658.

De Wied D (1977) Peptides and behaviour. *Life Sciences* **20**: 195–204.

Dohan F C (1966) Cereals and schizophrenia: data and hypothesis. *Acta Psychiatrica Scandinavica* **42**: 125–152.

Dohan F C (1969) Is celiac disease a clue to the pathogenesis of schizophrenia? *Mental Hygiene* **53**: 525–529.

Dohan F C (1978) Schizophrenia: are some food-derived polypeptides pathogenic? Coeliac disease as a model. In Hemmings G & Hemmings W A (eds) *The Biological Basis of Schizophrenia*, pp 167–178. Lancaster: MTP Press.

Dohan F C (1980) Hypothesis: genes and neuroactive peptides from food as cause of schizophrenia. In Costa E & Trabucchi M (eds) *Neural Peptides and Neuronal Communication*, pp 535–548. New York: Raven Press.

Dohan F C (1983) More on celiac disease as a model for schizophrenia. *Biological Psychiatry* **18**: 561–564.

Dohan F C & Grasberger J C (1973) Relapsed schizophrenics: earlier discharge from the hospital after cereal-free, milk-free diet. *American Journal of Psychiatry* **130**: 685–688.

Dohan F C Harper E H, Clark M H, Rodrigue R B & Zigas V (1984) Is schizophrenia rare if grain is rare? *Biological Psychiatry* **19**: 385–399.

Doherty M & Barry R E (1981) Gluten-induced mucosal changes in subjects without overt small-bowel disease. *Lancet* **1**: 517–520.

Edminson P D, Reichelt K L, Saelid G et al (1982) Biologically active peptides from the urine of schizophrenics. In Hemmings G (ed) *Biological Aspects of Schizophrenia and Addiction*, pp 21–33. Chichester: John Wiley.

Gardner M L G (1981) Amino acid analysis in the study of protein digestion and absorption. In Rattenbury J M (ed) *Amino Acid Analysis*, pp 158–187. Chichester: Ellis Horwood.

Gardner M L G (1983a) Evidence for, and implications of, passage of intact peptides across the intestinal mucosa. *Biochemical Society Transactions* **11**: 810–813.

Gardner M L G (1983b) Entry of peptides of dietary origin into the circulation. *Nutrition and Health* **2**: 163–171.

Gardner M L G (1984) Intestinal assimilation of intact peptides and proteins from the diet — a neglected field? *Biological Reviews* **59**: 289–331.

Hautefeuille M, Brantl V & Desjeux J F (1984) β-Casomorphin derivatives evoke a decrease in short-circuit current in rabbit ileum. *Abstracts of European Intestinal Transport Group, VIth meeting, Pamplona*, p 42.

Henschen A, Lottspeich F, Brantl V & Teschemacher H (1979) Novel opioid peptides derived from casein (β-casomorphins). II. Structure of active components from bovine casein peptone. *Hoppe-Seyler's Zeitschrift fur Physiologiche Chemie* **360**: 1217–1224.

Humphrey R R, Dermody W C, Brink H O, et al (1973) Induction of luteinizing hormone (LH) release and ovulation in rats, hamsters, and rabbits by synthetic luteinizing hormone-releasing factor (LRF). *Endocrinology* **92**: 1515–1526.

Iversen L L (1983) Nonopioid neuropeptides in mammalian CNS. *Annual Reviews of Pharmacology and Toxicology* **23**: 1–27.

Iversen L L (1984) Amino acids and peptides: fast and slow chemical signals in the nervous system. *Proceedings of the Royal Society of London, Series B* **221**: 245–260.

Jos J, Tand M F de, Arnaud-Battander F et al (1983) Separation of pure toxic peptides from a β-gliadin subfraction using high-performance liquid chromatography. *Clinica Chimica Acta* **134**: 189–198.

Kastin A J & Barbeau A (1972) Preliminary clinical studies with L-prolyl-L-leucyl-glycine amide in Parkinson's disease. *Canadian Medical Association Journal* **107**: 1079–1081.

Klee W A & Zioudrou C (1980) The possible actions of peptides with opioid activity derived from pepsin hydrolysates of wheat gluten and of other constituents of gluten in the function of the central nervous system. In Hemmings G (ed) *The Biochemistry of Schizophrenia and Addiction*, pp 53–76. Lancaster: MTP Press.

Kreil G, Umbach M, Brantl V & Teschemacher H (1983) Studies on the enzymatic degradation of β-casomorphins. *Life Sciences* **33** (Suppl. 1): 137–140.

Loukas S, Varoucha D, Zioudrou C, Streaty R A & Klee W A (1983) Opioid activities and structures of α-casein-derived exorphins. *Biochemistry* **22**: 4567–4573.

Masson M A, Moreau O, Debuire B et al (1979) Evidence for the resistance of thyrotropin-releasing hormone (TRH) and pseudo-hormone, pyroglutamyl histidyl amphetamine, to degradation by enzymes of the digestive tract in vitro. *Biochimie* **61**: 847–852.

Matthews D M (1975) Intestinal absorption of peptides. *Physiological Reviews* **55**: 537–608.

Matthews D M (1977) Memorial lecture: protein absorption — then and now. *Gastroenterology* **73**: 1267–1279.

Matthews D M & Payne J W (eds) (1976) *Peptide Transport in Protein Nutrition.* Amsterdam. North-Holland.

Morley, J E (1982) Food peptides. A new class of hormones? *Journal of the American Medica Association* 247: 2379–2380.

Morley J E, Levine A S, Yamada T et al (1983) Effect of exorphins on gastrointestinal function hormonal release, and appetite. *Gastroenterology* 84: 1517–1523.

Mycroft F J, Wei E T, Bernardin J E & Kasarda D D (1982) MIF-like sequences in milk and whea proteins. *New England Journal of Medicinel* 307: 895.

Nishi N, Arimura A, Coy D H, Vilchez-Martinez J A & Schally A V (1975) The effect of oral an vaginal administration of synthetic LH-RH and [D-Ala^6,des-Gly^{10}-NH$_2$]-LH-RH ethylamide o serum LH levels in ovariectomised, steroid-blocked rats. *Proceedings of the Society for Ex perimental Biology and Medicine* 148: 1009–1012.

Perry T L, Hansen S, Tischler B, Bunting R & Berry K (1967) Carnosinemia. A new metabolic disorde associated with neurologic disease and mental defect. *New England Journal of Medicine* 277 1219–1227.

Peters T J & Bjarnason I (1984) Coeliac syndrome: biochemical mechanisms and the missing peptidas hypothesis revisited. *Gut* 25: 913–918.

Petrilli P, Picone D, Caporale C et al (1984) Does casomorphin have a functional role? *FEBS Letter* 169: 53–56.

Polak J M & Bloom S R (1982) Peripheral regulatory peptides: a newly discovered control mechanism In Fink G & Whalley L J (eds) *Neuropeptides: Basic and Clinical Aspects*, pp 118–147. Edinburgh Churchill Livingstone.

Ross-Smith P & Jenner F A (1980) Diet (gluten) and schizophrenia. *Journal of Human Nutrition* 34 107–112.

Ryle A P & Auffret C A (1979) The specificities of some pig and human pepsins towards syntheti peptide substrates. *Biochemical Journal* 179: 247–249.

Schusdziarra V, Holland A, Schick R et al (1983a) Modulation of post-prandial insulin release b ingested opiate-like substances in dogs. *Diabetologia* 24: 113–116.

Schusdziarra V, Schick A, Fuente A de la et al (1983b) Effect of β-casomorphins and analogs on insuli release in dogs. *Endocrinology* 112: 885–889.

Snyder S H (1980) Brain peptides as neurotransmitters. *Science* 209: 976–983.

Spector W G (1958) Substances which affect capillary permeability. *Pharmacological Reviews* 10 475–505.

Szewczuk A & Kwiatkowska J (1970) Pyrrolidonyl peptidase in animal, plant and human tissues *European Journal of Biochemistry* 15: 92–96.

Takagi H, Shiomi H, Ueda H & Amano H (1979a) Morphine-like analgesia by a new dipeptide L-tyrosyl-L-arginine (kyotorphin), and its analogue. *European Journal of Pharmacology* 55 109–111.

Takagi H, Shiomi H, Ueda H & Amano H (1979b) A novel analgesic dipeptide from bovine brain is possible met-enkephalin releaser. *Nature, London* 282: 410–412.

Teschemacher H, Ahnert G, Umbach M, Kielwein G & Leib S (1980) β-Casomorphins — opiate-lik acting peptide fragments from β-casein: determination in various milk and tissue extracts b radioimmunoassay. *Naunyn-Schmiedeberg's Archives of Pharmacology* 311 (Suppl): R67.

Trygstad O E, Reichelt K L, Foss I et al (1980) Patterns of peptides and protein-associated peptid complexes in psychiatric disorders. *British Journal of Psychiatry* 136: 59–72.

Walsh J H (1981) Endocrine cells of the digestive system. In Johnson L R (ed) *Physiology of th Gastrointestinal Tract*, pp 59–144. New York: Raven Press.

Woodley J F (1972) Pyrrolidone carboxylyl peptidase activity in normal intestinal biopsies and thos from coeliac patients. *Clinical Chimica Acta* 42: 211–213.

Zioudrou C & Klee W A (1979) Possible roles of peptides derived from food proteins in brain functior In Wurtman R J & Wurtman J J (eds) *Nutrition and the Brain*, pp 125–158. New York: Rave Press.

Zioudrou C, Streaty R A & Klee W A (1979) Opioid peptides derived from food proteins. Th exorphins. *Journal of Biological Chemistry* 254: 2446–2449.

Chapter 10
The Relationship between Food, Nitrosamines and Gastric Cancer

P. I. Reed and C. L. Walters

Although gastric cancer has been on the decline world-wide over the past thirty years, even in high risk areas it still remains one of the major cancers, notably in Japan, the mountainous regions of central and western Latin-America, northern and eastern Europe and Iceland. It is the third most common cancer in males in Great Britain, while in the United States, even though fifth as a cause of death, it nevertheless accounts for approximately 24 000 cases annually with around 14 000 deaths (Gunby 1981). There is a south–north gradient in the southern hemisphere with a higher incidence in the cooler or mountainous zones. About twice as many men as women develop this disease in both high and low incidence areas, cancer of the distal stomach tending to have a sex ratio of unity but a pronounced excess of men having cancer of the cardia. There is a linear relationship between incidence and age as well as a clear association with socio-economic factors, disease mortality being 3–4 times greater in the poor than in the professional and managerial groups.

Geographical comparisons and patterns of disease incidence in migrants suggest that environmental factors predominate in influencing gastric cancer incidence. It is noteworthy, however, that migrants from high to low incidence areas seem to maintain part of their risk of developing gastric cancer, compared with colon cancer, whose incidence falls rapidly to that prevailing ordinarily in the adopted country as shown, for instance, among Japanese immigrants into California (Buell and Dunn 1965). This would suggest that childhood exposure is a critical component in gastric cancer incidence, even though the disease itself is predominantly seen in the aged. The mounting body of evidence would suggest that stem cells of the gastric mucosa are bombarded heavily with mutagens at two periods in the life span, in the very young and the elderly, and that the predominant mutagens involved are products of nitrosation reactions that are direct acting mutagens.

N-NITROSATION

Since the demonstration by Magee and Barnes (1956) of the carcinogenicity of *N*-nitrosodimethylamine (NDMA), extensive investigations have established that well over 200 compounds containing the *N*-nitroso group are carcinogenic in experimental animals. All 40 species so far tested, including mammals, birds, amphibia and fish (Bogovski and Bogovski 1981) and

135

reptiles (Schmähl and Scherf 1984) have shown varying degrees of susceptibility and in a variety of organs, including the oesophagus, stomach, intestines, liver, bladder, brain, lung and kidney. A marked degree of organ specificity, varying with their chemical structure and experimental conditions, has also been demonstrated for the *N*-nitroso compounds (*N*-NO). In addition to carcinogenicity, other biological actions demonstrated by them include toxicity, cytotoxicity, mutagenicity and teratogenicity.

N-Nitroso compounds are formed when secondary, tertiary and even primary amines or amides, guanidines, ureas, etc., react with nitrite or nitrogen oxides under either acidic, neutral or alkaline conditions, depending on the appropriate precursors and presence of catalysts. Such stimulators and catalysts of physiological importance include chloride, thiocyanate and micro-organisms. For instance, thiocyanate, which is capable of accelerating the rate of nitrosation of secondary amines several hundred-fold at acid pH, is present in saliva, particularly that of smokers. However, it does not catalyse the formation of *N*-nitrosamides. Other substances, including ascorbic acid and α-tocopherol, generally inhibit nitrosation by acting as anti-oxidants and nitrite scavengers.

There are two main groups of *N*-nitroso compounds: *N*-nitrosamines represent one type and *N*-nitrosamides, including guanidines and ureas, form the other. The *N*-nitrosamines are stable compounds, requiring biological activation to form the proximal carcinogen, whereas the *N*-nitrosamides are labile, especially at alkaline pH, and do not require metabolic activation for the methylation of nucleic acids, by which route they are considered to exert their direct carcinogenic action.

The in vitro nitrosation of a secondary amine occurs most readily at around pH 3.5 whilst that of a secondary amide continues to increase in rate with fall of pH. Whereas the rate of nitrosation of secondary amines is proportional to the square of the nitrite level, that of amides is directly related to the nitrite concentration; thus at a given nitrite concentration, the rate of formation of *N*-nitrosamides may be greater than that of *N*-nitrosamines (Mirvish 1975). In the presence of low nitrite concentrations this kinetic difference may become vitally important. The development in the early 1970s of a sensitive and specific analytical system employing the so-called thermal energy analyser (Fine et al 1974) has made possible not only more accurate measurements of *N*-nitrosamine concentrations but has also led to their characterisation. This instrument makes it possible to detect chromatographically separated simple dialkyl *N*-nitroso compounds at levels below 1 ppb. Although the analysis of non-volatile thermally labile compounds, such as the *N*-nitrosamides, has proved more difficult, with the development of new techniques employing a high-performance liquid chromatography system (HPLC), it is now possible to detect nanogram (10^{-9} g) amounts of *N*-nitrosamides and *N*-nitrosoureas in complex biological samples (Tannenbaum 1983). A large number of potential precursors to *N*-nitroso compounds are present in biological systems and hence a procedure has been developed for their selective determination as a group (Walters et al 1978). This method responds to all types of *N*-nitroso compounds so far examined, and can differentiate them from most of the many other types of compounds which can be formed from nitrite, such as the pseudonitrosites of lipids.

N-Nitroso compounds have been identified in many different environmental situations including water, alcoholic beverages, food products, drugs, cosmetics, tobacco products, human biological fluids, agricultural and industrial products (Preussmann 1984). Thus man is exposed to *N*-nitroso compounds which are formed in the environment and introduced through ingestion, inhalation or external contact, as well as those formed in the body from precursors ingested separately in food or water or produced by endogenous mechanisms.

NITROSAMINES IN FOOD

About twenty years ago an outbreak of a liver disease in sheep occurred in Norway, with many fatalities which appeared to be caused by feeds containing herring meal preserved with sodium nitrite. The possibility that *N*-nitrosamines were implicated was related to the knowledge that fish contain considerable quantities of amines, including dimethylamine (which is responsible for the smell of fish) and subsequently it was demonstrated that *N*-nitrosodimethylamine (NDMA) present in concentrations of up to 100 mg/kg were enough to explain the damage caused (Ender et al 1964; Sakshaug et al 1965). Malignant liver tumours were also demonstrated in commercially reared mink with nitrite-treated herring meal in the diet (Bohler 1962) and in Canadian mink fed similarly (Sen et al 1972). In these findings, the *N*-nitrosamines acted as dietary carcinogens and this has stimulated considerable interest in the possibility that the *N*-nitrosamines in the diet could also be a possible hazard to man. A number of volatile *N*-nitrosamines, including NDMA, *N*-nitrosopiperidine (NPip) and *N*-nitrosopyrrolidine (NPyr) have been detected analytically in foods at ppb levels.

The most consistent source of simple, volatile *N*-nitrosamines in the diet is that of fried bacon, the principal compounds involved being NPyr and NDMA. Over the past ten years measures, such as reduced input nitrite levels and the use of ascorbate as an inhibitor of *N*-nitrosation, have been introduced which have generally decreased, but not eliminated the formation of such contaminants (Sen et al 1973). Gough et al (1978) examined 50 samples of fried bacon and reported levels of NPyr ranging from 1 to 20 µg/kg rising occasionally to 200 µg/kg.

In addition, all samples contained NPip concentrations of up to 0.25 µg/kg and NDMA up to 5 µg/kg in content. A more recent finding for both raw and cooked smoked bacon has been that of *N*-nitrosothiazolidine but it is not yet known whether its formation, probably from cysteine, formaldehyde and nitrite, is sensitive to the addition of ascorbate. Use has been made recently (Massey et al 1984) of a modification of the procedure of Walters et al (1978) for the determination of total *N*-nitroso compounds as a group in a number of foods. The values obtained in bacon (470–6000 µg *N*-NO per kg raw and 360–2400 µg *N*-NO per kg cooked) and in canned cured meats (600–1400 µg *N*-NO per kg) were much higher than those in other foods (for instance, 10–15 µg *N*-NO per kg dried milk and 20–65 µg *N*-NO per kg cocoa and chocolate), although samples of uncured meats were not included in the survey. Of these totals, the volatile *N*-nitrosamines represent a very small proportion. Their likely daily intake from the normal diet in the UK, excluding beer, has been calculated by Gough et al (1978) to be 0.53 μg, of which approximately 80% is contributed by cured meats.

Because of its relatively high amine content, fish has been regarded as a likely source of *N*-nitrosamines, especially in oriental countries. Approximately 80% of uncooked and fried fish samples studied by Webb and Gough (1980) contained NDMA at levels of up to 10 μg/kg. Similar results were obtained in Japan (Kawabata et al 1979) for raw and broiled fish; in some samples NPyr was found as well as NDMA. Similar levels of NDMA were found in some cheeses (Webb and Gough 1980) but without any significant increase in the frequency of occurrence in those manufactured using nitrate.

Fruit and vegetables rarely, if ever, have detectable levels of nitrosamines. However, Webb and Gough (1980) reported finding NDMA in five of 12 samples of canned fruit (<0.1 μg/kg), and whereas 16 samples of different vegetables contained no volatile nitrosamines, three of 30 soups tested contained NDMA (<0.9 μg/kg).

Of recent years, beer and other beverages have represented a major source of dietary NDMA. This has arisen principally from the direct fired drying of malt, during which oxides of nitrogen in the combustion gases have reacted with alkaloids such as gramine and hordenine to form the *N*-nitrosamine. A survey of 158 samples of different types of beer in the Federal Republic of Germany (Spiegelhalder et al 1979) showed that 70% of them contained NDMA at levels of up to 68 μg/l and with a mean concentration of 2.5 μg/l. In addition, six out of seven brands of Scotch whisky, also made from malt, were reported by Goff and Fine (1979) to contain NDMA at levels ranging from 0.3 to 2.3 μg/kg. Measures which have been devised to reduce the contamination of beers include the addition of sulphur during the drying of malt and the development of burners operating at lower temperatures so as to reduce the formation of oxides of nitrogen.

Precursors of *N*-nitroso compounds in food

N-Nitroso compounds can be formed not only from secondary amines and amides but also from their tertiary amino counterparts and even from quaternary ammonium compounds. The reaction of a tertiary amine with nitrous acid can be accompanied by the nitrosative cleavage of an alkyl or other group with the formation of a *N*-nitrosamine(s) and a carbonyl compound. As an example, the nitrosation of the analgesic, aminopyrine, results in the nitrosative cleavage of the simple *N*-nitrosodialkylamine, NDMA, which takes place more readily than does its formation from its parent amine, dimethylamine, which is strongly basic.

The formation of *N*-nitrosamines can even occur from primary amines in which the formation of a carbonium ion from one such group with nitrous acid can result in its interaction with an unchanged primary amino group to form a secondary amine which is subsequently converted to its *N*-nitroso derivative. This is particularly true of a polyamine, such as putrescine, a component of foods subjected to bacterial decarboxylation, in which the intramolecular reaction of the carbonium ion and the unchanged primary amino group leads to the formation of a cyclic secondary amine (pyrrolidine in the case of putrescine). Similarly, the polyamines spermine and spermidine, which are widely distributed in foods, can react with nitrous acid to produce a mixture of *N*-nitrosamines, including NPyr.

Nitrosatable amino and amido compounds in foods are numerous in number and vary greatly in character. In general, foods which are produced by microbial fermentation or which have been subjected to spoilage contain high levels of amines. Whilst most of these are primary amines such as tyramine arising from bacterial decarboxylation, nitrosatable secondary amines such as dimethylamine, diethylamine, etc., are also formed in cheeses and other similar foods.

Marine and some freshwater fish often contain trimethylamine oxide which can be converted microbiologically post mortem to trimethylamine and dimethylamine, both of which are precursors of the volatile *N*-nitrosodialkylamine NDMA.

Some amino acids, such as proline, hydroxyproline and sarcosine, react with nitrous acid to form *N*-nitroso derivatives which can decarboxylate to form simpler *N*-nitrosamines. This probably represents the pathway by means of which NPyr and NDMA are formed during the frying of bacon. This is borne out by the fact that the amount of NPyr formed correlates better with the nitrite concentration used in the preservation of the meat rather than that prior to frying, implying thereby that a nitrosated intermediate(s) is formed rapidly on curing. Unexpectedly, NPyr formation occurs predominantly in the adipose tissue of bacon. This may result from the intermediate formation of a pseudo-nitrosite of unsaturated lipid(s), which are recognised to act as nitrosating agents, or of oxides of nitrogen such as N_2O_3 or N_2O_4, which are most active in the formation of *N*-nitrosamines in non-aqueous environments. Other probable precursors of NPyr in fried bacon include spermine and spermidine or collagen itself, a structural component of skeletal muscle which is particularly rich in proline in its molecular constitution.

Plant alkaloids may also be precursors of *N*-nitrosamines in foods and beverages, hence the high levels of NPyr and NPip found in mixtures used in the preservation of meats and including spices originated from sources of this type (Sen et al 1973). Piperine and chavicine in black pepper (*Piper nigrum*) provided the amine precursor to NPyr and paprika (*Capsicum annuum*) that to NPip. Similarly, the sources of NDMA in beer are probably gramine and hordenine.

Both animal and vegetable tissues contain metabolic intermediates which are potentially nitrosatable, such as the purine and pyrimidine bases, guanidine and related compounds, intermediates of the Krebs–Henseleit cycle such as citrulline, and so on. Whether or not the amide linkages of peptides and proteins are capable of forming *N*-nitroso derivatives under gastric conditions is still a matter of conjecture, but certainly the reaction of alanylalanine with nitrite at acid pH has led to a product exhibiting mutagenic activity without metabolic activation (Bartsch; reported by Walters et al 1982). Thus it is evident that there are many potential precursors of *N*-nitrosamines in the diet, which may give rise to *N*-nitrosamine formation either in food or after ingestion in vivo. Furthermore, dietary nitrosating agents may react with endogenous amines produced by gastro-intestinal microflora, enhancing the possibility of *N*-nitroso compound formation in the colonised hypochlorhydric stomach.

Nitrate and nitrite

Nitrate is present in most foods and particularly those of vegetable origin; its concentration is dependent on a number of factors, including the extent of use of fertilisers. The mean daily intake of nitrate in the U K and U S A has been estimated at 100–120 mg (Hill 1980). In beets and spinach, for instance, its concentration can reach several thousand parts per million as the nitrate ion (NO_3^-), sufficient to promote methaemoglobinaemia in some young infants in whom bacterial colonisation of the stomach has resulted from initial hypochlorhydria. In order to act as a nitrosating agent, nitrate must be reduced to either nitrite or oxides of nitrogen. This can be brought about by numerous bacteria and some metals and their salts. It has been suggested also that some mammalian tissues, notably the dorsum linguae, contain enzyme systems capable of reducing nitrate to nitrite although this is very difficult to prove with certainty. Walters et al (1967) found that the mitochondria of skeletal muscle are capable of utilising nitrate as a terminal electron acceptor, resulting thereby in its reduction to nitric oxide. However, no similar activity towards nitrate was observed.

Because of its greater reactivity with phenols, amines, thiols, etc., the levels of nitrite found in foods are generally much lower, except where it is used deliberately as an additive in preserved meats and some cheeses. In that capacity, it performs a very useful function in helping to prevent the outgrowth of spores of highly pathogenic micro-organisms, such as *Clostridium botulinum*. Ascorbate is commonly used as well as nitrite in the preservation of meat. Not only does it make the nitrite more effective in the curing process, but it also reduces the formation of *N*-nitrosamines in situ, although it rarely eliminates them altogether.

When nitrate is consumed in foods, particularly vegetables, and through the water supply, it is absorbed rapidly into the blood stream and is concentrated and secreted by the salivary glands in the mouth, the maximum concentration occurring approximately 1–2 hours after ingestion. While in the mouth, a part of the nitrate is reduced to nitrite. According to Tannenbaum et al (1976), this reduction occurs by microbiological intervention, but more recently Sasaki and Matamo (1979) have provided evidence that the dorsum linguae contains nitrate reductase enzyme(s) which contribute to the overall reduction of nitrate to nitrite. The extent to which a subject responds to a challenge of nitrate in terms of an increased nitrite level in the saliva is relatively constant (Walters and Smith 1981), but varies widely from individual to individual. The nitrite formed in the mouth is presumably swallowed into the acidic milieu of the stomach, in which the pH range covers that optimal for its reaction with amines, phenols, thiols, etc., of food and/or endogenous origin. White (1975) estimated that up to 68% of the daily intake of nitrite arose from in vivo reduction of nitrate. However, it should be remembered that many vegetables contain ascorbic acid in varying amounts, often dependent on the plant growth conditions, on the other hand it has not been established whether the pharmacokinetics are compatible, so that ascorbic acid is retained in the stomach whilst nitrite enters from the saliva.

When a meal containing nitrite is consumed, the concentration in the stomach increases whilst the pH rises as a result of the buffering action of the food. Following the consumption, for instance, of a meal containing nitrite at an overall level of 0.83 mM, the concentration in the gastric juice reached a maximum of close to 0.3 mM after about 50 minutes, at which time the pH had risen to around 4.5 (Walters et al 1979). As the pH fell subsequently, to around 3.2 after 100 minutes, the nitrite level dropped to about 0.15 mM as the result of its reaction with food and/or gastric components, disproportionation and/or absorption.

The fasting level of nitrite in the saliva has been reported (Tannenbaum et al 1974) to range generally from 6 to 10 mg $NaNO_2$ per litre (0.086–0.14 mM). It has been suggested that an individual secretes about 1.5 litres of saliva per 24 hours; this would represent a total daily output of nitrite from this source of about 9–15 mg. However, as already stated, the rate of nitrosation of a secondary amine is proportional to the square of the nitrite concentration, hence the maximum formation of *N*-nitrosamines in vivo may well occur following the intake of nitrite per se, as distinct from the background level derived from dietary nitrate.

In vivo formation of nitrosamines

There is now very strong evidence, based on many different types of studies, showing that nitrosamines are formed in vivo from dietary precursors after ingestion. In one type of study, Sander et al (1968) incubated homogenates containing amines of varying basicities with human gastric juice in vitro and demonstrated that the ease of nitrosamine formation depended on the basicity of the parent amine, while Sen et al (1969) showed that *N*-nitrosodiethylamine (NDEA) was formed when diethylamine and sodium nitrite were incubated with gastric juice from various animals as well as man. They also showed that more nitrosamine was formed in low pH gastric juice, as in man and the rabbit (pH 1–2), than in that of the rat (pH 4–5). These observations have since been confirmed by various other workers who also stressed the catalytic action of salivary thiocyanate for nitrosation, especially in smokers (Walters et al 1979). The same authors also showed that normal foods contain potential precursors of nitrosamines when incubated with nitrite and human gastric juice. Following up these in vitro studies, many in vivo experiments have confirmed that nitrosation may occur in the stomach after ingestion of dietary precursors. Walters et al (1979) detected trace amounts of NPip in gastric contents of volunteers, after ingestion of homogenised foods containing nitrite. Ohshima and Bartsch (1981) showed that certain *N*-nitrosamino acids, such as *N*-nitrosoproline (NPro), are excreted quantitatively almost unchanged in the urine and faeces. Furthermore, this compound is neither a carcinogen nor is it metabolised and thus the amount excreted is the amount synthesised (Chu and Magee 1981). Although nitrosation of L-proline occurs on both a low and a high nitrate diet, it is more marked when the nitrate intake is high. Ohshima and Bartsch (1981) were further able to show that the nitrosation inhibitors, ascorbic acid and α-tocopherol, both markedly reduced the excretion of NPro by blocking intragastric nitrosation. More recently, we have shown that greater amounts of the secondary amine thiazolidine-4-carboxylic acid, unlike that of proline, are nitrosated when gastric juice secretion is suppressed (Elder et al 1984).

Significant levels of N-nitrosamines have been found also in tissues and body fluids other than gastric juice. Wang et al (1978) detected NDMA and NDEA in normal human faeces in concentrations up to 1.5 μg/kg and 13 μg/kg respectively, together with lower levels of NPyr and N-nitrosomorpholine (NMor). Kakizoe et al (1979) demonstrated the presence of low concentrations of NDMA, NDEA and NMor in the urine of human volunteers. The presence of NDMA in blood has also been identified by Yamamoto et al (1980), interestingly in higher concentrations than in American subjects (Fine et al 1977), possibly due to the higher nitrate and secondary amine content of Japanese diets.

Since the demonstration by Sander (1968) that bacteria could catalyse the N-nitrosation reaction in vitro, it has been shown that N-NO could be formed in vivo whenever appropriate bacteria, nitrosatable amine and nitrate or nitrite co-exist in the body (Hill et al 1973). The presence of nitrate-reducing bacteria, increased concentrations of nitrite and of N-nitroso compounds, has been demonstrated in vivo in the human hypochlorhydric stomach (Ruddell et al 1976; Schlag et al 1980; Reed et al 1981a,b; Stockbrugger et al 1982), bacterial nitrate-reducing activity being noted particularly at or above pH 4. Furthermore, in vivo nitrosation has also been demonstrated both in the normal acidic as well as in the achlorhydric stomach, in the mouth, colon, urinary bladder and vagina (Hill 1981). Hill has stressed the fact that the bacterial flora at any given site determine the amount of nitrosation, both by affecting the amount of nitrite formed and also the rate of nitrosation. Thus the presence of a significant population of nitrate-reducing organisms, together with an adequate intake of nitrate which can be reduced to nitrite, forms the basis of an aetiological hypothesis for gastric cancer formation (Correa et al 1975), now supported by an increasing body of epidemiological data.

EPIDEMIOLOGY

Epidemiological studies have demonstrated an association between exposure to nitrate and gastric cancer in various countries including Chile (Armijo and Coulson 1975), Colombia (Cuello et al 1976), Japan (Thaler 1976) and China (Tsui 1979). For instance, a survey of water supplies in a high risk area of Colombia showed high nitrate concentrations in wells (Tannenbaum et al 1977); it is thought that the high incidence of gastric cancer in Chile is related to the intensive use of nitrate fertilisers (Thaler 1976) and in Japan, to a regular consumption of vegetables, with a high nitrite and nitrate content, and of fish which is a source of secondary amines (Thaler 1976). In contrast, the progressive reduction in the incidence of gastric carcinoma, even in high risk areas, has been associated in the case of Chile with an increased consumption of milk, animal protein (meat and fish) and sugar, fats, oils and butter (Zaldivar 1977), while in Japan it has been inversely related to the frequency of green-yellow vegetable intake (Hirayama 1981). Other earlier reports (Graham et al 1967, 1972; Haenszel et al 1972) have shown a similar inverse relationship, which has been interpreted as being due to a low intake of vitamin C, even though this has not been confirmed by dietary analyses.

However, all high risk regions have in common the consumption of foods low in vitamin C and raised intake of salt (Weisburger 1981). The former acts as an inhibitor of nitrosation (Mirvish et al 1972), whereas the latter exerts a promoting effect (Tatematsu et al 1975). This effect of salt is linked with epidemiological data from high risk areas for gastric cancer, in which there is also a high incidence of hypertension (Bjelke 1984; Armstrong et al 1979; Joossens et al 1979; Altschul and Grommet 1980; Ueshima et al 1981). In another study, Joossens and Geboers (1981) compared gastric cancer rates with stroke incidence in various countries. The good correlations found would suggest that the intake of salt or highly salted food may be the common link between the two conditions. They proposed the concept that a high salt intake leads to osmotic irritation of the gastric mucosa, with development of atrophic gastritis and eventually achlorhydria, which favours the formation of nitrite and *N*-nitroso compounds.

Table 10.1 lists the age-adjusted death rates for gastric cancer per 100 000 population in different countries, in males and females, as well as estimates of their nitrate and nitrite intake. These data indicate that ingestion of both nitrate and nitrite is generally higher in countries with a greater gastric cancer incidence. Epidemiological studies carried out in high risk areas in various countries, notably Chile, Colombia, China, Japan and England have reflected the relationship between cancer incidence and higher nitrate intake in water and/or food, often associated with higher salt consumption as well (Committee on Nitrite and Alternative Curing Agents in Food 1981). Furthermore, where gastric biopsy correlations have been studied, it was noted that individuals in high risk areas tend to develop atrophic gastritis at an earlier age and with greater frequency than in low risk areas, being associated with higher gastric juice pH and nitrite, but lower nitrate concentrations and higher counts of nitrate-reducing micro-organisms (Cuello et al 1976; Tannenbaum et al 1979) and in China a recent very extensive study in over 40 000 subjects has also demonstrated higher fungal counts, especially of *Aspergillus versicolor* and *nidulans* (Ru-fu et al 1984). The findings in the Colombian studies served as the basis for the gastric cancer models involving nitrate, one for the normal acidic and the other for an achlorhydric stomach, formulated by Tannenbaum et al in 1977 and brought up to date on the basis of further evidence (Tannenbaum 1983). These concepts are gaining increasing acceptance, even though the evidence is still essentially circumstantial.

MODIFYING FACTORS

Vitamin E (α-tocopherol)

Free α-tocopherol, the form in which it is found in food, is an anti-oxidant which has proved to be an effective inhibitor of *N*-nitrosation because of its ability to scavenge nitrite. Being lipid soluble, it is particularly effective in

Table 10.1. Age-adjusted death rate for gastric cancer and estimated daily consumption of nitrate and nitrite in different countries. After Committee on Nitrite and Alternative Curing Agents in Food (1981).

Country	Stomach cancer (age-adjusted death rate per 100 000 population)		Estimates of consumption (ranges and averages, mg/person/day)			
			Nitrate		Nitrite	
	Male	Female	Average	Range	Average	Range
Japan	56.6	29.0	297	380 – 490	1.5	0.7 – 10
			385	44 – 864		0.1–1.3
Czechoslovakia	33.3	16.6	218			
Federal Republic of Germany	27.1	14.1	388		3.3	
			271		1.7	
			142			
Yugoslavia	24.0	11.5	75		6.5	
Netherlands	21.4	9.7	49		2.8	
United Kingdom	19.7	9.0	156			
			110			
			58			
			115			
Switzerland	18.1	10.2	91		1.1	
Norway	17.4	9.8	32		0.11	
Sweden	16.3	8.3	48	24 – 68		0.5 – 5
			150	110 – 190	3.7	0.9 – 7.3
China	15.4		42			2 – 10
Denmark	14.8	8.1	54		0.74	
United States	7.2	3.7	75		0.78	

reducing *N*-nitrosation in non-aqueous systems such as the adipose tissue of bacon, in which the major part of the formation of *N*-nitrosopyrrolidine occurs during frying. It is worth noting that *dl*-α-tocopherol acetate, commonly found in food supplements, may not be an effective blocking agent. Ohshima and Bartsch (1981), in their studies confirming that endogenous nitrosation occurs in man, showed that nitrosation of the marker amine, L-proline, was significantly reduced by α-tocopherol, although to a lesser degree than that observed with ascorbic acid.

Vitamin C (ascorbic acid)

Since the serendipitous discovery by Mirvish et al (1972) of the nitrosation inhibiting action of ascorbic acid, many additional studies have confirmed that this occurs both in vitro and in vivo. Relatively low levels of vitamin C could block nitrosation of virtually all substrates in vitro. It has been shown in a series of animal experiments (Ivankovic and Preussmann 1970; Ivankovic et al 1975) that the simultaneous application of ascorbic acid with ethylurea and nitrite inhibited the induction of tumours typical of *N*-nitrosoethylurea, and also prevented of transplacental carcinogenesis, while more recently Ohshima and Bartsch (1981) showed in a human volunteer that vitamin C inhibited the formation of *N*-nitrosoproline from ingested L-proline and nitrate, in the form of beetroot juice. Weisburger and Rainieri (1975), using a model food system, showed that the formation of *N*-nitroso urea from added nitrate plus methylurea could be blocked either by the addition of excess vitamin C or by refrigerating the food which prevents the bacterial conversion of nitrate to nitrite. We have studied the effect of ascorbic acid administration on gastric juice nitrite and *N*-NO levels in achlorhydric subjects and showed that 4 g vitamin C daily for four weeks significantly reduced *N*-nitroso compound concentrations, especially in patients with partial gastrectomy, with a concurrent reduction in nitrite concentration which almost reached statistical significance (Reed et al 1984). This very high dose was employed in an attempt to maintain a significant level of ascorbic acid in the stomach over a prolonged period of time.

While it appears that vitamins C and E may be effective preventative agents in several cancers, including that of the stomach, possibly by acting primarily in the inhibition of *N*-nitroso compound formation, other mechanisms of action of these vitamins are possible. Furthermore, vitamins C and E are not necessarily the only nitrosation blockers in food, or perhaps even the most effective ones. To evaluate the effects of vitamin C and/or E supplementation on tumour or precursor incidence long term, large scale studies will be necessary. However, the many pitfalls of such projects must not be overlooked including the long latency for gastric cancer development, the difficulty and unreliability of obtaining information about the food intake, and the methodological problems which have to be overcome.

CONCLUSION

Man's contact with carcinogens in general is in the form of exposure to trace amounts. It has been shown by Druckrey et al (1967) that the efficiency of

NDEA as a carcinogen is markedly dependent on the mode of administration. Far less carcinogen is required for tumour induction when NDEA is applied in repeated small doses than is necessary when larger individual applications are made, even though the induction period is increased. As a number of *N*-nitroso compounds have been found to be carcinogenic to the grandular stomach of experimental animals (Homburger et al 1976; Sugimura and Fujimura 1976) and man is regularly exposed to potential carcinogens of this type and their precursors, it is not unreasonable to seek for evidence of any involvement of these compounds in human gastric cancer epidemiology. On the basis of the evidence presented in this chapter certain dietary factors can be identified which are related to the onset of gastric cancer. These include a food intake which is low in animal fat and protein, green and yellow vegetables and fresh fruit (especially of the citrus variety), and high in salt. Hopefully, the avoidance of these adverse factors should lead to a further reduction in the incidence of cancer of the stomach.

Acknowledgements

We wish to acknowledge the financial support of the Cancer Research Campaign and thank Mrs Pamela Gross for the secretarial work.

REFERENCES

Altschul A M & Grommet J K (1980) Sodium intake and sodium sensitivity. *Nutritional Review* 3 393–402.

Armijo R & Coulson A H (1975) Epidemiology of stomach cancer in Chile — the role of nitrog fertilizers. *International Journal of Epidemiology* 4: 301–309.

Armstrong B, Clarke H, Martin C et al (1979) Urinary sodium and blood pressure in vegetariar *American Journal of Clinical Nutrition* 32: 2472–2476.

Bjelke E (1974) Epidemiologic studies of cancer of the stomach, colon and rectum — with spec emphasis on the role of diet. *Scandinavian Journal of Gastroenterology* 9 (Suppl. 31): 1–235.

Bogovski P & Bogovski S (1981) Animal species in which *N*-nitroso-compounds induce cancer. Spec report. *International Journal of Cancer* 27: 417–474.

Bohler N (1962) Ondartet leversykdom hos pelsdyr: Norge. *Proceedings of IX Nordic Veterina Congress, Copenhagen* Vol. II, p. 774.

Buell P & Dunn J E (Jr) (1965) Cancer mortality among Japanese Issei and Nissei of California. *Canc* 18: 656–666.

Chu C & Magee P N (1981) The metabolic fate of nitrosoproline in the rat. *Cancer Research* 4 3653–3657.

Committee on Nitrite and Alternative Curing Agents in Food (1981) Adverse effects of nitrate, nitr and *N*-nitroso compounds. In *The Health Effects of Nitrate, Nitrite and* N-*Nitroso Compounds, P. I* pp 9/3–9/17. Washington DC: National Academy of Science Press.

Correa P, Haenszel W, Cuello C, Tannenbaum S & Archer M (1975) A model for gastric canc epidemiology. *Lancet* 2: 58–60.

Cuello C, Correa P, Haenszel W et al (1976) Gastric cancer in Columbia. I. Cancer risk and susp environmental agents. *Journal of the National Cancer Institute* 57: 1015–1020.

Druckrey H, Preussmann R, Ivankovic S & Schmähl D (1967) Organotrope carcinogene Winkungen 65 verschiedenen *N*-nitroso-Verbindungen an BD-Ratten. *Zeitschrift für Krebsforschung* 103–201.

Elder J B, Burdett K, Smith P L R, Reed P I & Walters C L (1984) The effect of H$_2$ blockers intragastric nitrosation as measured by the 24 hour urinary secretion of *N*-nitrosoproline. In O'N I K, von Borstel R C, Miller C T, Long J & Bartsch H (eds) N-*Nitroso Compounds: Occurren Biological Effects and Relevance to Human Cancer*, pp 969–974. IARC Scientific Publication N 57. Lyon: International Agency for Research on Cancer.

Ender F, Havre G, Helgebostad A et al (1964) Isolation and identification of a hepatotoxic factor in herring meal produced from sodium nitrate preserved herring. *Naturwissenschaften* **51**: 637–638.

Fine D H, Rufeh F & Lieb D (1974) Group analysis of volatile and non-volatile *N*-nitroso compounds. *Nature*, London **247**: 309–310.

Fine D H, Ross R, Rounbehler D P, Silvergleid A & Song L (1977) Formation in vivo of volatile *N*-nitrosamines in man after ingestion of cooked bacon and spinach. *Nature*, London **265**: 753–755.

Goff E U & Fine D H (1979) Analysis of volatile *N*-nitrosamines in alcoholic beverages. *Food and Cosmetic Toxicology* **17**: 569–573.

Gough T A, Webb K S & Coleman R F (1978) Estimate of the volatile nitrosamine content of UK food. *Nature*, London **272**: 161–163.

Graham S, Lilienfeld A M & Tidings J E (1967) Dietary and purgation factors in the epidemiology of gastric cancer. *Cancer* **20**: 2224–2234.

Graham S, Schotz W & Martino P (1972) Alimentary factors in the epidemiology of gastric cancer. *Cancer* **30**: 927–938.

Gunby P (1981) Nitrosoureas suspected in stomach cancer. *Journal of the American Medical Association* **245**: 1714.

Haenszel W, Kurihara M, Segi M & Lee R K C (1972) Stomach cancer among Japanese in Hawaii. *Journal of the National Cancer Institute* **49**: 969–988.

Hill M J (1980) Bacterial metabolism and human carcinogenesis. *British Medical Bulletin* **36**: 89–94.

Hill M J (1981) Nitrates and bacteriology. Are these important etiological factors in gastric carcinogenesis? In Fielding J W L, Newman C E, Ford C H J & Jones B G (eds) *Gastric Cancer*, pp 35–45. Oxford: Pergamon Press.

Hill M J, Hawksworth G & Tattersall U (1973) Bacteria, nitrosamines and cancer of the stomach. *British Journal of Cancer* **28**: 562–567.

Hirayama T (1981) Changing patterns in the incidence of gastric cancer. In Fielding J W L, Newman C E, Ford C H J & Jones B G (eds) *Gastric Cancer*, pp 1–15. Oxford: Pergamon Press.

Homburger F, Handler A H, Soto E et al (1976) Adenocarcinoma of the glandular stomach following 3-methylcholanthrene, *N*-nitrosodiethylamine or *N*-nitrosodimethylamine feeding in carcinogen susceptible inbred Syrian hamsters. *Journal of the National Cancer Institute* **57**: 141–143.

Ivankovic S & Preussmann R (1970) Transplazentare Erzeugung maligner Tumoren. *Naturwissenschaften* **57**: 460.

Ivankovic S, Preussmann R, Schmähl D & Zeller J W (1975) Prevention by ascorbic acid of in vivo formation of *N*-nitroso compounds. In Bogovski P & Walker E A (eds) *N-Nitroso Compounds in the Environment*, pp 101–102. IARC Scientific Publication No. 9. Lyon: International Agency for Research on Cancer.

Joossens J V & Geboers J (1981) Nutrition and gastric cancer. *Proceedings of the Nutritional Society* **40**: 37–46.

Joossens J V, Kesteloot H & Amery A (1979) Salt intake and mortality from stroke. *New England Journal of Medicine* **300**: 1396.

Kakizoe T, Wang T, Eng V W S et al (1979) Volatile *N*-nitrosamines in the urine of normal donors and of bladder cancer patients. *Cancer Research* **39**: 829–832.

Kawabata T, Ohshima H, Uibu J et al (1979) Occurrence, formation and precursors of *N*-nitroso compounds in the Japanese diet. In Miller E C, Miller J A, Hirons J, Sugimura T & Takayama S (eds) *Naturally Occurring Carcinogens — Mutagens and Modulators of Carcinogenesis*, pp 195–209. Tokyo: Japan Scientific Society Press.

Magee P N & Barnes J M (1956) The production of malignant primary hepatic tumours in the rat by feeding dimethylnitrosamine. *British Journal of Cancer* **10**: 114–122.

Massey R C, Key P E, McWeeny D J & Knowles M E (1984) The application of a chemical denitrosation and chemiluminescence detection procedure for estimation of the apparent concentration of total *N*-nitroso compounds in foods and beverages. *Food Additives and Contaminants* **1**: 11–16.

Mirvish S S (1975) Formation of *N*-nitroso-compounds: chemistry, kinetics and in vivo occurrence. *Toxicology and Applied Pharmacology* **31**: 325–351.

Mirvish S S, Wallcave L, Eagen M & Shubik P (1972) Ascorbate–nitrite reaction: Possible means of blocking the formation of carcinogenic *N*-nitroso compounds. *Science* **177**: 65–68.

Ohshima H & Bartsch H (1981) Quantitative estimation of endogenous nitrosation in humans by monitoring *N*-nitrosoproline excreted in the urine. *Cancer Research* **41**: 3658–3662.

Preussmann R (1984) Occurrence and exposure to *N*-nitroso compounds and precursors. In O'Neill I K, von Borstel R C, Miller C T, Long J & Bartsch H (eds) *N-Nitroso Compounds: Occurrence, Biological Effects and Relevance to Human Cancer*, pp 3–15. IARC Scientific Publication No. 57. Lyon: International Agency for Research on Cancer.

Reed P I, Haines K, Smith P L R, Walters C L & House F R (1981a) The gastric juice *N*-nitrosamines i health and gastroduodenal disease. *Lancet* **2**: 550–552.

Reed P I, Haines K, Smith P L R, Walters C L & House F R (1981b) The effect of cimetidine on gastri juice *N*-nitrosamine concentration. *Lancet* **2**: 553–556.

Reed P I, Smith P L R, Summers K et al (1984) The effect of gastric surgery for benign peptic ulcer an ascorbic acid therapy on gastric juice nitrite and *N*-nitroso compound concentrations. In Bartsch H O'Neill I K, Castegnaro M, Okada M & Davis M (eds) *N-Nitroso Compounds: Occurrence an Biological Effects*, pp 975–979. IARC Scientific Publication No. 57. Lyon: International Agency fc Research on Cancer.

Ruddell W S J, Bone E S, Hill J J, Blendis L M & Walters C L (1976) Gastric juice nitrite: a risk factor fc cancer in the hypochlorhydric stomach? *Lancet* **2**: 1037–1039.

Ru-fu Z, He-ling S, Mao-lin J & Song-nian L (1984) A comprehensive survey of etiological factors c stomach cancer in China. *Chinese Medical Journal* **97**: 322–332.

Sakshaug J, Sognen E, Hansen M A & Koppang N (1965) Dimethylnitrosamine; its hepatotoxic effect i sheep and its occurrence in toxic batches of herring meal. *Nature*, London **206**: 1261–1262.

Sander J (1968) Nitrosaminsynthese durch Bakterien. *Hoppe Seyler's Zeitschrift für Physiologische Chem* **349**: 429–432.

Sander J, Schweinsberg F & Menz H P (1968) Untersuchungen rüber die Enstehung cancerogenc Nitrosamine in Magen. *Hoppe-Seyler's Zeitschrift für Physiologische Chemie* **349**: 1691–1697.

Sasaki T & Matamo K (1979) Formation of nitrite from nitrate at the *dorsum linguae*. *Journal of the Foo and Hygiene Society of Japan* **20**: 263–269.

Schlag P, Ulrich H, Merkle P et al (1980) Are nitrite and *N*-nitroso compounds in gastric juice risk facto for carcinoma in the operated stomach? *Lancet* **1**: 727–729.

Schmähl D & Scherf H R (1984) Carcinogenic activity of *N*-nitrosodiethylamine in snakes (*Pytho reticulatus*, Schneider). In O'Neill I K, von Borstel R C, Miller C T, Long J & Bartsch H *N-Nitros Compounds: Occurrence, Biological Effects and Relevance to Human Cancer*, pp 677–682. IAR< Scientific Publication No. 57. Lyon: International Agency for Research on Cancer.

Sen N P, Donaldson B A, Iyengar J R & Panalaks T (1973) Nitrosopyrrolidine and dimethylnitrosamine i bacon. *Nature*, London **241**: 473–474.

Sen N P, Schwinghamer L A, Donaldson B A & Miles W H (1972) *N*-Nitrosodimethylamine in fish mea *Journal of Agricultural and Food Chemistry* **20**: 1280–1281.

Sen N P, Smith D C & Schwinghamer L (1969) Formation of *N*-nitrosamines from secondary amines an nitrite in human and animal gastric juice. *Food and Cosmetic Toxicology* **7**: 301–307.

Spiegelhalder B, Eisenbrand G & Preussmann R (1979) Contamination of beer with trace quantities c *N*-nitrosodimethylamine. *Food and Cosmetic Toxicology* **17**: 29–31.

Stockbrugger R W, Cotton P B, Eugenides B A et al (1982) Intragastric nitrites, nitrosamines and bacteri overgrowth during cimetidine treatment. *Gut* **23**: 1048–1052.

Sugimura T & Fujimura S (1967) Tumor production in glandular stomach of rat by *N*-methyl-*N*¹-nitro-*N* nitroso-guanidine. *Nature*, London **216**: 943–944.

Tannenbaum S R (1983) *N*-Nitroso compounds: a perspective on human exposure. *Lancet* **1**: 629–632.

Tannenbaum S R, Sinskey A J, Weisman M & Bishop W (1974) Nitrite in human saliva. Its possib relationship to nitrosamine formation. *Journal of the National Cancer Institute* **53**: 79–83.

Tannenbaum S R, Weisman M & Fett D (1976) The effect of nitrate intake on nitrite formation in huma saliva. *Food and Cosmetic Toxicology* **16**: 459–462.

Tannenbaum S R, Archer M C, Wishnok J S et al (1977) Nitrate and the etiology of gastric cancer. In Hia H H, Watson J D & Winsten J A (eds) *Origins of Human Cancer: Book C. Human Risk Assessmen* pp 1609–1625. New York: Cold Spring Harbor Laboratory.

Tannenbaum S R, Moran D, Rand W, Cuello C & Correa P (1979) Gastric cancer in Colombia. IV. Nitri and other ions in gastric contents of residents from a high-risk region. *Journal of the National Canc Institute* **62**: 9–12.

Tatematsu M, Takahashi M, Fukushima S, Hanaouchi M & Shirai T (1975) Effects in rats of sodiu chloride on experimental gastric cancers induced by *N*-methyl-*N*¹-nitro-*N*-nitrosoguanidine or nitroquinoline-1-oxide. *Journal of the Natonal Cancer Institute* **55**: 101–104.

Thaler H (1976) Nitrates and gastric carcinoma. *Deutsche Medizinische Wochenschrift* **101**: 1740–1742.

Tsui K W (1979) Situation of prevention and treatment of gastric cancers in China. *Zhonghua Zhong. Zazhi* **1**: 223–227.

Ueshima H, Tanigaki M, Iida M et al (1981) Hypertension, salts and potassium. *Lancet* **1**: 504.

Walters C L & Smith P L R (1981) The effect of water-borne nitrate on salivary nitrite. *Food and Cosme. Toxicology* **19**: 297–302.

Walters C L, Casselden R J & Taylor A McM (1967) Nitrite metabolism by skeletal muscle mitochondria in relation to haem pigments. *Biochimica et Biophysica Acta* **143**: 310–318.

Walters C L, Downes M J; Edwards M W & Smith P L R (1978) Determination of a non-volatile *N*-nitrosamine on a food matrix. *Analyst* **103**: 1127–1133.

Walters C L, Carr F P A, Dyke C S et al (1979) Nitrite sources and nitrosamine formation in vitro and in vivo. *Food and Cosmetic Toxicology* **17**: 473–479.

Walters C L, Smith P L R & Reed P I (1982) Endogenous amines in human gastric juice. In Magee P N (ed) *Banbury Report 12: Nitrosamines and Human Cancer*, pp 445–452. New York: Cold Spring Harbor Laboratory.

Wang T, Kakizoe T, Dion P et al (1978) Volatile nitrosamines in normal human faeces. *Nature*, London **276**: 280–281.

Webb K S & Gough T A (1980) Human exposure to preformed environmental *N*-nitroso compounds in the UK. *Oncology* **37**: 195–198.

Weisburger J H (1981) *N*-Nitroso compounds: Diet and cancer trends. An approach to the prevention of gastric cancer. In Scanlan R A & Tannenbaum S R (eds) N-*Nitroso Compounds*, ACS Symposium Series, No. 174, pp 305–317. New York: American Chemical Society.

Weisburger J H & Rainieri R (1975) Dietary factors and the etiology of gastric cancer. *Cancer Research* **35**: 3469–3474.

White J W (1975) Relative significance of dietary sources of nitrate and nitrite. *Journal of Agricultural and Food Chemistry* **23**: 886–891.

Yamamoto M, Yamada T & Tanimura A (1980) Volatile nitrosamines in human blood before and after ingestion of a meal containing high concentration of nitrate and secondary amines. *Food and Cosmetic Toxicology* **18**: 297–298.

Zaldivar R (1977) Decline in stomach cancer mortality rates in a high risk geographical area. *Österreichische Zeitschrift der Onkologie* **3**: 115–116.

Chapter 11
Diet and Cancer of the Digestive Tract

M. J. Hill

Cancers of the gastro-intestinal tract show wide variations in incidence between countries (Table 11.1) and this has been postulated as being due to dietary differences. Many human cancers are associated with dietary factors (Armstrong and Doll 1975) including the hormone-related cancers (breast, endometrium, ovary, prostate) as well as those of the digestive tract. The evidence that diet is important in the causation of these cancers is derived from studies of migrants, comparisons of racial or religious groups within countries, case-control studies and temporal changes in incidence.

In migrant studies the incidence of the disease in a population group living in their original homeland is compared with that in a subsection of the population that has migrated to a region with a different disease pattern. For example, Japanese living in Japan have a high incidence of cancer of the stomach and a low incidence of colorectal and of breast cancer. When they migrate to the United States (which has a low incidence of gastric cancer and a high incidence of colorectal and of breast cancer) the incidence of all three diseases approaches that of the new homeland whilst amongst the children of the migrants the diseases show a similar incidence to that in native-born Americans. This indicates that the incidence of all three cancers is largely determined by environmental factors and that genetic factors are unimportant in determining the risk of these diseases in populations.

Environmental factors can be divided into two classes: the physical and the cultural environment. The physical environment includes climate, geography, altitude, air pollution, etc. and is made up of factors shared by all members of a population living in a particular location. The cultural environment includes those items chosen by the individual, such as diet, habits of personal hygiene, smoking and use of other drugs etc., and is unique to the individual (and like-minded persons). The effect of these two classes of environmental factor can be distinguished by studying, for example, the different religious subgroups of Bombay or California, or the different racial subgroups in Johannesburg, Singapore, London. In all such studies it is found that different racial or religious subgroups have different risks of cancers of the digestive tract, despite having a shared physical environment.

Case-control studies should help in distinguishing between the effects of various aspects of the cultural environment (such as various items of the diet, alcohol, and tobacco). However, there are problems associated with case-control studies of the effect of diet in studying digestive tract cancers and these are described below.

The diet of most populations varies with time as a result of improved methods of food preservation, food supply and marketing, as well as

150

Table 11.1. The incidence (per annum per 100 000, age adjusted) of cancers of the digestive tract in various countries.

	Oesophagus		Stomach		Colon-rectum	
	Male	Female	Male	Female	Male	Female
Europe						
England (S. Thames)	5.1	2.7	18.5	8.1	28.0	23.5
Finland	4.0	3.1	29.3	15.3	17.0	16.0
Sweden	2.9	1.1	18.3	9.5	27.2	22.3
Germany (Saarland)	5.3	0.9	29.8	13.2	37.8	29.2
Poland (Cracow)	4.0	0.8	35.1	15.6	21.4	13.6
Hungary	1.2	0.2	28.5	12.2	13.2	12.4
Italy	7.8	1.4	38.5	19.1	35.6	26.0
Asia						
Japan (Miyagi)	13.8	3.2	88.0	42.0	17.5	13.8
China (Shanghai)	24.7	8.0	55.7	21.0	15.7	11.7
Singapore (Chinese)	18.9	4.1	43.7	17.6	29.1	20.9
India (Bombay)	15.7	10.7	9.7	5.9	8.0	6.6
South America						
Brazil	14.1	2.8	45.7	19.0	19.3	16.6
Colombia	3.1	1.7	46.3	27.3	7.9	7.7
Antilles	16.7	8.7	27.5	9.5	11.5	8.2
Africa						
Senegal	0.2	0.2	3.7	2.0	2.1	1.7
North America						
US (Connecticut)	5.3	1.7	11.1	5.1	50.0	37.5
Canada (Ontario)	4.2	1.7	16.3	7.9	41.0	35.9
Jamaica	7.1	3.0	17.7	9.3	12.4	11.3
Australasia						
Australia (NSW)	4.4	2.0	13.7	6.7	34.3	26.4
New Zealand	5.3	2.3	16.3	7.0	41.6	38.1

increased prosperity and increased communication about the food habits of other countries. The major problem associated with correlating such changes with the changing disease pattern is to guess the latency between an effect on the causation of a disease and its manifestation in cases of disease (especially of cancers, where the latency may be 20–50 years if initiation is being considered, or 0–10 years if the effect of diet is promotional).

The simple relationship between diet and cancer may be studied by comparing populations, by case-control studies or by prospective studies. However, the consumption of the various components of the diet are interrelated and so a correlation may either indicate a causal (or protective) relationship, or it may be coincidental. It is therefore necessary to postulate a plausible mechanism to rationalise any observed relationship; absence of such a mechanism leaves an epidemiological observation highly suspect. It is important to recognise that science, however well carried out, is unable to *prove* a hypothesis but can only either refute it or be compatible with it. Epidemiological studies alone cannot even suggest causality, but can only indicate a correlation. It is wrong, therefore, to state that a study shows a causal or protective effect of a dietary item; it can only show a positive or an inverse correlation.

In this review I will first discuss the types of epidemiological study and their pitfalls. The various mechanisms by which diet might cause or promote carcinogenesis will be described. Finally, the evidence relating diet to cancers of the oesophagus, stomach and large bowel will be discussed.

TYPES OF EPIDEMIOLOGICAL STUDY AND THEIR PITFALLS

The epidemiological relation between diet and cancer can be examined in populations and in case control studies as well as in large prospective studies. Major criticisms may be made of all three types of study in the context of digestive tract carcinogenesis.

People do not consume specific classes of nutrients (e.g. fat, protein, dietary fibre); they eat foods which usually contain a complex mixture of all classes of nutrient. Since a number of individual food items are major sources of more than one nutrient, coincidental correlations are inevitable. For example, in Western populations meat is the major source of both protein and of fat; a causal correlation with fat will therefore produce a coincidental correlation with animal protein and vice versa. Similarly, a correlation with milk might be due to its content of fat or of calcium; a correlation with fresh vegetables might be due to fibre or to vitamins C or E. In all types of study it is difficult to distinguish between these causal and coincidental correlations.

In population studies the data on food consumption are normally taken from data from the Food and Agriculture Organizaton (FAO) which is based on food sales. Food which is not bought (such as home grown vegetables, or fruits from wild sources) is not included; in contrast, food which is wasted is not excluded. Thus although the data are likely to be qualitatively correct, they cannot be assumed to be accurate quantitative guides to food intake and this is a major criticism of population comparisons.

Diseases of the digestive tract usually lead to loss of appetite and often to a change in the diet in an attempt to palliate symptoms. Therefore, in case-control studies, the determination of the current diet gives no information on the possible causal role of diet in carcinogenesis and dietary recall has to be attempted. This is notoriously difficult and the data obtained by dietary recall methods are of no use unless the item being sought is one which is easy to recall and is consumed in large amounts by some, and not at all by others. Alcohol consumption is always underestimated by those completing dietary questionnaires. There is a major problem also in the choice of suitable controls. Because of the effect of gastro-intestinal symptoms on diet, the best controls would include those with matched gastro-intestinal symptoms but with diseases other than the malignancy being studied or its precurser lesions. This is very rarely attempted and the controls are usually healthy persons matched only for age and sex and, on occasions, location of residence. These difficulties make case-control studies of gastro-intestinal cancer of very little value.

Prospective studies should be the best and most reliable means of assessing the role of diet in carcinogenesis. Current diet is relatively simple to assess accurately and the data of cohorts of persons can be regularly updated to monitor changes in diet over a long time period. However, such studies are extremely expensive in time and in money and are therefore rarely attempted.

A very common mistake in discussing epidemiological studies is to describe inverse correlations as showing a 'protective' effect and positive correlations as indicating a 'causal' effect. This is wrong; it suggests a total misunderstanding of the strengths and weaknesses of such studies.

In studying the relation between diet and human cancer the requirements are that different types of study should point to the same dietary item with a measure of unanimity, that a dose–response relationship should be detectable, that a plausible mechanism explaining the relationship should be available and that this mechanism should have a measure of scientific confirmation. If all of these criteria are satisfied, then the observed relationship can be tested in a dietary intervention study; if this produced the expected result then the 'causal' (or 'protective') nature of the observed relationship can be accepted with some confidence. Unfortunately this does not apply to any of the cancers of the digestive tract.

MECHANISMS

Diet might affect the risk of carcinogenesis by acting as a source of carcinogens, or of tumour promoters or inhibitors; it might also act as a source of substrates for the endogenous production of any of these. Alternatively, diet might affect the activity of enzymes responsible for carcinogen activation or influence the effectiveness of the host immune defence mechanisms; it might also affect the gut bacterial flora and so interfere with the enterohepatic circulation of carcinogens, or the solubility and transport of carcinogens.

Dietary carcinogens

The diet is a rich source of carcinogens which may be naturally present, produced during food processing or cooking, or as a result of food spoilage. Some of the carcinogens present in food are listed in Table 11.2.

Polycyclic aromatic hydrocarbons (PAHs) are normal products of thermal decomposition of organic matter and so are present in the smoke used in food preservation, in the charred parts of grilled or toasted foods and in the cooking oil used in frying of foods (especially if the oil is reused many times). They are at highest concentrations in traditional wood-smoked products.

N-Nitroso compounds are found in all cured meat products containing added nitrite (which is added as a food preservative either as nitrite or as a component of sea salt). They are also present in beers and alcoholic beverages where the malt or hops are roasted before fermentation (see Chapter 10).

Table 11.2. Carcinogens present in food, their sources and their possible association with human cancer.

Carcinogen	Source	Site of associated cancer
Polycyclic aromatic hydrocarbons (PAHs)	Smoking or grilling of food	Stomach
N-Nitroso compounds	Nitrite preservative	Stomach, oesophagus
Aflatoxin and mycotoxins	Fungal contamination	Liver
Harman, norharman, etc.	Pyrolysis products formed during cooking	?
Cycasin, etc.	Naturally occurring	Colon in animals
Alkyl hydrazines	Present in mushrooms	Colon in animals

Aflatoxins and other mycotoxins are detectable in most foods as a result of contamination of the food with *Aspergillus* spp. (for aflatoxins), *Fusarium* spp. and other fungi. They are present in greatest amounts in food which have been badly stored and in hot and humid climates.

A number of products of the pyrolysis of amino acids have been shown to be extremely potent mutagens (e.g. harman, norharman) particularly those produced from aromatic amino acids. These are present in grilled foods, the amount rising with increasing temperature of cooking.

Cycasin is a naturally occurring carcinogen present in cycad nuts; cycads are a major starch source in south-east Asia and are only consumed after prior removal of the cycasin. However, on occasions raw cycads are consumed following natural disasters which disrupt normal communications and food supplies. In animals cycasin is a potent colon carcinogen.

A range of alkylhydrazines have been detected in mushrooms and fungi, and in animals many of these have been shown to give tumours of the large bowel, also of the ear duct.

Dietary anti-carcinogens or tumour inhibitors

Much less attention has been given to tumour inhibitors and anti-carcinogens. The major anti-cancer agents in the diet are vitamins A, C and E, tannins, substances present in cruciferous vegetables and the anti-oxidants used as food preservatives. Most of these act as scavengers for proximate carcinogens; their action has been reviewed and described by Wattenberg (1980).

Endogenously produced carcinogens/tumour promoters

The endogenous production of carcinogens or tumour promoters by the bacterial flora of the gastro-intestinal tract has been discussed at length by Hill (1980) and is summarised in Table 11.3. N-Nitroso compounds are

Table 11.3. Substrates for the endogenous production of carcinogens, tumour promoters, mutagens, co-mutagens, etc.

Product	Substrate
N-Nitroso compounds	Nitrate in vegetables
	Secondary amines, produced from meat
Nonapentene glycerol ether (and related compounds)	Fat
Secondary amines for *N*-nitrosation	
Piperidine	Lysine, from protein
Pyrrolidine	Arginine, from protein
Dimethylamine	Lecithin
Volatile phenols	Tyrosine, from protein
Range of metabolites	Tryptophan, from protein
Deoxycholic and lithocholic acids	Bile acids, in response to fat
Cholesterol	Fat and meat

formed by the action of nitrite on secondary amino groups; the reaction can be catalysed by hydrogen ions with a pH optimum of 2, and can also be catalysed by bacterial enzymes (Leach et al 1985). Nitrosatable amines are present in the diet in only small amounts, but considerable amounts of dimethylamine, piperidine and pyrrolidine are produced in the colon by bacterial action on protein or fat of either dietary or endogenous origin. In addition, very large amounts of urea and alkylureas are produced endogenously by the liver.

Phenol and *p*-cresol are produced in the colon by the bacterial flora from tyrosine; they have been shown to promote the development of tumours on the rodent skin initiated by dimethylbenzanthracene (DMBA). Most of the phenol and *p*-cresol is absorbed from the colon and excreted in the urine.

A range of metabolities of tryptophan, produced by the liver and by bacteria in vitro, has been shown to be co-carcinogenic (Table 11.4) using the bladder implantation test (Bryan 1971). Although it has yet to be demonstrated that such metabolites are produced in vivo they have been detected in the colon.

A number of bile acids have been shown to be co-carcinogenic in the rat colon and co-mutagenic in the Ames test (Table 11.5), as well as by a range of other tests. The bile acids on which there is most information are deoxycholic and lithocholic acids; recent studies by Wilpart et al (1984) have characterised the structure–activity relationships in the co-mutagenicity of bile acids (Table 11.5) and their results suggest that the highest activity would be found in a 3β-hydroxy-5α-cholanoic acid (although this compound has still to be tested).

Cholesterol has been shown to be a solid state carcinogen by a number of workers but it is unlikely that this is of importance in human carcinogenesis. It may be oxidised to cholesterol α-epoxide but, although this binds to DNA in vitro, it was not carcinogenic or tumour promoting in the rat colon (Reddy and Watanabe (1979).

Table 11.4. Metabolites of tryptophan which have been shown to be co-carcinogenic.

Metabolite	Test system showing co-carcinogenicity
Quinaldic acid	Bladder implantation test
8-Hydroxyquinaldic acid	Bladder implantation test
3-Hydroxyanthranilic acid	Bladder implantation test, mammalian cell mutation
3-Hydroxykynurenine	Bladder implantation test, mammalian cell mutation
Xanthenuric acid	Bladder implantation test
Indole	Aceto-amido fluorene (AAF) treated rats
Indoleacetic acid	AAF treated rats

Table 11.5. Evidence that bile acids can act as tumour promoters or co-mutagens.

Test system	Observation
Rectal instillation in initiated rodents	Deoxycholic and lithocholic acids are promoters; primary bile acids are inactive
Skin painting in oily vehicle	Active bile acids: deoxycholic, apocholic, and bis-nor-5-cholenic acids
Mouse kidney embryo cell transformation test	Lithocholic acid is mutagenic
Bacterial mutagenesis	Primary bile acids are inactive; deoxycholic and lithocholic acids are co-mutagens; 5α-isomers are more active than 5β-isomers; 3β-hydroxyl are more active than 3α-hydroxyl

Other mechanisms

All carcinogens need to be activated to a proximate carcinogen and this is usually carried out by the mixed function oxidases. A number of studies of the hepatic microsomal enzymes have shown that their activity is very sensitive to diet, being inducible by a wide range of foreign compounds. The role of immune surveillance in controlling or preventing the growth of human cancers has still to be determined; however, it is established that immunoglobulins and the activity of the cellular immunity system is decreased in persons on a low protein diet and is impaired in protein malnutrition. The enterohepatic circulation of foreign compounds is dependent in part on the metabolic activity of the ileal and caecal bacterial flora which, in turn, is dependent on the diet. It is known that many classes of lipophilic carcinogens (e.g. PAHs) undergo enterohepatic circulation and increased retention time within the body might increase the risk of carcinogenesis by such compounds.

OESOPHAGEAL CANCER

Oesophageal cancer is relatively common in Asia and relatively rare in North America and Europe. Such a generalisation masks huge variations in incidence which occur within countries, over very short distances; these variations are far greater for oesophageal than for any other cancer. In general, the disease is more common in men than in women, but the relative proportion of female cases increases with the overall frequency of the disease. Most of the areas where the disease is common are very poor and their populations suffer malnutrition. Population studies show that, together with alcohol, dietary deprivation is the major risk factor for this disease.

An early study by Wynder and Bross (1961) showed that both alcohol and tobacco were important risk factors, that their effect was multiplicative rather than additive, and that the two factors together accounted for 76% of the total risk of the disease. Consumption of spirits carried a greater risk than beer drinking. The study confirmed many early case-control studies showing that alcohol and tobacco were important risk factors in Western populations.

Case-control studies suggest that these two main risk factors predominate in different areas, with alcohol being the more important in Europe and the West, and dietary deprivation in Asia. However, they do not act alone, but in concert with some known carcinogen. In a case-control study in Brittany, Tuyns et al (1977) found that alcohol consumption and cigarette smoking were risk factors, with multiplicative combined action. In this study the joint dose–response relationship could be expressed as

$$\text{Relative risk} = (\text{tobacco} + 1)^{0.45} \cdot \exp(\text{alcohol}/4)$$

where tobacco usage is in grams, as is alcohol consumption. The equation makes clear that as alcohol consumption increases, its relative importance as a risk factor increases disproportionately. In the Brittany study, alcohol consumption of more than 40 g/day and/or cigarette smoking of more than 10 g/day accounted for more than 83% of the total risk.

As is clear from the above equation, giving up smoking should have a major effect on oesophageal cancer rates; studies of various groups that have given up smoking suggest reductions in incidence of 20–60%; religious groups in the United States which do not permit either smoking or drinking have a much lower risk of the disease than the general population (Enstrom 1980; Phillips 1980).

In the Third World, smoking and alcohol are relatively unimportant, the main risk factor being malnutrition. Although most populations with a high incidence of the disease are poor, the converse is not necessarily true, suggesting that poor nutrition makes a population susceptible to some other factor such as thermal irritation, N-nitroso compounds, etc. In Transkei, China and Hong Kong, N-nitroso compounds have been implicated in the causation of the disease, whilst in other populations the consumption of very hot food and drink, the consumption of mouldy or spicy food, or cigarette smoking, correlate with the disease.

In summary, poor nutrition, either in the form of excessive alcohol intake, undernutrition, or food deprivation, is strongly associated with a high risk of

Table 11.6. The relation between diet and oesophageal cancer in various countries or populations.

Population	Predisposing diet	Carcinogen source
Brittany	Alcohol	Tobacco
United States	Alcohol, poor nutrition	Tobacco
Puerto Rico	Alcohol, poor nutrition	Tobacco
Japan	Poor nutrition	Hot food, tobacco
China	Poor nutrition	N-Nitroso compounds?
Chile	Poor nutrition	N-Nitroso compounds?
Transkei	Poor nutrition	N-Nitroso compounds?
Iran	Poor nutrition	?
Singapore	Poor nutrition	Hot drinks

oesophageal cancer (Table 11.6), acting together with some 'carcinogen', such as tobacco smoke, N-nitroso compounds or moulds. The epidemiology of cancer of the oesophagus has been well reviewed by Day (1975) and by Day et al (1982). It is suggested that alcohol and very hot food may aid the transport of carcinogens into the mucosal tissues; they may also act as irritants, so promoting the development of cancers that have been already initiated.

GASTRIC CANCER

Gastric cancer has a similar world distribution to that of oesophageal cancer, being very common in eastern Asia and the Andean countries of South and Central America and relatively rare in north-west Europe, North America and Australasia. Within Europe, the disease is more common in the south and east; within the British Isles it is more common in the north and west. In Western Europe and North America the stomach was the commonest site of cancer before 1940, but since then the disease has declined in importance and is now less common than lung, colorectal or breast cancer.

Migrant studies suggest that environmental factors acting during the first 20–30 years of life are crucial determinants of the risk of the disease, suggesting that the most important stage in carcinogenesis is the establishment of a precancerous state (since the disease itself is rare in persons aged less than 50). Since the stomach is the first place of residence for food and food-borne carcinogens, there have been a vast number of studies attempting to relate diet to the disease, but none has produced any conclusive evidence incriminating any particular food item. In general the food items which appear to correlate with the disease are staple foods (bread, cereal foods, potatoes, rice) or fried foods (Table 11.7), although fresh vegetables and salads appear to be inversely correlated with the disease in many studies. The conclusion of Haenszel and Correa (1975) was that the mode of food preparation or storage was more important than the actual diet; an alternative explanation is that the correlation with staple foods reflects a lack of variety in the diet and is a measure of dietary deprivation.

Table 11.7. The relationship between diet and gastric cancer in various studies.

Population studied	Dietary item correlated with gastric cancer risk
Finland	Grain products
Norway	Salted or smoked foods Cereals
Iceland	Smoked fish and birds
Holland	Bacon
Wales	Fried foods
United States	Starchy foods and vegetables
Japan	Rice
China	Vegetables
Colombia	Corn
Slovenia	Potatoes

Gastric cancers have been divided into two histological classes by Lauren (1965), namely the diffuse and intestinal types. The diffuse type has an incidence which is even throughout the world and and is associated with genetic factors; the intestinal type is responsible for the differences in incidence between countries and is associated with environmental factors. This latter type has received considerable attention and a histopathological sequence has been postulated (Correa et al 1975) in which the first step is gastric atrophy; this has been associated with high salt intake and with protein malnutrition. The second stage is atrophic gastritis followed by the development of intestinal metaplasia. Dysplasia of increasing severity develops in the areas of intestinal metaplasia and finally culminates in cancer.

The mechanism of this histopathological sequence has been discussed by Hill (1984). The proposed mechanism is based on the common observation that gastric atrophy is accompanied by bacterial overgrowth of the gastric mucosa and lumen; this bacterial flora reduces nitrate to nitrite and may also promote the formation of N-nitroso compounds. These N-nitroso compounds (or some other metabolite of nitrite) cause the progression from gastric atrophy to gastric cancer; there have now been many studies demonstrating that progression along the sequence from gastric atrophy through intestinal metaplasia and dysplasia to carcinoma correlates with the numbers of bacteria and the nitrite concentration in the lumen of the stomach.

If this mechanism is valid, then in countries where gastric atrophy is common in young adults, a correlation between nitrate exposure and gastric cancer risk should be observed and this is so (Table 11.8); a weaker correlation might be expected where gastric atrophy is less common and this too has been noted. The correlation with staple foods would then reflect the type of diet consumed by populations still using salt as a preservative or living on vegetables which were rich in nitrate because of mineral deficiencies in the soil or the excessive use of nitrate fertiliser.

Table 11.8. Correlation between nitrate intake and gastric cancer in various populations.

Population studied	Prevalence of gastric atrophy	Source of high nitrate exposure
China	High	Vegetables, due to low molybdenum content of soil resulting in nitrate build-up
Chile	High	Vegetables, due to use of high amounts of nitrate fertiliser
Colombia	High	Vegetables, due to high nitrate content of soil; also drinking water
Japan	Moderate	Vegetables, due to high nitrate content of the soil
Italy	Moderate	Drinking water
Denmark	Low	Drinking water
Israel	?	Drinking water
England	Low?	Drinking water

The data relating diet to gastric carcinogenesis have been reviewed by Correa and Haenszel (1982) and Hill (1983, 1984).

LARGE BOWEL CANCER

The epidemiological studies of diet and large bowel cancer include population studies, case-control studies and one prospective study. A good review is that by Zaridze (1981).

Population studies

There have been many studies of the relation between diet and colorectal cancer in populations (Table 11.9) and they nearly all suggest a relationship between the disease and the intake of meat (or its component animal fat and animal protein) or of total calories. Such correlation studies imply a dose–response relationship, which in many cases is very strong. For example, in the study by Drasar and Irving (1973) the intake of bound fat (that fat which is 'hidden' in the meat, as distinct from the 'visible fat' which may be removed) was correlated with colorectal cancer incidence in 37 populations with a correlation coefficient of 0.88.

In an attempt to avoid the problems of coincidental correlations, a number of groups have attempted to estimate the partial correlation coefficients. For example, Armstrong and Doll (1975) observed strong correlations with total energy intake, fat, meat and protein but only energy intake and meat remained strong when the others were controlled. Similarly, Liu et al (1979) noted a strong correlation with fat and cholesterol intake and an inverse correlation with dietary fibre; only cholesterol had a strong partial correlation coefficient, the other two appearing to be secondary or coincidental relationships.

When all of the studies are put together the strongest correlations are for fat, meat and total energy intake. Although dietary fibre is only very weakly correlated in most of these studies, it has been suggested that this is due to the weakness of the data. In a comparison of the English hospital regions, an inverse correlation with the pentosan fraction of dietary fibre was observed (Bingham et al 1979) and this was supported by the results of a comparison of four Scandinavian regions (Cummings et al 1982). However, more recent information which indicates low fibre intakes for Japanese and Indians (Bingham 1985) has clouded the issue, as has the observation by Walker (1985) of a *positive* correlation with dietary fibre when white, black, coloured and Indian populations in South Africa were compared.

Table 11.9. The correlations between diet and colorectal cancer in populations.

Dietary item	Description of the study
Meat	Study of 23 countries
Animal protein	Study of 23 countries
	Study of 28 countries
	Study of 37 countries
Fat	Study of 23 countries
	Study of 28 countries
	Study of 37 countries
Beer	Study of 47 countries
Cholesterol	Study of 20 countries
Fibre (positive)	Study of 3 populations in Hong Kong
	Study of 4 racial groups in South Africa
Fibre (inverse)	Study of hospital regions in England and Wales
	Study of 4 populations in Scandinavia
Milk (inverse)	Study of 2 Scandinavian populations

Table 11.10. Dietary items which appear to be related to colorectal carcinogenesis in case-control studies (most studies showed no correlations).

Dietary item positively related	Country	Dietary item inversely correlated	Country
Meat String beans	Hawaii	Crude fibre	Israel
Fat (dose–response relationship)	Canada	Vitamins A and C	Norway
Fat	Finland		
Fat	United States		

Case-control studies

As would be expected from the difficulties discussed previously (p. 152), case-control studies have incriminated almost every item of the diet (Table 11.10). However, it is notable that, although the majority of studies showed no correlation with any dietary item, a number have produced positive correlation with fat or meat, and in one case (Jain et al 1980) a dose–response relationship was detected.

Prospective study

A single large scale prospective study has been undertaken by Hirayama in Japan (Hirayama 1981). Unfortunately the population examined (which is being used to study a wide range of cancers) has a very low incidence of colorectal cancer and may not, therefore, provide useful clues to the causation of the disease in countries where the incidence is high.

Postulated mechanisms

The risk of colorectal cancer cannot be correlated with any of the carcinogens commonly found in foodstuffs, but two suggestions have been made involving the production of bacterial metabolites in the colon. The first is that large bowel carcinogenesis is promoted by a diet rich in fat because of the action of bile acids (Hill et al 1971; Hill 1981). The second is that the disease is caused by lack of dietary fibre (Burkitt, 1971). The evidence suggesting a role for bile acids in colorectal carcinogenesis is summarised in Table 11.11, and has

Table 11.11. Evidence of a role for bile acids as tumour promoters in the causation of large bowel cancer (for more details see Hill 1984).

Type of study	Observation
Population studies	Faecal bile acid concentration is correlated with the incidence of colorectal cancer
Dietary studies	Faecal bile acid concentration increases with increasing dietary fat and with decreasing bran intake
High-risk patient groups	Faecal bile acid concentration correlates with the severity of epithelial dysplasia in adenoma and in long term ulcerative colitis patients
	Bile acid turnover and absorption from the colon is higher in adenoma patients than in controls
Mucosal studies	Bile acids cause epithelial dysplasia in rodents, in humans and in cultured adenoma cells
Bile acid receptors	Bile acid receptors are present in the colonic mucosa of a high proportion of colon cancer patients and a very small proportion of controls
Mutagenicity/carcinogenicity	Bile acids are tumour promoters in the rodent colon and co-mutagens in the bacterial mutagenesis assay (Ames test); bile acids cause DNA strand breakages

recently been reviewed by Hill (1985); the relationship between faecal bile acid concentration and diet is summarised in Table 11.12.

The hypothesis that large bowel cancer is a disease of fibre depletion was put forward by Burkitt (1971). In summary (Table 11.13), a decrease in the amount of dietary fibre was thought to produce hard small stools with a slow colonic transit. Slow transit would allow more time for the bacterial production of carcinogens and more time for such products to exert their action on the colon mucosa. An increase in dietary fibre intake would reverse these processes; in addition the stool bulking would dilute any carcinogens formed. A major problem with the fibre hypothesis is that so few groups of workers have attempted to validate it; apart from the notable exception of the Cambridge group, whose work in this field has been summarised by Cummings (1981) and Bingham (1985), most of the proponents of this hypothesis have simply repeated it unquestioningly. It is certainly true that cereal fibre (although not pectin gums and lignin) increases stool bulk and dilutes a range of faecal components. Recent evidence (Berghouse et al 1984) also suggests that a high fibre diet modifies the bacterial flora of the right colon (see Chapter 5). However there is little evidence that fibre has any effect on the metabolism of a range of substrates and the argument that slow colonic transit provides more time for a carcinogen to act is fallacious (Hill 1974). In summary, Burkitt's hypothesis remains largely untested.

Table 11.12. The relation between diet and faecal bile acid concentration in humans.

Dietary change		Effect on faecal bile acid concentration
Increase fat		Increase
Increase protein		Small increase
Supplement with	bran	Decrease
	pectin	Small increase
	lignin	No change
	lactulose	Decrease

Table 11.13. The postulated effects of a decrease in the amount of dietary fibre in relation to colorectal carcinogenesis.

Effect	Consequence
Modify the gut bacterial flora	Increase carcinogen/co-carcinogen production
Decrease stool bulk	Increase the concentration of carcinogens/co-carcinogens
Increase colonic transit time	Allow more time for carcinogen production; allow more time for carcinogens to act on the mucosa

CONCLUSIONS

There has been a recent spate of articles and reports giving advice to the nation on how to prevent cancer by dietary change. In my opinion this is largely misguided. Although the incidence of cancer of the digestive tract is high and must be reduced, more than 90% of people will *not* develop such a tumour. People consume foods because they like them or because they cannot afford other more palatable foods. Those whose diets are determined economically are in a poor position to change and the advice is therefore directed at those whose diet is determined by choice; in those persons a change from the diet of choice must decrease the pleasure of eating and so it is essential that we have *very* good reasons for advising such a change.

The evidence relating specific dietary items to cancer of the digestive tract is still weak. Furthermore, most of the items that are strongly correlated with colorectal cancer are inversely correlated with gastric and oesophageal cancer and vice versa. Since colorectal cancer has a much better prognosis than either gastric or oesophageal cancer, a shift in diet away from that correlated with cancer of the latter sites is more sensible. In my opinion the current guidelines proposed in the United States are premature and ill-advised.

Nevertheless, during the last 10–15 years much progress has been made in our understanding of the mechanism of both gastric and of colorectal carcinogenesis. If groups of people at high risk of either disease could be identified, dietary advice could be given in the confidence that the likely benefit would greatly exceed the likely risk. This is the correct way forward.

Acknowlegement

The work of my laboratory is generously supported by the Cancer Research Campaign.

REFERENCES

Armstrong B & Doll R (1975) Environmental factors and cancer incidence and mortality in different countries with special reference to dietary practices. *Inernational Journal of Cancer* **15**: 617–631.

Berghouse L, Hori S, Hill M, Hudson M et al (1984) Comparison between the bacterial and oligosaccharide content of ileostomy fluid in subjects taking diets rich in refined or unrefined carbohydrate. *Gut* **25**: 1071–1077.

Bingham S (1985) Epidemiology of colon cancer. In Kritchevsky D & Vahouny G (eds) *Dietary Fiber in Health and Disease*. New York: Plenum Press.

Bingham S, Williams D R, Cole T J & James W P T (1979) Dietary fibre and regional large bowel cancer mortality in Britain. *British Journal of Cancer* **40**: 456–463.

Bryan G T (1971) The role of urinary tryptophan metabolites in the etiology of bladder cancer. *American Journal of Clinical Nutrition.* **24**: 841–847.

Burkitt D P (1971) Epidemiology of cancer of the colon and rectum. *Cancer* **28**: 3–13.

Correa P, Haenszel W, Cuello C, Tannenbaum S & Archer M (1975) A model for gastric cancer epidemiology. *Lancet* **2**: 58–60.

Correa, P & Haenszel, W (1982) Epidemiology of gastric cancer. In Correa P and Haenszel W (eds). *Epidemiology of Cancer of the Digestive Tract*, pp 59–84. The Hague: Martinus Nijhoff.

Cummings J H (1981) Dietary fibre and large bowel cancer. *Proceedings of the Nutrition Society* **40**: 7–14.

Cummings J H, Branch W J, Bjerrum L et al (1982) Colon cancer and large bowel function in Denmark and Finland. *Nutrition and Cancer* **4**: 61–66.

Day N E (1975) Some aspects of the epidemiology of oesophageal cancer. *Cancer Research* **35**: 3304–3307.

Day N E, Munoz N & Ghadirian P (1982) Epidemiology of esophageal cancer: A review. In Correa P & Haenszel W (eds) *Epidemiology of Cancer of the Digestive Tract*, pp 21–58. The Hague: Martinus Nijhoff.

Drasar B S & Irving D (1973) Environmental factors and cancer of the colon and breast. *British Journal of Cancer* **27**: 167–172.

Enstrom I E (1980) Cancer mortality among Mormons in California during 1968–75. *Journal of the National Cancer Institute* **65**: 1073–1082.

Haenszel W & Correa P (1975) Developments in the epidemiology of stomach cancer over the past decade. *Cancer Research* **35**: 3452–3459.

Hill M J (1974) Colon cancer: a disease of fibre depletion or dietary excess? *Digestion* **11**: 289–306.

Hill M J (1980) Bacterial metabolism and human carcinogenesis. *British Medical Bulletin* **36**: 89–94.

Hill M J (1981) Metabolic epidemiology of large bowel cancer. In De Cosse J & Sherlock P (eds) *Gastrointestinal Cancer*, pp 187–226. The Hague: Martinus Nijhoff.

Hill M J (1983) Environmental and genetic factors in gastrointestinal cancer. In Sherlock P, Morson B C, Barbara L & Veronesi U (eds) *Precancerous Lesions of the Gastrointestinal Tract*, pp 1–22. New York: Raven Press.

Hill M J (1984) Aetiology of gastric cancer. *Clinics in Oncology* **3**: 237–250.

Hill M J (1985) Biochemical approaches to the interventions in large bowel cancer. In Ingall J & Mastromarino A (eds) *Carcinoma of the Large Bowel and its Precursers*. New York: Alan Liss.

Hill M J, Drasar B S, Aries V C et al (1971) Bacteria and the aetiology of large bowel cancer. *Lancet* **1**: 95–100.

Hirayama T (1981) A large-scale cohort study on the relationship between diet and selected cancers of digestive organs. In Bruce W R, Correa, Lipkin M, Tannenbaum S R & Wilkins T D (eds) *Gastrointestinal Cancer: Endogenous Factors*, pp 409–430. New York: Cold Spring Harbor.

Jain M, Cook G M, Davis F G et al (1980) A case-control study of diet and colorectal cancer. *International Journal of Cancer* **26**: 757–768.

Lauren P (1965) The two main types of gastric cancer: diffuse and so called intestinal type. *Acta Pathologica Microbiologica Scandinavica* **64**: 31–49.

Leach S A, Challis B, Cook A R, Hill M J & Thompson M H (1985) The bacterial catalysis of the *N*-nitrosation of secondary amines. *Biochemical Society Transactions* (in press).

Liu N, Stamler J, Moss D et al (1979) Dietary cholesterol, fat and fibre and colon cancer mortality. *Lancet* **2**: 782–785.

Phillips R L (1980) Cancer among Seventh Day Adventists. *Journal of Environmental Pathology and Toxicology* **3**: 157–169.

Reddy B S & Watanabe K (1979) Effect of cholesterol metabolites and promoting effect of lithocholic acid in colon carcinogenesis in germ-free and conventional F344 rats. *Cancer Research* **39**: 1521–1524.

Tuyns A J, Pequignot G & Abbatucci J S (1977) Le cancer de l'oesophage en Ille-et-Vilaine en fonction des niveaux de consommation d'alcohol et de tabac. Des risques qui se multiplinet. *Bulletin de Cancer* **64**: 45–60.

Walker A (1985) Cancer patterns in inter-ethnic South African populations. In Kritchevsky D and Vahouny G (eds) *Dietary Fiber in Health and Disease*. New York: Plenum.

Wattenberg, L (1980) Inhibitors of chemical carcinogens. *Journal of Environmental Pathology and Toxicology* **3**: 35–52.

Wilpart M, Mainguet O, Maskens & Roberfroid M (1984) Structure–activity relationships among biliary acids showing co-mutagenic activity towards 1,2-demethylhydrazine. *Carcinogenesis* **5**: 1239–1241.

Wynder E L & Bross I J (1961) A study of the etiological factors in cancer of the oesophagus. *Cancer* **14**: 389–413.

Zaridze D G (1981) Diet and cancer of the large bowel. *Nutrition and Cancer* **2**: 241–249.

Chapter 12
Cow's Milk Intolerance and Other Related Problems in Infancy

J. A. Walker-Smith

A number of foods have now been associated with gastro-intestinal problems in childhood, particularly in early infancy. Cow's milk is the food most often associated with these problems which are typically temporary disorders of early infancy, apart from coeliac disease which is a state of permanent intolerance to gluten and is not discussed here.

The syndromes of food intolerance may be grouped into those disorders where intolerance is chiefly due to an enzyme deficiency, e.g. secondary lactase deficiency, and those where an allergic mechanism is believed to be involved, e.g. cow's milk protein intolerance. The former are largely syndromes of carbohydrate intolerance and the latter protein intolerance, although often an infant may be both protein- and carbohydrate-intolerant, e.g. cow's milk protein sensitive enteropathy with secondary lactase deficiency (Walker-Smith 1982). Either way, cow's milk intolerance producing acute or chronic diarrhoea is the most important food intolerance problem in infancy.

In this chapter, disorders causing carbohydrate intolerance will be reviewed first, followed by those associated with protein intolerance.

CARBOHYDRATE INTOLERANCE

Carbohydrate intolerance, occurring in infants and children, is characterised by diarrhoea and/or vomiting and failure to thrive. Such intolerance may result from a congenital defect, for example glucose–galactose malabsorption, or it may be a secondary phenomenon whereby temporary damage to the mucosa of the small intestine leads to carbohydrate malabsorption, as occurs in acute rotavirus enteritis.

There are two major syndromes of carbohydrate intolerance in childhood: monosaccharide intolerance and disaccharide intolerance.

Monosaccharide intolerance

In infancy, the simplest clinical way to make the diagnosis of monosaccharide intolerance is to demonstrate the presence of excess amounts of reducing substances (i.e. $1-5\%$) in the typically watery stools while the child is having a feed known to contain only monosaccharide, for example a glucose–electrolyte solution. The importance of collection of the watery portion of the stool cannot be overstressed. If there is doubt about which feed may be responsible for the child's continuing diarrhoea, stool chromatography will identify the sugar present and so the likely cause of the carbohydrate intolerance. More recently, the breath hydrogen test has been used for diagnosis of monosaccharide as well as disaccharide intolerance. This test may be used to measure fermentation of carbohydrate reaching the colon by estimating peak breath hydrogen levels. About 5% of children have an enteric flora incapable of producing hydrogen and therefore may produce a falsely negative response to the test. There is no clear evidence that the hydrogen breath test offers any diagnostic advantage over testing properly collected stools for reducing substances.

The second aspect of the diagnosis is the clinical response to the removal of monosaccharide from the diet, with relief of diarrhoea. When this does not occur it means that other mechanisms are contributing to the diarrhoea.

An example of temporary monosaccharide intolerance is indicated in Figure 12.1.

Congenital glucose–galactose malabsorption

Congenital glucose–galactose malabsorption is a rare, genetically determined disorder. It is inherited as an autosomal recessive trait. The absorptive defect is confined to the two structurally similar hexoses, glucose and galactose. The active sodium-coupled co-transport system for these two monosaccharides is either absent or does not function. Fructose is absorbed normally.

Gastro-intestinal symptoms are profuse watery diarrhoea, abdominal distension and abdominal pain, following the ingestion of most sugar solutions or milk in the neonatal period. Mild renal glycosuria is often present. Elimination of foods containing glucose and/or galactose from the diet may be life-saving. Severe dehydration, neurological complications, and even death, have occurred in young infants with this disorder. Although severe symtoms usually lead to a diagnosis during the early months of life, some patients are sufficiently mildly affected to escape diagnosis until they reach adult life.

The diagnostic criteria for congenital glucose–galactose malabsorption include the following: watery diarrhoea which is present from soon after birth; clinical improvement on withdrawal of dietary glucose and galactose; relapse on reintroduction of glucose or galactose to the child; morphologically normal small intestinal mucosa with normal disaccharidase activities and an absorptive defect confined to glucose and galactose which is permanent.

Apart from correction of water and electrolyte deficits during the acute phase, management consists of elimination of glucose- and galactose-containing foods from the diet. Fructose is used as a substitute for glucose and sucrose. During the first year of life, a fructose-containing, modified milk is used. Galactomin 19 is available in Britain. It is essential for the child's adequate growth and health that, when such a markedly modified milk is used, the diet is assessed to ensure adequate vitamins, minerals and trace elements. These normally require supplementation.

Secondary monosaccharide intolerance

A temporary defect of monosaccharide absorption was first described in a group of newborn infants following surgery to their gastro-intestinal tracts,

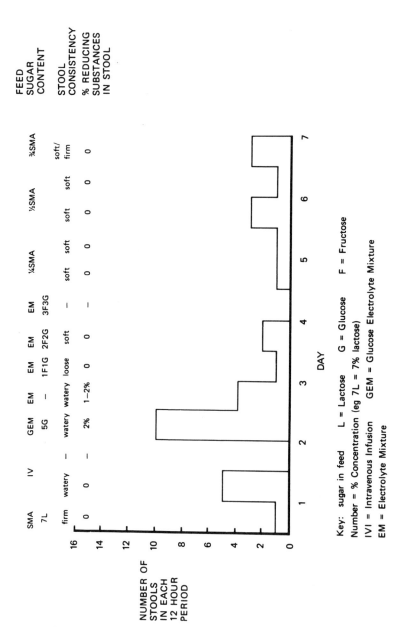

Figure 12.1. Example of stool findings related to dietary intake in an infant with temporary monosaccharide intolerance.

but it is also seen in infants who are temporarily unable to absorb any monosaccharide after an enteritis (Burke and Anderson 1966; Burke and Danks 1966). Thus it is clear that extensive damage to the small intestinal epithelium can impair glucose and galactose transport. It has also been suggested that bacterial overgrowth can in some way contribute to monosaccharide malabsorption.

Intolerance to monosaccharide may be brief and of little consequence when associated with an enteritis, e.g. rotavirus infection. However, a longer lasting syndrome may occur in a variety of circumstances including: severe chronic malnutrition: surgery of the gut in the neonatal period; after severe enteritis, often with severe mucosal damage in the small intestine.

The main symptom is severe watery diarrhoea. It may present immediately after an acute attack of gastro-enteritis or its onset may be delayed, presenting as an apparent sequel to disaccharide intolerance in an infant given a lactose-free, monosaccharide-containing feed. In some cases, this problem may be part of the intractable or protracted diarrhoea syndrome. Excoriation of the buttocks is usually a problem, probably because of the high organic acid content of the stools.

Management will depend upon the clinical severity and duration of the problem, in particular upon the degree of dehydration. If dehydration is significant, intravenous fluids will be required to correct water and electrolyte disturbances. Then management proceeds, as for those who are not dehydrated, to a period of carbohydrate restriction followed by the gradual reintroduction of carbohydrate. In practice a carbohydrate-free oral solution or formula may be given for a short period after which small amounts of carbohydrate are added, usually as increasing increments of 1% glucose and 1% fructose daily until a level of 5% carbohydrate is reached. At this stage, these infants must be observed carefully for signs of hypoglycaemia as they are often of low weight or severely malnourished. If signs of intolerance reappear (i.e. return of diarrhoea and vomiting) increments of carbohydrate cease for a time, but in most cases may be restored again within a day or two. However, when such intolerance lasts for more than a few days special formulae, such as the fructose free formula Galactomin 19, or a comminuted chicken based formula with added fructose, can be used. For more severe cases, oral feeding may not be possible for a time and parenteral nutrition is indicated. The child may then be graded back onto carbohydrate in the manner outlined above.

Disaccharide intolerance

Sucrase–isomaltase deficiency

Sucrase–isomaltase deficiency is an inherited enzyme deficiency of the small intestinal mucosa; it is an autosomal recessive characteristic (Weijers et al 1965). The exact incidence of this condition in Western countries is unknown; a high incidence has been observed in the Eskimo population of Greenland where sucrase–isomaltase deficiency has been reported in 10% of the population.

Symptoms will not appear until solids that contain sucrose are introduced into the child's diet, at about three months of age. The severity of symptoms will depend upon the amount of sucrose added to the infant's diet. Severe watery diarrhoea may occur in these infants and is usually associated with poor weight gain. In the older child and adults the symptoms may be much less severe. The condition may present with intermittent watery diarrhoea and sometimes with incontinence; there may be intermittent abdominal distension and cramping abdominal pain in the older child. Abdominal distension and excoriation of the buttocks are common.

Diagnosis is based upon the demonstration of a flat sucrose tolerance curve, coupled with the development of diarrhoea after an oral load of sucrose, and an enzyme assay which demonstrates the characteristic sucrase–isomaltase deficiency in the small intestinal mucosa, which is morphologically normal. An abnormal breath hydrogen test is a useful screen for this disorder, but diagnosis must be established by enzyme assay.

Children with this deficiency will respond clinically within 24 hours to a sucrose-free diet. There is no need to limit intake of starch because of the small percentage of 1→6 linkages in the amylopectin of starch. The need for dietary restriction appears to be permanent. Although it has been claimed that, with time, increasing tolerance to sucrose may occur, this apparent increasing tolerance is due to the patient's unconscious restriction of sucrose intake, even though he usually imagines he is still having a normal diet.

Congenital alactasia

This rare primary congenital syndrome, the very existence of which has been queried, is characterised by diarrhoea from a few days after birth (Launiala et al 1966; Levin et al 1970). Mucosal disaccharidase activities have actually been measured in only a few children with this disorder. In these, lactase activity has not always been completely absent, i.e. there is hypolactasia rather than complete alactasia. Congenital alactasia appears to be recessively inherited.

The disorder may easily be confused with secondary lactase deficiency which is a far commoner condition; some of the earlier reports of congenital alactasia may have confused this secondary type of lactase deficiency with primary alactasia. In primary alactasia the mucosa is morphologically normal and there is a specific depression of lactase activity, whereas in secondary lactase deficiency the mucosa is abnormal and the other disaccharides also have reduced activity. True congenital alactasia, unlike secondary alactasia, is a permanent disorder.

Secondary disaccharide intolerance

Disaccharide intolerance may occur as a transient phenomenon in a wide variety of diseases of the small intestine in childhood (Table 12.1). Very premature infants tend to have lactase deficiency because lactase is the last enzyme to attain mature levels during fetal development. Therefore, lactose intolerance complicates enteritis more frequently in premature newborn infants than in full-term babies.

Table 12.1. Causes of secondary lactose intolerance.

Infective enteritis, e.g. rotavirus infection
Coeliac disease
Giardiasis
Protein-calorie malnutrition
Neonatal surgery
Cow's milk protein intolerance
Immunodeficiency syndromes
Massive resection of small intestine

The pathogenesis of this syndrome is believed to be based on a temporary deficiency, chiefly of lactase, but sometimes of sucrase, both deficiencies being secondary to mucosal damage. A lack of correlation between mucosal damage as assessed by light microscopy and disaccharidase levels has been described.

Secondary disaccharide intolerance should be suspected whenever diarrhoea, especially watery diarrhoea, develops following a change or increase in the proportion of carbohydrate in an infant's feed, or in association with one of the disorders listed in Table 12.1. Diagnosis is based upon the finding of excess reducing substances in a watery stool or an abnormal lactose hydrogen breath test, followed by a clinical improvement on a lactose-free diet.

Carbohydrate intolerance complicating gastro-enteritis

Most often gastro-enteritis is a short lived illness which responds to a brief period of therapy with oral glucose–electrolyte mixture and a relatively rapid graded return to the infant's normal cow's milk based feed. In some cases, however, there is a temporary intolerance to glucose which complicates the acute phase of the illness, i.e. a temporary monosaccharide intolerance, whilst in other cases diarrhoea returns as lactose is reintroduced. The incidence of these problems relate both to the aetiological agent causing the gastro-intestinal infection and to the carbohydrate and protein composition of the infant feed. Rotavirus is most often associated with carbohydrate intolerance. The use of glucose–electrolyte mixtures containing higher levels of glucose is more likely to be complicated by monosaccharide intolerance. Likewise, partly modified cow's milk feeds are more sensitising, and so more likely to produce post-enteritis cow's milk sensitive enteropathy which may be accompanied by secondary lactose intolerance, than modern adapted formulae (Walker-Smith 1982).

A prospective study of the incidence of monosaccharide intolerance and disaccharide intolerance occurring as a sequel to acute gastro-enteritis in infancy was undertaken in 200 children admitted to the Queen Elizabeth Hospital for Children, London (Trounce and Walker-Smith 1985). All were managed with a glucose–electrolyte solution (Dioralyte) regraded onto an adapted cow's milk formula (SMA): 31 children (15.5%) developed carbohydrate intolerance; 7.5% (15) of these were lactose intolerant, and 8% (16)

were glucose intolerant. Rotavirus was the most frequent cause of the gastro-enteritis; 51.7% of the children with carbohydrate intolerance had rotavirus compared with 27.1% of the group as a whole. Fifteen of 45 children with rotavirus (33%) developed carbohydrate intolerance; none of them were monosaccharide intolerant and six were disaccharide intolerant. Three children with lactose intolerance had the persistent condition and proved to have cow's milk sensitive enteropathy.

In all cases food intolerance was temporary. In the case of monosaccharide intolerance it was usually brief in duration and could be regarded almost as part of the natural history of the disease. Lactose intolerance was sometimes both more persistent and associated with cow's milk sensitive enteropathy.

Treatment is dietary with the temporary need of a lactose-free diet. Lactose-free formulae, as listed in Table 12.2 may be used.

Late-onset lactose intolerance

An isolated deficiency of lactase is common in adults; genetic aetiology has been suggested for this type of lactose malabsorption which may present in late childhood or adult life. It has been shown to be common in Africans, Greek Cypriots, Indians, Chinese, American Negroes, natives of New Guinea and Australian Aborigines; indeed Caucasians are one of the few racial groups to maintain lactase levels into adult life. This has been explained either on the basis of genetically determined decline in lactase activity, or as an acquired defect resulting from the lack of continued substrate challenge.

Table 12.2. Lactose-free milk formulae.

Special milk	Carbohydrate	Amount g per 100 ml
Nutramigen (Australia)	Glucose	5.8
	Starch	2.6
Nutramigen (UK and USA)	Sucrose	6.1
	Starch	2.7
Pro-Sobee	Sucrose	4.1
	Corn sugars	2.7
Velactin	Glucose	3.0
	Corn sugars	2.4
	Sucrose	0.3
	Soy starch	1.7
Galactomin 17	Glucose	1.25
	Maltose, dextrins and higher sugars	5.0
Galactomin 19	Fructose	7.3
Pregestimil	Glucose	6.3
	Starch	2.3
Isomil	Sucrose	3.1
	Corn sugars	3.7

Secondary damage to intestinal mucosa from enteritis, protein-calorie malnutrition or parasitism could contribute to the severity of such a defect, thus hastening the onset of a genetic tendency for lactase levels to fall. The demonstration of an abnormal lactose tolerance test, based on blood glucose levels, does not prove that milk intolerance is present or indicate the need for dietary restriction. Evidence of lactose malabsorption was found in 80% of a group of Ethiopian children based on lactose tolerance tests, yet milk consumption in normal quantities (250 ml) was tolerated in all these school children, including those who were shown to have 'flat' lactose tolerance test. Some initially had transient symptoms with the ingestion of milk but all were able subsequently to tolerate the milk without any symptoms. The practical importance of this 'racial' lactose intolerance may thus have been exaggerated in the past. Nonetheless, the older child of any race who has a history of watery diarrhoea with the passage of excess flatus and abdominal pain following milk ingestion should be investigated for possible lactose intolerance. The diagnosis is established either by means of a lactose tolerance test, combining studies of blood glucose rise with observations of the stools for the onset of diarrhoea and the presence of excess reducing substances, or by hydrogen breath test. Treatment is then simple and highly effective.

Glucose polymer intolerance

Occasionally an infant may be briefly intolerant to glucose polymer given as Caloreen or in a formula such as Pregestimil (Meadows et al 1985).

PROTEIN

Food protein intolerance is most often due to gastro-intestinal food allergy. Gastro-intestinal food allergic diseases may be defined as those clinical syndromes following food ingestion, where the underlying mechanism is an immunologically mediated reaction within the gastro-intestinal tract. These symptoms may be accompanied by other manifestations outside the alimentary tract, such as in the skin or the respiratory tract.

Clinical syndromes

The range of adverse reactions to foods is wide, from an acute anaphylactic reaction, even leading to death, to relatively minor symptoms which are difficult to distinguish from other disorders such as toddler's diarrhoea, or psychological disorders with gastro-intestinal symptoms.

Frequently more than one system is involved in an adverse reaction to a food and the reported patterns of clinical symptoms vary considerably from one author to another. Gastro-intestinal manifestations have been reported in the majority of children in most studies, and often gastro-intestinal symptoms were seen alone. The large variations between observers can probably be explained by the differences in criteria used to establish the diagnosis, the preselection bias of the investigators, the age of the patients, and the pattern of infant feeding, as well as the antigenicity of the milk feeds in a particular community.

The proteins of cow's milk and soy have been highlighted as the major causes of food allergic syndromes in infancy and early childhood, although wheat (in individuals in whom coeliac disease has been excluded), egg, rice, fish, chicken, and corn, as well as tomatoes, oranges, bananas and chocolates, have been reported as producing gastro-intestinal symptoms in some individuals (Bleumink 1974). The adverse responses to some of these foods have been much better documented than others as causes of gastro-intestinal food allergic disease. There is not always a consistent association between specified food and a particular symptom or complex of symptoms. While, in some individuals, a single food may cause an adverse response, in others there may be clinical intolerance to many foods. Furthermore, in any individual with cow's milk protein intolerance, the symptoms may change with increasing age. For example, a child who developed diarrhoea and lethargy in infancy might later develop abdominal pain and irritability, although eventually becoming completely tolerant to cow's milk.

The incidence of gastro-intestinal food allergic diseases is greatest in the first months and years of life and decreases with age. The natural history of gastro-intestinal food allergic disease is best documented for reactions to cow's milk, with most such children developing their adverse symptoms within the first three months of life. The reported age of onset ranges from one day to 15 months. The age at which these children were first exposed to cow's milk will, of course, influence this to some extent. Adverse symptoms to milk become less severe with increasing age, and most children have become fully tolerant to milk by two years of age. Adequate catch-up growth has usually occurred by this time, if there had been a period of growth failure. Verkasalo et al (1981) found that after clinical tolerance to cow's milk had developed, one-third of their patients had persistent minor symptoms which did not seem to be associated with milk intake. These symptoms included occasional abdominal pains, a tendency to have loose stools or constipation, eczema, and recurrent respiratory infections, particularly otitis media. It is not known whether or not these symptoms are related to an underlying gastro-intestinal food allergy.

Gastro-intestinal syndromes of food intolerance

The major adverse gastro-intestinal reactions to cow's milk are vomiting, diarrhoea, and abdominal pain. These symptoms are frequently seen in many childhood illnesses, such as generalised infections, gastro-enteritis, parasitic infestation, sugar malabsorption, and stress-related psychosomatic illnesses. Symptoms must therefore be accurately assessed in relation to milk ingestion, and careful guidelines used for the diagnostic differentiation of gastro-intestinal food allergic disease from other conditions.

Broadly, gastro-intestinal food reactions may be divided into those that are apparent within minutes or up to an hour after taking the food and those in which the onset is slower, taking several hours and even days to become manifest (Ford et al 1983). The former syndromes are usually easy to diagnose on historical grounds and levels of food–specific IgE antibodies are usually raised. By contrast, the slow onset reactions are often difficult to diagnose clinically and the currently available diagnostic investigations may be impractical for general use.

Rapid-onset reactions

Acute anaphylaxis is the most serious of the rapid-onset gastro-intestinal food reactions. Anaphylaxis results from a generalised, immediate, IgE mediated reaction, following the introduction of a sufficient amount of antigen into a previously sensitised individual, releasing histamine and other biologically active mediators from sensitised mast cells. It represents the most severe extreme of the clinical spectrum of gastro-intestinal food allergic disease (Goldman et al 1963; de Peyer and Walker-Smith 1979) and may even result in death (Finklestein, 1905). Acute vomiting with or without diarrhoea, frequently accompanied by involvement of other systems, is commonly the presenting feature of rapid onset gastro-intestinal reactions. These reactions occur within minutes to an hour of the food being ingested, with often only small amounts of food needed to precipitate such a reaction. These reactions may occur at the first exposure to the food, the child having been previously sensitised via the breast milk or in utero. Many foods may produce such reactions.

Some entirely breast-fed infants are extremely sensitive to cow's milk (Jacobssen and Lindberg 1978). Small amounts of cow's milk, given as a complement feed or in solids, may lead to a rapid onset of vomiting which will cease when cow's milk is completely withdrawn from the diet. Often such vomiting may be accompanied by the onset of eczema. In some infants the lips and tongue may swell immediately upon contact with cow's milk and this oedema is sometimes associated with urticaria and angio-oedema which may in fact be the major presenting clinical problem. Characteristically these children have increased levels of total serum IgE and elevated milk specific IgE antibodies (Ford et al 1983) which can be demonstrated by skin prick test and RAST responses. They also tend to have lower titres of IgG, IgA and IgM milk antibodies than do infants who develop cow's milk protein intolerance some months after they have been fed with cow's milk (Firer et al 1981).

Vomiting a few minutes to an hour after egg ingestion is seen in about a quarter of children with egg hypersensitivity. Diarrhoea, abdominal pain and nausea may also occur (Ford and Taylor 1982). However, skin and respiratory manifestations also frequently occur and are ususally a more important part of the clinical presentation than gastro-intestinal symptoms. Again, skin prick test and RAST responses to egg are usually positive.

Acute abdominal pain seems to be a particular feature of fish hypersensitivity (Nizami et al 1977), whilst peanuts often produce immediate reactions of the oral mucosa (Wraith et al 1979) as well as abdominal pain.

Some individuals have gastro-intestinal and other symptoms related to a wide variety of foods. Such patients characteristically have a number of quick onset symptoms such as vomiting, urticaria or wheezing upon exposure to many foods. They often have a personal and family history of atopy, with peripheral eosinophilia, elevated total serum IgE and positive RAST and skin tests to specific foods. Diets involving the elimination of a number of foods may be impractical or ineffective on their own. However, treatment with oral disodium cromoglycate may be highly effective in children already on an elimination diet, as has been shown in the group of children described by Syme (1979) and also in older patients reported by Wraith et al (1979) but the therapeutic dose is empirical at present (Kochoshis and Gryboski 1979). Curiously, if oral sodium cromoglycate alleviates the symptoms, then these may not relapse when the drug is subsequently discontinued. These patients need to be distinguished from those with eosinophilic gastro-enteritis.

Slow-onset reactions

Slow-onset reactions are much more difficult to diagnose because of the problem of associating symptoms with a food taken hours or even days before. However, in general, the pathology is more site-specific. The problem is usually one of confirming whether or not the observed gastro-intestinal pathology is caused by an adverse immunological response to a food. Here elimination of the suspected food or foods and their subsequent reintroduction into the diet as food challenge provides the basis for the diagnostic approach.

Transient food-sensitive enteropathies

Abnormalities of the mucosa of the small intestine have been reported in children suffering temporary intolerances to cow's milk protein, soy protein, gluten, eggs, chicken, ground-rice and fish. The evidence that the enteropathy is directed related to a particular food is based on biopsy studies combined with dietary challenge, as in coeliac disease. The enteropathy is not usually as severe as that seen in coeliac disease, although a flat mucosa occasionally occurs. These disorders usually resolve by the age of 18 months to two years.

Clinically the reaction to these, and other foods, may be rapid (i.e. within an hour) or slow, (hours to days after food ingestion). In some cases, acute anaphylactic reactions have occurred. In other cases children appear to develop food intolerance after an acute episode of gastro-enteritis. Few morphological studies have been performed on individuals showing rapid reactions.

It is thought that the underlying causes of these illnesses is a transient sensitisation of the child to dietary antigens. The precise mechanisms which cause the enteropathy are unclear, although the application of the Gell and Coombs (1963) classification of hypersensitivity reaction provides a basis for investigation. For the reactions to occur, the offending antigen must enter the mucosa in appropriate amounts to cause sensitisation. There are two hypotheses regarding this process: one suggests sensitisation caused by overstimulation of the immune system by excess antigen entry; the other a minimal entry of antigen which stimulates a reaginic response, because of failure of the normal suppression reclusion. It is possible that both hypotheses are correct. Post-enteritis food-sensitive enteropathies are thought to arise from excess antigen entry in susceptible individuals, following gut damage. Children reacting quickly are presumably responding to small amounts of antigen which, in the normal individual, cause no abnormality. From animal studies it is clear that, apart from some oedema, there is no obvious histological abnormality in the mucosa of the small intestine when a Type I reaction occurs. An hypothesis relating acute gastro-enteritis and cow's milk sensitive enteropathy is illustrated in Figure 12.2. It is known from the observations of Gruskay and Cook (1955) that excess antigen absorption (in their studies, egg albumin) occurs in infants with acute gastro-enteritis. Later studies have shown increased entry of small molecular weight sugars in acute gastro-enteritis (Ford et al 1984), and larger molecular weight protein in post-enteritis and food-sensitive enteropathies (Jackson et al 1983). Their observations indicate that damage to the mucosa of the the small intestine will result in a local increase in antigen entry. This excessive antigen entry may, in some susceptible individuals, be of pathogenetic importance.

It remains to be established whether mucosal damage due to food ingestion occurs in adults, other than after gluten ingestion in patients with coeliac disease.

Cow's milk protein intolerance

Cow's milk ingestion may cause a variety of extra-intestinal features in infancy, such as eczema and asthma. There are also a number of gastro-intestinal problems associated with cow's milk protein intolerance (Table 12.3). This account will be confined to those disorders where milk has caused

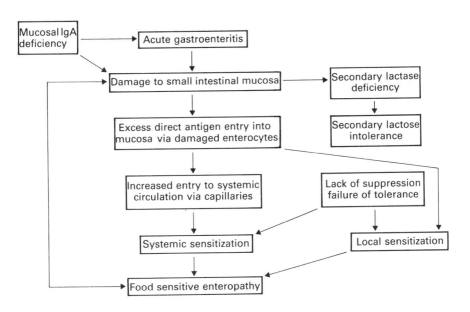

Figure 12.2. Hypothesis relating acute gastro-enteritis to cow's milk sensitive entero-pathy.

Table 12.3. Clinical manifestations attributed to cow's milk protein intolerance.

Gastrointestinal symptoms:	Syndromes:
Vomiting	Immediate onset of symptoms
Diarrhoea	Cow's milk sensitive enteropathy
Abdominal pain	Protein-losing enteropathy
Rectal bleeding	Cow's milk-induced colitis
(gross or occult)	

damage to the mucosa of the small intestine, i.e. cow's milk sensitive enteropathy or colonic mucosal damage and cow's milk induced colitis.

There appear to be two syndromes, a primary disorder of immunological origin and a secondary disorder, a consequence of mucosal damage which in turn produces an immunological abnormality. It seems probable that abnormal handling of dietary antigens across the intestinal mucosa occurs in infants with this disorder. This may be related to a temporary immunodeficiency state, such as transient IgA deficiency (Taylor et al 1973), or to non-specific mucosal damage from any cause. There is evidence that acute enteritis may be followed, not only by lactose intolerance but also by more persistent and longer lasting cow's milk protein intolerance (Harrison et al 1976).

Unlike coeliac disease, HLA status is normal in this disorder, suggesting that environmental factors are more important than genetic ones (Kuitunen et al 1975).

In the vast majority of patients with slow onset of symptoms after cow's milk ingestion, the architecture of the mucosa of the proximal small intestine is abnormal but the severity of the enteropathy is variable (Figure 12.3). In some early reports the mucosa was said to be flat and indistinguishable from that seen in coeliac disease (Kuitunen et al 1975). More recent reports from the same centre show that less severe mucosal damage has been characteristic. Typically the mucosa in untreated cow's milk sensitive enteropathy is thin (Maluenda et al 1984) and the pathological changes are patchy (Manuel et al 1979). The intra-epithelial lymphocytes are increased, although not to the levels found in untreated coeliac disease (Phillips et al 1979). There is also often a dense accumulation of fat in the epithelium which is a particular feature of this disorder and the post-enteritis syndrome (Variend et al, 1984) (Figure 12.4) The mucosa rapidly returns towards normal, or to near normal, on withdrawal of milk, only to relapse following challenge with milk (Walker-Smith et al 1978). However, unlike coeliac disease, the mucosa remains thin throughout (Maluenda et al 1984) and the intra-epithelial lymphocytes fall to levels below normal on a milk free diet, rising to levels within normal limits after cow's milk challenge (Phillips et al 1979).

Cow's milk protein intolerance may present as an acute syndrome with vomiting and diarrhoea, or as a chronic syndrome characterised by less severe vomiting and chronic diarrhoea with failure to thrive. The majority of cases present with acute symptoms under the age of six months. The clinical features may be indistinguishable from acute infective enteritis. Only electron

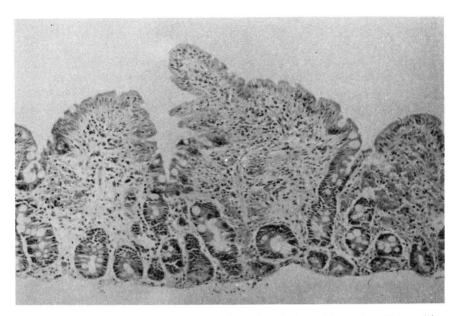

Figure 12.3. Biopsy from the small intestine of an infant with cow's milk sensitive enteropathy.

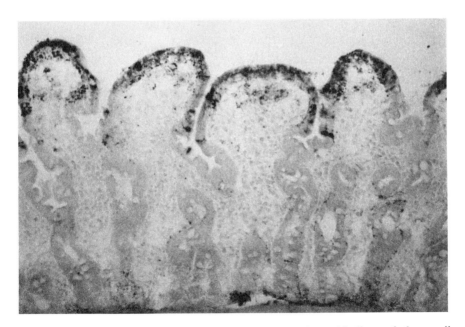

Figure 12.4. Scharlack R stain demonstrating fat in the epithelium of the small intestine of an infant with cow's milk enteropathy.

microscopy for viruses in the stool may enable a distinction to be made. Lactose intolerance may accompany protein intolerance, but it is relatively short lived.

There is usually a latent interval between the introduction of cow's milk to an infant's diet and the onset of symptoms. Occasionally violent reactions, such as anaphylactic shock, may immediately follow the infant's first contact with cow's milk. The chronic syndrome may present in a very similar fashion to coeliac disease, with loose stools and failure to thrive. Cow's milk protein intolerance may also be associated with iron deficiency anaemia, due to intestinal blood loss (either occult or overt). This is related to an associated colitis (Gryboski 1967; Jenkins et al 1984). Indeed, presentation as chronic bloody diarrhoea in infancy is an important clinical syndrome of cow's milk protein intolerance. Curiously, children with cow's milk colitis often have a normal small intestinal mucosa and those with a small intestinal enteropathy a normal colon. However, it is most important to remember that chronic inflammatory bowel disease can present in infancy in a similar way (Chong et al 1984).

The transient nature of cow's milk sensitive enteropathy may make it difficult to fulfil all the diagnostic criteria, as for coeliac disease; nevertheless accurate diagnosis is important. It is important to exclude an infective cause of the enteropathy. As with all dietary protein intolerances, diagnosis is based upon the response to withdrawal and reintroduction of the offending protein, there is no specific laboratory test, apart from serial biopsy related to elimination and challenge. The finding of a patchy enteropathy with a thin mucosa in an infant fed with cow's milk, who responds rapidly to a cow's milk elimination diet, provides firm presumptive evidence for this diagnosis. Such children may be described as having a 'milk elimination responsive entero-pathy'. The transient nature of this disorder, as well as the desire to avoid early milk challenge (because of the potential risk of acute anaphylaxis), leads in practice to a late milk challenge between the age of nine months and one year. These children may be milk intolerant no longer and challenge merely establishes that it is safe to introduce cow's milk in the diet. It does not confirm the diagnosis of cow's milk sensitive enteropathy. The initial biopsy is important to include other causes of the syndrome, such as giardiasis, but it is not essential to have serial biopsies to make a diagnosis.

Cow's milk colitis is diagnosed by means of endoscopy and biopsy. Typically there is an infiltration with eosinophils in the mucosa, i.e. an eosinophilic colitis.

Treatment involves substituting natural cow's milk feeds with commercially available cow's milk protein free formula feeds. Cow's milk substitutes fall into three categories, those based on: (i) casein hydrolysate, e.g. Pregestimil for infants under six months and Nutramigen for infants over six months (preferred options); (ii) soya protein, e.g. Cow and Gate formula S, Prosbee liquid, Prosbee powder, Wysoy; (iii) comminuted chicken, which requires supplements with the complete range of vitamins and minerals and may be required when the other formulae are not tolerated. Only those formulae which are nutritionally complete (if necessary with vitamin supplementation) are recommended. Those with a low osmolality should be chosen for young infants or infants with small bowel disease. It is important to ensure that both liquid and solid feeds are free of cow's milk proteins. Disaccharide intolerance may accompany the protein intolerance, and in such circumstances disaccharides should also be withdrawn from the diet. The necessity for dietary treatment is always temporary, and reintroduction of a normal diet is normally nearly always possible by the age of one to two years. This may be done at home, but a history of severe reactions, such as urticaria or anaphylactoid shock, is an absolute indication for reintroduction of a normal diet under very close medical supervision.

Soy protein intolerance

It has been shown that soy protein can induce enteropathy of the small intestine, which resolves with soy elimination and which reappears when soy protein is reintroduced into the diet (Ament and Rubin 1972). These workers described a flat mucosal lesion, indistinguishable from that found in coeliac disease, but more usually the damage is less severe and is similar to cow's milk sensitive enteropathy (Perkkio et al 1981). Kuitunen et al (1975) described the clinical findings in 54 children with cow's milk intolerance. Thirty-five of these children were given soya protein as a cow's milk substitute: four developed soya protein intolerance. The symptoms were vomiting, diarrhoea and weight loss; three had partial villous atrophy on biopsy and the fourth had a flat mucosa. The frequency of soy protein intolerance may well be increasing with the more widespread use of soy protein-based infant feeds.

Transient gluten intolerance

Firm evidence for a syndrome of transient gluten intolerance, based upon serial small intestinal biopsies related to dietary elimination and challenge, only been described in one patient (Walker-Smith and Phillips 1979). However, a number of children have been reinvestigated following a diagnosis of coeliac disease (based on the finding of a flat mucosa and a clinical response to a gluten-free diet), who have remained clinically well with a normal small intestinal mucosa for more than two years after the reintroduction of a gluten-containing diet. A clinical response to the initial withdrawal of dietary gluten cannot be regarded as proof of temporary gluten toxicity; this can only be established by early reinvestigation, with the demonstration of gluten toxicity and the finding that such toxicity disappears after a time interval. Such early reintroduction is not routine practice. Hence there is still controversy regarding this clinical entity. This emphasises the necessity to reinvestigate, by means of gluten challenge and intestinal biopsy, infants diagnosed as coeliac disease when under the age of two years, before recommending a life-long diet. The difficulties in diagnosing transient gluten intolerance relate to the varying time intervals between gluten challenge and relapse which may be more than two years. A scheme outlining an approach to the differential diagnosis of transient gluten intolerance is illustrated in Figure 12.5 (Walker-Smith et al 1984). Early introduction of gluten into the diet (more common in the early 1970s than the 1980s) is associated both with the development of transient gluten intolerance and the earlier onset of coeliac disease (Figure 12.6).

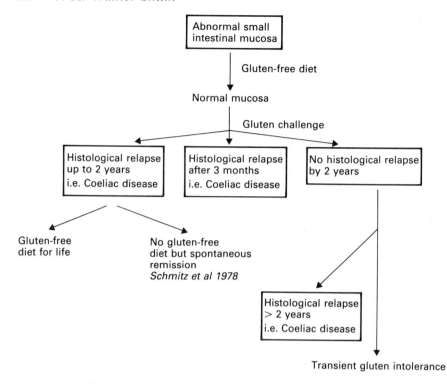

Figure 12.5. Scheme outlining approach to diagnosis of transient gluten intolerance.

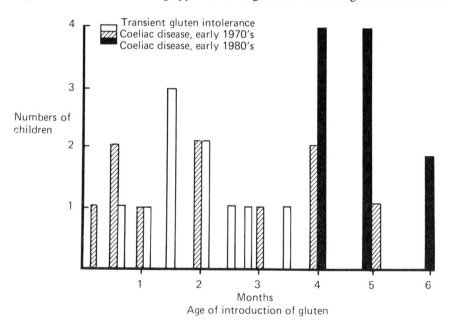

Figure 12.6. Age of introduction of gluten into the diet of the children with transient gluten intolerance, coeliac disease in early 1970s and coeliac disease in early 1980s.

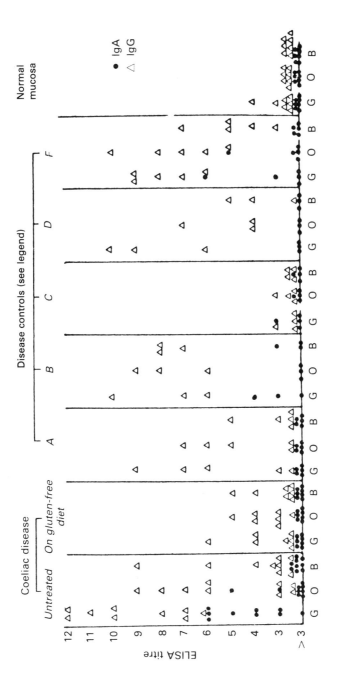

Figure 12.7.

ELIZA titres of serum antibodies to food in infants with coeliac disease: (A) transient gluten intolerance (B & C) cow's milk sensitive enteropathy untreated and treated; (D) multiple food protein intolerance; (F) Crohn's disease. On horizontal axis, then, G = gliadin, O = ovalbumin, B = beta-lactoglobulin. From Unsworth et al (1983) with kind permission of the authors and the editor of *Lancet*.

Other food-sensitive enteropathies

It has now been established, by means of serial biopsy and dietary elimination and challenge, that egg protein (Iyngkaran 1982), ground rice, chicken and fish (Vitoria et al 1982) may all temporarily damage the mucosa of the small intestine in infancy. In this latter study, all infants were also cow's milk intolerant and under the age of six months.

Food antibodies and food intolerance

Circulating food antibodies have been considered to be pathogenetically significant in children with temporary food intolerance syndromes. IgA and IgG or food antibodies have been examined in 70 children with syndromes of food intolerance, and compared with the antibodies found in children with coeliac disease and chronic inflammatory bowel disease. Elevated antibody levels were found particularly in untreated coeliac disease but were also found in children with food intolerance and chronic inflammatory bowel disease (Table 12.3 and Figure 12.7) (Unsworth et al 1983). Their role in pathogenesis of temporary food intolerance remains to be established.

CONCLUSION

Over the past decade a number of temporary syndromes of food intolerance in infancy have been well described. Much is still unknown of their pathogenesis, but temporary food elimination under dietetic supervision is usually highly effective therapy.

REFERENCES

Ament M E & Rubin C (1972) Soy protein — another cause of the flat intestinal lesion. *Gastroenterology* **62**: 277–234.
Bleumink E (1974) Allergies and toxic protein in food. In Hekkens W Th J M & Pena A S (eds) *Coeliac Disease*, pp. 46–55. Leyden: Kroese.
Burke V & Anderson C M (1966) Sugar intolerance as a cause of protracted diarrhoea following surgery of the gastrointestinal tract in neonates. *Australian Paediatric Journal* **2**: 219.
Burke V & Danks D M (1966). Monosaccharide malabsorption in young infants. *Lancet* **1**: 1177.
Chong S K F, Sanderson I R, Wright V & Walker-Smith J A (1984) Food allergy and infantile colitis. *Archives of Disease in Childhood* **59**: 691.
Peyer E de & Walker-Smith J A (1977) Cow's milk intolerance presenting as necrotizing enterocolitis. *Helvetica Paediatrica Acta* **32**: 509.
Finkelstein H (1905) Kuhmilch als ursache akuter Ernathrungstorungen bei Sauglingen. *Monatsschrif Kinderheilkunde* **4**: 65–72.
Firer M A, Hosking C S & Hill D J (1981) Effect of antigen load on development of milk antibodies in infants allergic to milk. *British Medical Journal* **283**: 693–696.
Ford R P K & Taylor B (1982) Natural history of egg hypersensitivity in childhood. *Archives of Disease in Childhood* **57**: 649–652.
Ford R P K, Hill D J & Hosking C S (1984) Cows milk hypersensitivity: immediate and delayed onset clinical patterns. *Archives of Disease in Childhood* **58**: 856–862.

Gell R G H & Coombs R R A (1963) Classification of allergic reactions. In Gell R G H & Coombs R R A (eds), *Clinical Aspects of Immunology*. Oxford: Blackwell Scientific Publications.

Goldman A S, Anderson D W, Sellers W et al (1963) Milk Allergy. *Pediatrics* 32: 425–443.

Gruskay F L & Cook R E (1955) The gastrointestinal absorption of unaltered protein in normal infants and in infants recovering from diarrhoea. *Pediatrics* 16: 763–767.

Gryboski J D (1967) Gastrointestinal milk allergy in infants. *Pediatrics* 40: 354–362.

Harrison M, Kilby A, Walker-Smith J A, France N E & Wood C B S (1976) Cow's milk protein intolerance: A possible association with gastroenteritis, lactose intolerance, and IgA deficiency. *British Medical Journal* 1: 1501–1504.

Iyngkaran N, Abidain Z, Meng L L & Yadav M (1982) Egg-protein-induced villous atrophy. *Journal of Pediatric Gastroenterology and Nutrition* 1: 29–35.

Jackson D, Walker-Smith J A & Phillips A D (1983) Macromolecular absorption by histologically normal and abnormal small intestinal mucosa in childhood: An in vitro study using organ culture. *Journal of Pediatric Gastroenterology and Nutrition* 2: 235–248.

Jacobsson I & Lindberg T (1978) Cow's milk as a cause of infantile colic in breast fed infants. *Lancet*: 2 437–439.

Jenkins H R, Milla P J, Pincott T R, Soothill J F & Harries J T (1984) Food allergy: the major cause of infantile colitis. *Pediatric Research:* 431 (Abstract).

Kochoshis S & Gryboski J D (1979) Use of cromolyn in combined gastrointestinal allergy. JAMA 242: 1169–1173.

Kuitunen P, Visakorpi J K & Hallman N (1965) Histopathology of duodenal mucosa in malabsorption syndrome induced by cow's milk. *Annales de Pediatrie* 205: 54–63.

Kuitunen P, Rapola J, Savilahti E & Visakorpi J K (1972) Light electron microscopic changes in the small intestinal mucosa in patients with cow's milk induced malabsorption syndrome. *Acta Paediatrica Scandinavica* 61: 237.

Kuitunen P, Visakorpi J K, Savilahti E & Pelkonen P (1975) Malabsorption syndrome with cow's milk intolerance clinical findings and course in 54 cases. *Archives of Disease in Childhood* 50: 351.

Launiala K, Kuitunen P & Visakorpi J K (1966) Disaccharidases and history of duodenal mucosa in congenital lactose malabsorption. *Acta Paediatrica Scandinavica* 55: 257.

Levin B, Abraham J M, Burgess E A & Wallis P G (1970) Congenital lactose malabsorption. *Archives of Disease in Childhood* 45: 173.

Maluenda C, Phillips A D, Briddon A & Walker-Smith J A (1984) Quantitative analysis of small intestinal mucosa in cow's milk sensitive enteropathy. *Journal of Pediatric Gastroenterology and Nutrition* 3: 349–356.

Manuel P D, Walker-Smith J A & France N E (1979) Patchy enteropathy. *Gut* 20: 211.

Meadows N J, Oberholzer V & Walker-Smith J A (1985) Glucose polymer intolerance in infants. *Journal of Pediatric Gastroenterology and Nutrition* (in press).

Nizami R M, Lewin P K & Baloo M T (1977) Oral cromolyn therapy in patients with food allergy: a preliminary report. *Annals of Allergy* 39: 102–105.

Perkkio M, Savilahti E & Kuitunen P (1981) Morphometric and immunochemical study of jejunal biopsies from children with intestinal soy allergy. *European Journal of Pediatrics* 137: 63–69.

Phillips A D, Rice S J, France N E & Walker-Smith J A (1979) Small intestinal lymphocyte levels in cow's milk protein intolerance. *Gut* 20: 509–512.

Schmitz J, Jos J & Rey J (1978) Transient mucosal atrophy in confirmed coeliac disease. In McCarthy and McNicholl (eds) *Perspectives in Coeliac Disease. Proceedings of Third International Coeliac Symposium, Galway*, p 259. Lancaster: MTP Press.

Syme J (1979) Investigation and treatment of multiple intestinal food allergy in childhood. In Pepys J & Edwards A M (eds) *The Mast Cell: Its Role in Health and Disease*, pp 438–442. Tunbridge Wells: Pitman Medical.

Taylor B, Norman A P, Orgel H A et al (1973) Transient IgA deficiency and pathogenesis of infantile atopy. *Lancet*: 22: 111.

Trounce J Q & Walker-Smith J A (1985) A prospective study of the incidence of aetiological associations and managements of sugar intolerance complicating acute gastroenteritis. *Archives of Disease in Childhood* (in press).

Unsworth J, Walker-Smith J A & Holborow E J (1983) Gliadin and reticulin antibodies in childhood coeliac disease. *Lancet* 2: 874–875.

Variend S, Placzek M, Raafat F & Walker-Smith J A (1984) Small intestinal mucosal fat in childhood enteropathies. *Journal of Clinical Pathology* 37: 373–377.

Verkasalo M, Kuitunen P, Savilahti E & Tilikainen A (1981) Changing pattern of cow's milk intolerance. An analysis of the occurence and clinical course in the 60's and mid-70's. *Acta Paediatrica Scandinavica* 70 (3): 289–295.

Vitoria J C, Camarero C, Sojo A, Ruiz A & Rodriguez-Soriano J (1982) Enteropathy related to fish, rice and chicken. *Archives of Disease in Childhood* **57**: 44–48.

Walker-Smith J A (1982) Cow's milk intolerance as a cause of post-enteritis diarrhoea. *Journal of Pediatric Gastroenterology and Nutrition* **1**: 163–175.

Walker-Smith J A & Phillips A D (1979) The pathology of gastrointestinal allergy. In Pepys J and Edwards A M (eds) *The Mast Cell: Its Role in Health and Disease*, pp 31–39. Tunbridge Wells: Pitman Medical.

Walker-Smith J A, Harrison M, Kilby A, Phillips A D & France N E (1978) Cow's milk sensitive enteropathy. *Archives of Disease in Childhood* **53**: 375–380.

Walker-Smith J A, Phillips A D, Rossiter M & Wharton B E (1984) Transient gluten intolerance. *Gut* **25**: A1191.

Weijers H A, Van de Kamer J H, Dicke W K & Ijsseling J (1961) Diarrhoea caused by deficiency of sugar splitting enzymes. 1. *Acta Paediatrica Scandinavica,* **50**: 55.

Wraith D G, Young G V W & Lee T H (1979) The management of food allergy with diet and Nalcrom. In Pepys J and Edwards A M (eds) *The Mast Cell: Its Role in Health and Disease*, pp 443–446. Tunbridge Wells: Pitman Medical.

Chapter 13
Mechanisms of Gluten Toxicity in Coeliac Disease

Alice Bullen

In 1888, Samuel Gee gave a remarkably accurate clinical description of the disease which is today recognised as coeliac disease and suggested that 'To regulate the food is the main part of treatment.'

Following the crucial observations made by Dicke (1950), it was realised that the part of the diet which causes damage in coeliac disease is the gluten component of wheat flour. Soon afterwards, the essential morphological features of the small intestinal mucosa in coeliac disease were recognised (Paulley 1954) and the introduction of peroral biopsy (Shiner 1956) enabled these features to be readily detected. Thus, coeliac patients can now generally be offered an accurate diagnosis, and effective treatment by strict adherence to a gluten-free diet.

Over the last thirty years, much interest and research has been stimulated by the discoveries made in the 1950s, but the mechanism whereby gluten exerts its toxic effect is still not understood. Increased understanding might lead to improvements in the methods of prevention, diagnosis or treatment of the condition. In addition to this incentive to research, coeliac disease is a fascinating and still mysterious illness. What is special about gluten, out of the many substances which humans eat, that it can so relatively commonly cause the mucosal lesion of coeliac disease? And what is special about coeliac patients, that they develop a mucosal lesion, when most humans do not? Partial answers to some aspects of these questions have been provided, while other aspects remain largely unexplained. The evidence which has so far been accumulated has led to the development of several theories about the mechanism of gluten toxicity in coeliac disease.

THEORIES CONCERNING THE MECHANISM OF GLUTEN TOXICITY

The theories put forward to explain the toxic effect of gluten in coeliac disease fall into two main groups. The first group postulates that coeliac disease occurs because there is a primary abnormality of the epithelium. This may be either an increase or decrease of the activity of a mucosal enzyme, which causes the accumulation of a product of gluten degradation which is toxic to the cell (*enzyme theory*). Alternatively, there may be abnormal glycoproteins on the enterocyte membrane, to which gluten or a gluten product binds because of its lectin properties, and thereby initiates cell damage (*lectin theory*). A third possibility is that the epithelial layer is more permeable than normal and thus increased entry of a gluten product into or between the enterocytes occurs, causing direct cell damage or initating damage by a secondary mechanism (*permeability theory*).

The second group of theories relates to various postulated primary abnormalities of immune response to gluten in coeliac disease (*immunologic-al theory*). According to these theories, antigenic gluten products initially enter the mucosa in a similar way in both coeliac patients and normal subjects, but in the coeliac patients an exaggerated immune response is triggered which causes secondary mucosal damage.

These theories of the mechanism of gluten toxicity are not necessarily mutually exclusive. For example, it is possible that an abnormality of mucosal resistance to gluten needs to be combined with an abnormal immune response in order to produce and perpetuate mucosal damage.

In this chapter, information relating to the mechanism of gluten toxicity will be reviewed in relation to the theories outlined above. However, it is appropriate to consider first some gaps in knowledge and difficulties of interpretation of results which affect several types of investigation of the primary abnormality in coeliac disease.

Some problems in investigating mechanisms of gluten toxicity

In order to define the mechanism of gluten toxicity in coeliac disease, it is necessary to understand the nature of the essential difference between coeliac patients and subjects without coeliac disease. Before the introduction of gluten into the diet, a potential coeliac has a presumably normal small intestinal mucosa, apart from the latent 'essential difference'. At some point after gluten feeding starts, the combination of gluten and the 'essential difference' must trigger a series of events causing mucosal damage.

Unfortunately the conditions operating before and during the introduction of gluten, and during the development of the mucosal lesion (events which may not coincide) (Egan-Mitchell et al 1981; Doherty and Barry 1981; Rolles et al 1981), are difficult to study because the diagnosis of coeliac disease is made on the basis of a mucosal lesion having already occurred. In the presence of a mucosal lesion, it may be uncertain whether an observed abnormality is of primary importance in pathogenesis, or merely secondary to the mucosal damage. Even when treated patients are studied, there remains the possibility of subtle persisting damage, particularly in adults, and the extent to which this difficulty can be overcome by studying only those patients with completely normal histological appearances of the mucosa is speculative. Certainly anything less than this leads to problems of interpretation of abnormal findings.

In such well-treated patients, there is the further difficulty that differences from controls might relate to the fact that the coeliacs are taking a strict gluten-free diet, whereas controls are generally on diets containing gluten. For example, differences in the mucosal digestive capacity for gluten (Cornell and Rolles 1978) or cell surface glycoconjugates (Weiser and Douglas 1978; Vasmant et al 1982) might be partly caused by dietary differences between treated coeliacs, coeliac relatives and healthy controls. In animals, intestinal enzyme adaptation to diets of different composition has been shown to occur

(McCarthy et al 1980; Biol et al, 1981, 1984; Goda et al 1983) and it is possible that a mucosa which has not recently encountered gluten may handle it less efficiently, simply because the normal mechanisms for its metabolism have not been stimulated recently. In addition, a gluten-free diet is usually different from the normal diet in ways other than gluten restriction; for example, fibre content is often different (Barry et al 1978). Experimental evidence suggests that the fibre or lectin content of the diet may normally affect mucosal cell proliferation or brush border turnover (Ecknauer et al 1981; Lorenzsonn and Olsen 1982; Fairweather-Tait et al 1983), but observations of the response of the normal human small intestine to diets of different gluten content are relatively scanty (Rubin et al 1962; Levine et al 1966; Weinstein 1974; Doherty and Barry 1981). Indeed, the way in which wheat flour and gluten are degraded, bound, absorbed and metabolised in normal subjects, let alone coeliac patients, is poorly understood (Anderson et al 1981; Peters and Bjarnason 1984). In studies attempting to define a primary abnormality in treated coeliac patients, some of these uncertainties could probably be eliminated by the inclusion of control subjects on a strict gluten-free diet, but again, this is difficult to arrange.

Further difficulties occur because of the differing genetic backgrounds of coeliac patients and unselected controls. Since the possession of certain genetic markers is associated with differences in some aspects of cell function, patients and non-coeliac controls should ideally be matched for genetic status in order to be satisfied that an observed difference between the two groups is related to the coeliac disease itself rather than to genetic disparity.

The above considerations should be kept in mind when evaluating evidence which suggests that an observed abnormality is of primary importance in the pathogenesis of coeliac disease. Not surprisingly, many studies have not taken these factors into account, and it is difficult to know how important this is.

An alternative method of investigation, by attempting to identify 'potential coeliacs' among genetically predisposed relatives of coeliac patients, and looking for abnormalities in these subjects, might be feasible. If an abnormality could be identified before mucosal damage developed, such evidence might be a very useful pointer to a primary mechanism, but the 'potential coeliacs' would have to be followed for a long time to determine whether environmental stresses ultimately caused any of them to develop coeliac disease. Alternatively, challenge with a high gluten diet might be suggested (Doherty & Barry 1981; Strober 1981) but there are ethical problems associated with investigations of coeliac relatives (Shmerling et al 1981).

FACTORS INFLUENCING THE DEVELOPMENT OF COELIAC DISEASE

Any explanation of the mechanism of gluten toxicity in coeliac disease must take into account the factors in the host and in the environment, which are thought to influence the development of the disease. Host factors include genetic make-up and IgA deficiency. Environmental factors include the dose and quality of gluten and the effect of transient mucosal inflammation and infant feeding.

Host factors

Genetic factors in the development of coeliac disease

Coeliac disease is familial, with an incidence in first degree relatives of coeliac patients of 5–19% reported in different studies (Stokes et al 1973, 1976; Rolles et al 1974).

HLA-B8. Further evidence of a genetic factor has been shown by the association of coeliac disease and the histocompatibility antigen HLA-B8, first reported in 1972 and confirmed many times since (Falchuk et al 1972; Stokes et al 1972). Approximately 80% of coeliacs are positive for HLA-B8, compared with approximately 25% of control subjects. However, the mechanism by which this genetic factor influences the development of the disease is not known. One possibility is that there is a linkage between an immune response gene for gluten and the HLA-B8 gene.

Immune response genes, which modulate humoral and cellular immune responses to specific antigens, have been described in several species and are commonly linked to genes of the major histocompatibility systems (Benacerraf and McDevitt 1972; Balner 1976). HLA status has been shown to affect the immune response to several antigens in man and HLA-B8 is associated with a range of diseases in which abnormalities of immune function are thought to be important, including insulin-dependent diabetes mellitus, thyrotoxicosis, myasthenia gravis, Addison's disease and hepatitis B negative chronic active hepatitis (Dausset et al 1974; Vladutiu and Rose 1974; Svejgaard et al 1975; Galbraith et al 1976). Patients with HLA-B8 also have increased survival after development of neoplasia (Osoba and Falk 1978). These associations suggest that the possession of HLA-B8 confers a general increase in immune responsiveness.

Supporting evidence includes the finding that HLA-B8 is associated, in healthy subjects, with an increased mixed leucocyte reaction (Osoba and Falk 1978), strong responses to flagellin immunisation and skin test antigens (Morris 1973) and decreased suppressor activity of blood mononuclear cells (Robertson et al 1982).

With respect to HLA status and immunity to gluten, it has been shown that HLA-B8 positive individuals, with a variety of conditions, have higher titres of serum gluten antibody than HLA-B8 negative individuals (Scott et al 1974). HLA-B8 is also associated, in healthy subjects, with increased lymphocyte transformation (Cunningham-Rundles et al 1978a) and increased leucocyte migration inhibition (Simpson et al 1981) in the presence of gluten. These findings are compatible with the suggestion that there is an immune response gene for gluten in linkage disequilibrium with HLA-B8. The presence of the postulated immune response gene may be necessary but not sufficient for the development of coeliac disease. It has been suggested that HLA-B8 itself may directly contribute to the mechanism of gluten toxicity, perhaps by providing a binding site for gluten on the enterocyte membrane, since Falchuk et al (1980) found that the damaging effect of gluten on coeliac mucosa in tissue culture was related to the presence of HLA-B8. This has not been confirmed by others (Howdle et al 1981; Arnaud-Battandier et al 1983).

The suggestion that altered immune responses are of fundamental importance in the pathogenesis of the disease remains speculative. Since there are known to be alterations in various tests of immunity in non-coeliacs with HLA-B8, adequate matching of controls or analysis of results taking genetic markers into account is necessary.

The HLA antigens are coded at loci on the sixth chromosome (Woodrow 1981) and individual HLA specificities are inherited as co-dominant alleles. Loci A, B and C are defined by serological methods. The products of the A, B and C genes are attached to nucleated cell membranes as single glycosylated polypeptide chains. The cell membrane antigens determined by D locus alleles are demonstrated by mixed lymphocyte culture. Closely associated with (and possibly identical to) the D locus is the DR locus, whose gene products are present on B lymphocytes and macrophages, induce strong allo-antibody production and are identified by serological methods. B cell antigens are thought to be analogous to the murine Ia (immune response associated) antigens, which are important in determining the type and magnitude of immune responses in the mouse.

HLA-D/DR3. It has been found that there is a stronger association between HLA-D3 and coeliac disease than HLA-B8 and coeliac disease (Keuning et al 1976). There is a similar strong association between the B cell allo-antigen DR3 and coeliac disease (Ek et al 1978; McKenna et al 1981) and also an association with DR7 in some populations (Scholz et al 1981). In the west of Ireland, 88% of coeliacs were found to possess DR3, compared with 44% of controls; for HLA-B8 the incidence was 81% and 45% respectively (McKenna et al 1981). The complexity of proposed hereditary factors has increased with increasing knowledge (Mearin et al 1983; De Marchi et al 1983).

It is not known whether HLA-D/DR antigens are directly involved in the development of coeliac disease, but it has been shown that HLA-DR-like antigens are present in the epithelial cells of normal and coeliac mucosa (Scott et al 1981). HLA-D/DR antigens are thought to be important in antigen presentation and the induction of T cell responses, and in interactions between T and B cells. Evidence is accumulating for a close association between the intestinal immune system and epithelial cell function and growth (Castro 1982; Kay and Ferguson 1984; Walker 1984). In rats, it has been shown that intra-epithelial lymphocytes may modulate the expression of Ia antigens on epithelial cells (Cerf-Bensussan et al 1984). In coeliac disease, transport of exogenous antigens in association with HLA-DR determinants might affect local T cell responses (Scott et al 1983c).

HLA-DC3. Recently, by using monoclonal antibodies, another locus, DC (recently renamed 'DQ' by the WHO Nomenclature Committee), closely linked to DR, has been found to have an allelic specificity, DC3, in strong linkage disequilibrium with DR3 and DR7 (Tosi et al 1983). There is evidence that DC3 is the HLA specificity most closely associated with coeliac disease, in that $DR3^+ DC3^+$ and $DR7^+ DC3^+$ haplotypes were associated with coeliac disease, whereas $DR3^+ DC3^-$ and $DR7^+ DC3^-$ were not. In the group studied by Tosi et al, the one $DR3^- DR7^-$ coeliac patient was $DC3^+$. There is a suggestion that DC locus alleles may control the induction of cytotoxic T cells; such a mechanism could be involved in the pathogenesis of coeliac disease.

Although immunologists and geneticists appear to be getting closer and closer to the HLA locus specificity primarily associated wtih coeliac disease, it is apparent from family studies that the inheritance of coeliac disease is difficult to explain on the basis of a single major gene. Multifactorial modes of inheritance and a two locus model have been proposed (Greenberg and Rotter 1981).

Gluten sensitive enteropathy-associated B cell antigen. In 1976, Mann et al reported the detection of another antigen associated with coeliac disease, the 'GSE-associated B cell antigen', identified with antisera obtained from D3 positive mothers of coeliac patients. The cell surface antigen reacting with the maternal antisera was found only on B cells and not T cells. Data obtained from family studies (Pena et al 1978) suggested that the HLA locus antigens and GSE-associated B cell antigen were inherited separately. The presence of GSE-associated B cell antigen was detected in 13 out of 18 (72%) unrelated coeliac patients and three out of 13 (18%) control subjects. Pena et al concluded that at least two genes are necessary for the development of coeliac disease.

The finding of GSE-associated B cell antigens led to the speculation (Strober 1978) that this gene codes for a binding site on B cells. The antigen was present on too large a proportion of B cells to be present solely on cells producing gluten antibody. The presence of such a receptor might ensure a disproportionately strong immune response to gluten protein.

Further evidence to support the existence of a surface receptor for gliadin on B lymphocytes has been provided (Verkasalo 1982). Adherence of gliadin did not appear to be related to HLA status. However, Stern and Dietrich (1982) demonstrated that some immunoglobulin-containing cells of the lamina propria in coeliac children also contained gliadin, but found no evidence to support the existence of a local gliadin receptor, either on enterocyte or lymphocyte membranes.

Immunoglobulin heavy chain markers. In the past five years, several immunologically mediated diseases have been found to be associated with a combination of HLA genes and other unrelated genetic markers (Welsh 1981; Bodmer and Bodmer 1984). Kagnoff (1982) showed that two separate genetic loci control the murine antibody response to gliadin, one locus in the major histocompatibility complex, and the other at the immunoglobulin heavy chain allotype locus. Subsequently, immunoglobulin G heavy-chain (Gm) markers located on chromosome 14 have been found to be associated with coeliac disease and the immune response to gliadin (Carbonara et al 1983; Kagnoff et al 1983; Weiss et al, 1983). Out of 30 coeliac patients, five lacking HLA-B8 and DR3 had the Gm phenotype (f; n; b). Thus both HLA and immunoglobulin heavy-chain linked genes appear to determine susceptibility to coeliac disease. Among 30 unrelated coeliac patients, 83% were positive for DR3 and 80% were positive for G2m(n). None of the patients had neither marker. Of unrelated healthy controls, 61% were positive for G2m(n). Carbonara et al (1983) have suggested that Gm markers and gender influence the risk of development of coeliac disease in those with susceptible HLA-DR genotypes. Among coeliacs on a gluten-free diet, persistently raised IgG antigliadin antibody was found only in those having the G2m(n) marker. Antigliadin antibody could mediate mucosal damage by Type II or Type III reactions in the mucosa, and thus the possession of G2m(n) could be of importance in the pathogenesis of coeliac disease.

Since 1972, the genetic background of coeliac disease has been the subject of much research; the genetic associations are becoming more clearly defined and at the same time more complex. Partly by analogy with other immunologically mediated diseases, it is postulated that the possession of HLA-B8/DR3 determines the predisposition to an exaggerated immune response, but disease susceptibility and organ specificity are determined by other factors, such as the presence of genes unique for each disease, genes determining antibody specificity, the site of antigen encounter and factors in the environment. HLA and immunoglobulin genes are active throughout the immune response from recognition to control (Welsh 1981) and there is ample evidence of abnormalities of the immune response to gluten in coeliac disease. Nevertheless, the primary event triggering the mucosal damage is not known and may be wholly or partially related to some non-immunological phenomenon, such as altered permeability of the mucosa or abnormal binding of gluten to the enterocyte membrane.

There may be an intrinsic difference between the epithelial cell surface of coeliacs and non-coeliacs (Weiser and Douglas 1978; Vasmant et al 1982; Bjarnason and Peters 1984). There is, as yet, little information about the relationship of genetic markers to epithelial cell surface characteristics. It is possible that the genetic factor in coeliac disease also acts by coding for a 'mucosal receptor' for gluten (Falchuk 1983). The surface expression of genetic markers on lymphocytes and epithelial cells has attracted increasing interest. With advances in technology, such as the use of monoclonal antibodies and lectin probes, molecular biologists, immunologists and membrane chemists are beginning to define the surface expression of HLA antigens (Dobberstein et al 1982; Bodmer and Bodmer 1984). Gluten may modify cell surface components of the genetic markers associated with coeliac disease and perhaps this is recognised immunologically as a 'non-self' target (Kimura and Ersson 1981). Greater understanding of the relationship of major histocompatibility antigens and T lymphocyte receptors is developing rapidly and is likely to clarify some aspects of the pathogenesis of coeliac disease (Leading article, *Lancet* 1984).

However, it must be remembered that HLA-B8, DR3, DC3, G2m(n) and GSE-associated B cell antigens occur in many healthy individuals. It is possible that eventually a combination of the presence (and absence) of various antigens (Albert et al 1978; Pena et al 1978) might be found which would be common to all patients with coeliac disease. If so, it would be important to know what proportion of the non-coeliac population had a similar genetic background. Considering HLA-B8 alone, it has been estimated that for every 3000 individuals in the West of Ireland, eight coeliacs and 600 non-coeliacs would be HLA-B8 positive (Asquith and Haeney 1979).

Whatever the mechanism of action of the genetic factor, it is unlikely that the development of the disease can ever be explained entirely on the basis of genetics. Coeliac disease has been reported in only one member of some pairs of identical twins. Polanco et al (1981) reviewed six out of 21 monozygotic twin pairs discordant for the disease. Coeliac disease may be more common in women (McConnell 1981), and many clinical and epidemiological observations suggest that environmental factors are important in putting stress on a genetically determined susceptibility.

IgA deficiency

There is an increased incidence of IgA deficiency in coeliac disease; approximately one in 40 coeliacs have IgA deficiency (Ross and Asquith 1979). Possibly a weakening of the immunological barrier to antigen absorption caused by IgA deficiency predisposes to the development of coeliac disease (Cunningham-Rundles et al 1978b; Walker 1981; Scott et al 1983a), but IgA deficiency can also occur when the mucosa is normal (Asquith 1970).

Environmental factors in the development of coeliac disease

Ingestion of gluten is, of course, a necessary environmental factor for the development of coeliac disease. Other environmental factors might influence the amount of gluten absorbed or bound to proposed epithelial surface receptors and thus affect the chance of initiating cell damage.

The quantity and type of gluten (Stevens et al 1981; Aurrichio et al 1982) and the period over which it is eaten may partly determine its toxicity. There is a marked variation in sensitivity to the amount ingested (Weinstein 1974; Price et al 1975). Some challenged patients relapse months or years after reintroduction of gluten, and the degree of mucosal abnormality in untreated patients may vary with age (McNeish 1980). It has been suggested that the interplay between genetic susceptibility and environmental influences leads to a spectrum of abnormality within coeliac disease (Stokes et al 1976).

Doherty and Barry (1981) have shown that a high gluten intake can induce mucosal changes in susceptible individuals who do not have overt coeliac disease (notably HLA-B8 positive relatives of coeliac patients). Coeliac disease may present after gastric surgery, possibly because of a change in the characteristics of the gluten load entering the intestine (Franklin 1970; Losowsky et al 1974).

Transient mucosal inflammation, perhaps due to virus infections, may temporarily increase the amount of gluten absorbed or bound. In animals, various causes of mucosal cell damage can produce a susceptibility to gluten toxicity as shown by altered permeability of the mucosa (Sandhu and Fraser 1983). Intercurrent infection may also impair some protective mechanism, perhaps by upsetting the checks and balances of the immune system. Strober (1981) described a monozygotic twin pair discordant for coeliac disease in whom the coeliac twin had a severe infection prior to the development of the disease, whereas the normal twin did not have the infection.

In recent years, the incidence of childhood coeliac disease has decreased (Littlewood et al 1980; Dossetor et al 1981; Logan et al 1984). Since about 1974 there have been a number of changes in infant feeding practices. Breast feeding, avoidance of hyperosmolar feeds and later introduction of cereals have all been encouraged, and gluten has been removed from some widely used baby foods. The intestinal mucosa is thought to be more permeable during the first months of life and the IgA producing system is not fully developed (Savilahti 1972). Animal studies suggest that there are structural differences in microvillus membranes depending on age (Pang et al 1983) which could explain the increased intestinal permeability to macromolecules in young animals (Udall et al 1981). It seems likely that the intestinal mucosa of infants is more vulnerable to the toxic effect of gluten than that of older subjects and this may explain the recent fall in incidence of coeliac disease since gluten is now introduced later and in smaller amounts. A mucosal lesion of similar severity and extent to that of coeliac disease has not yet been produced in adult experimental animals (which presumably have no genetic predisposition to gluten sensitivity) by administration of cereals or lectins (Lorenzsonn and Olsen 1982; Sandhu and Fraser 1983), but a lesion very like that of coeliac disease has been induced by feeding gluten to three week old pre-ruminant calves (Kilshaw and Slade 1982).

Cooke and Holmes (1984a) have suggested that patients with a strong genetic predisposition become symptomatic soon after introduction of gluten into the diet, but in those with a weaker genetic predisposition, other environmental factors are more important. There is some evidence that low-risk genotypes induce a later presentation of disease (De Marchi et al 1983). Whether the recent decline in incidence of childhood coeliac disease represents prevention, postponement or decline in severity of the disease is not known. However, recent evidence tends to suggest that gluten is less toxic to a healthy, fully developed epithelium, with fully developed mucosal immunity, than to one which is immature, or has been damaged by some environmental factor.

Nature of the toxic component of gluten

Gluten is the fraction of wheat flour which is insoluble in water. It is´ a heterogeneous material and much research has concerned attempts to isolate the toxic component. This involves the preparation of the smallest fragment of gluten protein that is toxic to coeliac patients, in the hope that it can be purified to homogeneity and its structure determined. Unfortunately, identification of the toxic fragment has been hampered by the technical difficulties encountered in breaking down and separating the many proteins involved. In addition, establishing toxicity by feeding fractions of gluten digests, perhaps over a period of time, may be impracticable for small amounts of material. As a preliminary to feeding experiments, in vitro studies based on organ culture of jejunal biopsies may be helpful, and have recently been used to show that all gliadins are toxic (Howdle et al 1984); 43% of gliadin is composed of glutamine, and Van de Kamer and Weijers (1955) suggested that a bound form of glutamine might cause the toxicity. Phelan et al (1978) suggested that a side-chain component of carbohydrate might be the cause. Jos et al (1982) and Cornell and Maxwell (1982) suggested that toxicity resides in fractions containing peptides of 5000 to 8000 molecular weight, rich in proline and glutamine. Offord et al (1978) reported that they had extracted some toxic fragments of much smaller molecular weight.

The search continues, but whether the toxic fragment is a pure peptide, a glycopeptide, or some other material is not known, and much work remains to be done. Most experimental studies have used Frazer's gluten fraction III (Frazer et al 1959), gliadin or α-gliadin. Although relatively crude, these fractions have been shown to be toxic in coeliac patients and large amounts of material are available.

With respect to the various theories of gluten toxicity, it is relevant that gluten subfractions are cytotoxic to several types of cell in tissue culture (Hudson et al 1976), a gluten component can act as a lectin (Douglas 1976), and there is ample evidence that gluten is antigenic.

Theories of gluten toxicity

Enzyme theory of gluten toxicity. This theory is the oldest of the theories, and postulates that coeliac mucosa is deficient in an enzyme which normally digests a toxic component of gluten. In the absence of the enzyme, the increased local concentration of this substance causes mucosal damage.

In 1956, Frazer reported that the toxicity of gluten could be abolished by prior incubation with hog intestinal mucosa. Since then, the search for a missing peptidase has produced much conflicting evidence. Many abnormalities of enzyme levels are found in untreated coeliac mucosa, but these tend to return to normal after treatment (Peters et al 1978; O'Grady et al 1984). Persisting abnormalities of brush border enzymes, for example β-glucosidase or lactase, may be related to a primary defect, or merely represent a slow or incomplete response of the mucosa. A recent study showed no difference between treated coeliacs and controls in the breakdown of gliadin peptides by intestinal brush borders (Bruce et al 1984). Douglas and Booth (1970) found no difference between treated coeliacs and controls in the liberation of amino acids from gluten peptides by jejunal mucosal homogenates. However, Cornell and Rolles (1978) found an increased amount of residual peptides after digestion of gluten with mucosa from treated coeliacs compared with controls, lending support to the enzyme deficiency hypothesis. The increased amount of peptides was found after incubation of mucosa for two hours (Cornell and Townley 1973). Non-specific cytotoxicity of gluten fractions in tissue culture was shown during 24 hours incubation (Hudson et al 1976). Thus, if an undigested gluten product exerts a direct effect on the epithelial cells in coeliac disease, the result might be expected to be apparent after culture of treated coeliac mucosa for 24 or 48 hours in the presence of gluten. Falchuk et al (1974a) were unable to show such a toxic effect on treated mucosa, and it has therefore been suggested that a primary enzyme deficiency is unlikely. However, Howdle et al (1981) found evidence of minor toxicity to treated mucosa. Whatever the mechanism of gluten toxicity, it is possible that the length of time necessary to produce cytotoxicity in well treated mucosa in an organ culture system is longer than the period of viability of the tissue. Alternatively, the early changes of toxicity in mature epithelial cells may be difficult to detect by measurement of either alkaline phosphatase activity (Falchuk et al 1974a) or enterocyte height (Howdle et al 1981).

More subtle defects than the simple missing brush border enzyme have been suggested. Peters and Bjarnason (1984) discussed the possibility of defects of peptide transporters, and the suggestion that the toxicity of gluten is caused by increased activity of an enzyme, for example transglutaminase, which might facilitate gluten binding to membrane components.

Other workers have suggested that the toxicity of gluten might reside in a glycoprotein side-chain and that the deficient enzyme is a carbohydrase, but the evidence is incomplete (Phelan et al 1978; Stevens et al 1978).

Much remains to be discovered about the biochemical handling of gluten in the small intestine. Whether a primary enzyme abnormality contributes to gluten toxicity in coeliac disease is not known.

Lectin theory of gluten toxicity. The regulation of cell growth and differentiation is mediated primarily by the surface of the cell, and particularly by the branching sugar molecules on its surface. Lectins are proteins which bind to specific groups of sugar molecules (Sharon 1977). They are widely distributed in plants and it has been proposed that gluten is toxic to coeliac mucosa because it contains a lectin which binds to abnormal epithelial surface membrane glycoproteins (Weiser and Douglas 1976).

Glycoproteins of the cell membrane are synthesised by the addition of sugars in sequence to the oligosaccharide chain, under the control of a series of glycosyl transferases. Some glycoprotein chains will be incomplete, particularly in immature cells (Etzler 1979). The binding of gluten to altered, exposed, incomplete cell-surface glycoproteins might induce cytotoxicity by altering membrane permeability or transport systems (Li and Kornfeld 1977). If there are few incomplete glycoproteins, damage might be confined to the microvillus membrane, with increased vesiculation and shedding (Lorenzsonn and Olsen 1982; Matsudaira 1983), but adequate replacement, so that the mucosa remains morphologically normal. Indeed, it has been suggested that membrane glycoproteins are normally shed in defence of the gastro-intestinal tract (Fox 1979).

In coeliac patients, the greater number of incomplete glycoproteins would cause increased binding and more extensive damage, with epithelial cell loss, increased cell turnover, an increased mitotic index and lengthened crypts (Kosnai et al 1980). Immature cells have more incomplete glycoproteins, and so damage would be perpetuated. Environmental factors such as high gluten intake (Doherty and Barry 1981) and transient mucosal damage (Sandhu and Fraser 1983) might increase susceptibility to gluten toxicity by converting a steady state of membrane shedding to more rapid cell loss. This theory would also explain why morphologically normal treated coeliac mucosa might be relatively resistant to damage with gluten in some subjects. It is interesting to speculate whether coeliacs who relapse slowly after gluten challenge have a weaker genetic predisposition, perhaps related to fewer incomplete membrane glycoproteins in healthy epithelium.

Vasmant et al (1982) have shown that the localisation of lectin (concanavalin A) receptors on the brush border differs in controls, in treated and in untreated coeliacs, suggesting that there is abnormal glycosylation of the brush border in coeliac disease, but whether the changes indicate a primary abnormality or are merely secondary to membrane damage, is unknown; for example, a local immune response may not only influence crypt cell turnover (Ferguson and Jarret 1975) but also affect the degree of differentiation of the microvillus surface (Castro 1982; Castro and Harari 1982). A gluten product which acts as a lectin also acts as an antigen and can induce T cell proliferation (Scott et al 1983b).

Lectins are commonly present in food (Nachbar and Oppenheim 1980) and can resist intestinal degradation (Brady et al 1978). They may cause intestinal damage through various mechanisms (Lorenzsonn and Olsen 1982; Banwell et al 1983). It is of interest that there are similarities between intestinal damage induced by soy protein and coeliac disease, since a lectin is present in soy beans (Kilshaw and Slade 1982; Poley and Klein 1983).

Although the lectin theory is attractive, and circumstantial evidence in its favour is accumulating (Kottgen et al 1983; Weiser 1983), much more information is needed to evaluate the relevance of the theory in coeliac patients. Weiser and Douglas (1978) were able to show an increase in epithelial cell surface galactosyltransferase activity in coeliac compared with control mucosa and suggested that this may be a primary abnormality in coeliac disease. The authors stressed that the results were preliminary and that strong conclusions could not be drawn because of methodological problems. Nevertheless, their suggestion has stimulated interest in the effect of plant lectins on the gastro-intestinal tract and offered new approaches to the study of coeliac disease.

Permeability theory of gluten toxicity. Abnormal permeability of the intestinal mucosa to sugars occurs in untreated coeliac disease (Hamilton et al 1982). The recent demonstration that there is a persistent increase in permeability in histologically normal treated coeliac mucosa to inert probes of molecular weight lower than 1500 has led to the suggestion that a primary abnormality of permeability may allow access of a toxic gluten product to the mucosa and initiate mucosal damage (Bjarnason et al 1983; Bjarnason and Peters, 1984). Whether the increased permeability revealed using [57Co]cyanocobalamin and 51Cr-EDTA (edetic acid) represents enhanced entry of material into the enterocyte, or between the enterocytes via disorganised tight junctions or in areas of cell loss, is not known. Madara and Trier (1980) have shown that in untreated coeliac disease the expanded population of crypt cells and the damaged surface cells have defective tight junction structure, and this abnormality may contribute to the increased permeability to molecules which are sufficiently large to be normally excluded. Permeability to molecules which normally cross the mucosa is more difficult to assess because of the effect of reduction in surface area, which decreases absorption, and also because secretion by the mucosa may be increased.

Increased permeability to 51Cr-EDTA in treated coeliacs might reflect a primary abnormality in coeliac disease, or merely be associated with subtle persisting damage. Since increased permeability also occurs in various types of mucosal damage not related to coeliac disease (Bjarnason et al 1984), factors additional to the permeability abnormality, as demonstrated by this test, would be necessary to explain the production of villous atrophy. In rat mucosa subjected to mild epithelial cell damage, gluten induced an increase in permeability to sugars after 24–48 hours. There was no evidence that the mucosal damage itself had affected permeability, as measured by sugar absorption, suggesting that the permeability defect in coeliac disease may be secondary to gluten toxicity (Sandhu and Fraser 1983).

The factors which affect uptake from the gut of intact proteins and other macromoloecules which may be antigenic are more complex than those affecting an inert substance. Ingested antigenically intact proteins and peptides gain access to the systemic circulation (Bernstein and Ovary 1968; Thomas and Parrott 1974; Walker 1981; Gardner 1983; Gardner et al 1983) and immune reactions against a protein may have marked effects on function of the small intestine and antigen distribution and absorption (Pang et al 1981; Walker 1984). In the presence of an enteropathy (Jackson et al 1983) or immaturity of the mucosa (Udall et al 1981) an increase in mucosal permeability to macromolecules may occur. The presence of gluten antibody in patients with various gastro-intestinal disorders, and of other food antibodies in coeliac patients, probably reflects increased antigen absorption because of mucosal damage (Taylor et al 1964; Ferguson and Carswell 1972).

Immunological theory of gluten toxicity. In recent years there has been increasing emphasis on the immunological theory of gluten toxicity. According to this theory, the primary factor causing mucosal damage in coeliac disease is an abnormal immune response to gluten. The gut is a major lymphoid organ, and it would be surprising if there was not evidence of secondary immune reactions occurring in association with mucosal damage. There is ample evidence for an immunological basis for some of the features of the disease. The difficulty lies in distinguishing a primary immunological abnormality, in some way directed against gluten, unique to coeliac disease, and capable of initiating mucosal damage. No such primary abnormality has yet been clearly identified, although understanding of the mucosal immune system has increased dramatically over the last fifteen years.

Gluten fractions have been shown to be antigenic in many in vivo and in vitro tests. However, wheat proteins may be antigenic and yet not enterotoxic (Stern et al 1978). That is, immunogenicity does not necessarily imply pathogenicity.

The nature of the target for immune-mediated cytotoxicity in coeliac disease is not known. In view of the marked epithelial cell damage, several groups have suggested that the target is gluten bound in some way to the epithelium. The possibility of a genetically determined receptor site for gluten has been raised (Strober 1978; Falchuk 1983; Scott et al 1983a). Gluten binding might allow persistence of the antigen and thus facilitate immune reactions (Ferguson and MacDonald 1977). However, direct evidence for epithelial binding of gluten is limited (Rubin et al 1965) and has not been confirmed in later immunofluorescence studies (Brandtzaeg and Baklien 1976; Stern and Dietrich 1982).

Marsh (1983) has described a series of experiments in which very small doses of gluten were administered to treated coeliacs. A dose-dependent rise in the number of epithelial lymphocytes occurred between 12 and 48 hours later, with increased blastogenic and mitotic responses, increased turnover of lymphocytes and an increased number of perforations of the basement membrane. The epithelial lesion developed as a result of the formation of multiple intra-epithelial blebs, with separation of the epithelium and basement membrane and subepithelial oedema, not present in control specimens.

From detailed light and electron microscopic examinations of post-challenge biopsies, he concluded that there was no evidence in support of enzyme deficiency or direct lymphocytotoxic attack affecting the enterocytes, but rather that epithelial cell loss occurred because of the extensive inflammatory component accompanying T lymphocyte–gluten interactions within the mucosa. He suggested that the cytological abnormalities could be best accounted for by subsequent recruitment through lymphokines of numerous other mechanisms of response, including B cell activation, mast cell degranulation, increase in vascular permeability and anoxia of the enterocytes. The increased loss of enterocytes would lead to increased crypt cell mitosis and ultimately villous atrophy and crypt hypertrophy (Kosnai et al 1980). Evidence from experimental production of local T cell mediated immune reactions in animal mucosa also suggests that epithelial cell damage might be viewed as a result of the generation of humoral enteropathic factors, such that the gut is damaged as an 'innocent bystander', and not by immunocompetent cells interacting directly with the epithelium (Elson et al 1977; Kay and Ferguson 1984). Local immune reactions might produce a spectrum of damage, from increased enterocyte loss but a steady state of replacement (such that morphological changes do not occur), to the development of subtotal villous atrophy.

Although many abnormalities of humoral and cellular immunity to gluten have been demonstrated by blood tests in coeliac patients, and to a lesser extent in control subjects (reviewed by Asquith and Haeney 1978; Cooke and Holmes 1984b), these give indirect and possibly distorted evidence of abnormalities in the mucosa. A more specific indication of an immunological basis for gluten toxicity may be obtained by study of small bowel biopsies in organ culture. By this means, gluten toxicity to untreated or post-challenge coeliac mucosa has been demonstrated, whereas toxicity to treated coeliac or control mucosa is minimal (Falchuk et al 1974a; Howdle et al 1981). It has been suggested that gluten toxicity is not demonstrated in treated mucosa because the effector mechanism involves an aspect of the mucosal immune system which cannot be brought into activity in isolated tissue, not recently stimulated with gluten. Possibly cells directly involved in the immune response to gluten are not present in the mucosa of patients on a gluten-free diet, but may be present in the blood (Holmes et al 1976; Bullen and Losowsky 1978; Howdle et al 1982). Addition of autologous blood lymphocytes to treated coeliac biopsies cultured with gluten increases mucosal damage (Simpson et al 1983). In untreated or post-challenge coeliac mucosa, culture with gluten leads to increased synthesis of gliadin antibody and secretion of a humoral factor which inhibits leucocyte migration (possibly a lymphokine, secreted as a result of a local cell-mediated immune reaction) (Falchuk and Strober 1974; Ferguson et al 1975; Howdle et al 1982). Falchuk et al (1974b) also reported that a humoral factor released from untreated mucosa cultured in the presence of gluten was toxic to treated mucosa. These experiments cannot precisely define the immune mechanism involved in gluten toxicity (damage by cytotoxic T cell, lymphokine production, immune complex deposition or antibody-dependent cellular cytotoxicity), but they support the immunological theory. In the fully developed mucosal lesion, it is likely that several types of immune reaction are occurring together.

The mucosal immune system is subject to powerful regulatory mechanisms which usually induce and maintain secretory immunity and systemic tolerance, via suppressor T cell activation, to an ingested antigen (Strober 1982; Clancy et al 1984). In coeliac disease there may be an imbalance of the local immune response to gluten, related to the presentation of antigen in association with certain genetic markers (Scott et al 1983c). An antigen-specific suppressor-T-cell defect has been postulated in two other diseases associated with HLA-B8 (How et al 1984; Vento et al 1984). In animals, feeding of an antigen after cyclophosphamide pretreatment, which produces suppressor cell inhibition, can cause a local cell mediated reaction, though the mucosal lesion is not as marked as in coeliac disease (Mowat and Ferguson 1981). Abrogation of the normal mechanism for production of tolerance might be particularly likely to occur in neonatal animals, because of increased permeability of the mucosa to antigens (Udall et al 1981) and immaturity of the mucosal immune system and IgA response (Savilahti 1972). Production of a cell-mediated immune reaction in the mucosa of neonatal mice by feeding ovalbumin (Kay and Ferguson 1984) and of villous atrophy and crypt hyperplasia in calves by feeding gluten (Kilshaw and Slade 1982), may be related to the possibly increased susceptibility of children to gluten toxicity if gluten is introduced early (Logan et al 1984). Increased understanding of the inter-relation between genetic markers on B and T cells, and the immune response (Leading Article 1984) is likely to help in the understanding of the balance between helper and suppressor function and the mechanism of gluten toxicity in coeliac disease.

CONCLUSION

Coeliac disease develops because of the effect of environmental factors combined with genetic susceptibility. None of the theories of gluten toxicity is completely proven, and elements of each theory may provide part of the explanation. However, on current evidence, the genetic effect is best explained in association with the immunological theory. Understanding of genetics and its relation to immune responses is increasing and may clarify the mechanism of gluten toxicity, but identification of the toxic component of gluten remains a difficult challenge.

Acknowledgements

Thanks are due to Mrs. Margaret Cullingworth for typing the manuscript and the staff of the George Eliot Library, Nuneaton, for help with obtaining references.

REFERENCES

Albert E, Harms K, Bertele R et al (1978) B-cell alloantigens in coeliac disease. In McNicholl B, McCarthy C F & Fottrell P F (eds) *Perspectives in Coeliac Disease*, pp 123–129. Lancaster: MTP Press.

Anderson I H, Levine A S & Levitt M D (1981) Incomplete absorption of the carbohydrate in all-purpose wheat flour. *New England Journal of Medicine* **304**: 891–892.

Asquith P (1970) Adult coeliac disease. A clincal, morphological and immunological study. MD thesis University of Birmingham.

Asquith P & Haeney M R (1979) Coeliac disease. In Asquith P. (ed) *Immunology of the Gastrointestine Tract*, pp 66–94. Edinburgh: Churchill Livingstone.

Arnaud-Battandier F, Schmitz J, Muller J, Jos J & Rey J (1983) HLA and gluten cytotoxicity in vitro *Gastroenterology* **84**: 201.

Auricchio S, De Ritis G, De Vincenzi M, Occorsio P & Silano V (1982) Effects of gliadin-derive peptides from *Bread* and *Durum* wheats on small intestine cultures from rat fetus and coelia children. *Pediatric Research* **16**: 1004–1010.

Balner H (1976) Histocompatibility-linked genes controlling Ia-like antigens in rhesus monkeys *Transplantation Proceedings* **8**: 417–421.

Banwell J G, Boldt D H, Meyers J et al (1983) Phytohemagglutinin derived from red kidney bea (*Phaseolus vulgaris*): A cause for intestinal malabsorption associated with bacterial overgrowth the rat. *Gastroenterology* **84**: 506–515.

Barry R E, Henry C & Read A E (1978) The patient's view of a gluten-free diet. In McNicholl B McCarthy C F & Fottrell P F (eds) *Perspectives in Coeliac Disease*, pp 487–493. Lancaster: MT Press.

Benacerraf B & McDevittt H O (1972) Histocompatibility linked immune response genes. *Science* **179** 273–279.

Bernstein I D & Ovary Z (1968) Absorption of antigens from the gastrointestinal tract. *Internation Archives of Allergy and Applied Immunology* **33**: 521–527.

Biol M-C, Martin A, Oehninger C, Louisot P & Richard M (1981) Biosynthesis of glycoprotein in th intestinal mucosa. II Influence of diets. *Annals of Nutrition and Metabolism* **25**: 269–280.

Biol M-C, Martin A, Paulin C et al (1984) Glycosyltransferase activities in the rat intestinal mucosa comparison between standard commercial and semi-synthetic diets. *Annals of Nutrition an Metabolism* **28**: 52–64.

Bjarnason I & Peters T J (1984) In vitro determination of small intestinal permeability: demonstratio of a persistent defect in patients with coeliac disease. *Gut* **25**: 145–150.

Bjarnason I, Peters T J & Veall N (1983) A persistent defect in intestinal permeability in coeliac diseas demonstrated by a ^{51}Cr-labelled EDTA absorption test. *Lancet* **1**: 323–325.

Bjarason I, Peters T J & Veall N (1984) ^{51}Cr-EDTA test for intestinal permeability. *Lancet* **2**: 523.

Bodmer J G & Bodmer W F (1984) Monoclonal antibodies to HLA determinants. *British Medic Bulletin* **40**: 267–275.

Brady P G, Vannier A M & Banwell J G (1978) Identification of the dietary lectin, wheat gerr agglutinin, in human intestinal contents. *Gastroenterology* **75**: 236–239.

Brandtzaeg P & Baklien K (1976) Immunohistochemical studies of the formation and epithelia transport of immunoglobulins in normal and diseased human intestinal mucosa. *Scandinavia Journal of Gastroenterology* **11** (Suppl. 36): 1–45.

Bruce G, Woodley J F & Swan C H J (1984) Breakdown of gliadin peptides by intestinal brush border from coeliac patients. *Gut* **25**: 919–924.

Bullen A W & Losowsky M S (1978) Cell-mediated immunity to gluten fraction III in adult coelia disease. *Gut* **19**: 126–131.

Carbonara A O, De Marchi M, van Loghem E & Ansaldi N (1983) Gm markers in celiac disease *Human Immunology* **6**: 91–95.

Castro G A (1982) Immunological regulation of epithelial function. *American Journal of Physiolog* **243**: G321–329.

Castro G A & Harari Y (1982) Intestinal epithelial membrane changes in rats immune to *Trichinell spiralis*. *Molecular and Biochemical Parasitology* **6**: 191–204.

Cerf-Bensussan N, Quaroni A, Kurnick J T & Bhan A K (1984) Intraepithelial lymphocytes modulate I expression by intestinal epithelial cells. *Journal of Immunology* **132**: 2244–2252.

Clancy R, Cripps A & Chipchase H (1984) Regulation of human gut B lymphocytes by T lymphocytes *Gut* **25**: 47–51.

Cooke W T & Holmes G K T (1984a) *Coeliac Disease*, p 272. Edinburgh: Churchill Livingstone.

Cooke W T & Holmes G K T (1984b) *Coeliac Disease*, pp 247–263. Edinburgh: Churchill Livingstone

Cornell H J & Maxwell R J (1982) Amino acid composition of gliadin fractions which may be toxic t individuals with coeliac disease. *Clinica Chimica Acta* **123**: 311–319.

Cornell H J & Rolles C J (1978) Further evidence of a primary mucosal defect in coeliac disease. *Gut* **19** 253–259.

Cornell H J & Townley R R W (1973) Investigation of possible intestinal peptidase deficiency in coeliac disease. *Clinica Chimica Acta* **43**: 113–125.

Cunningham-Rundles S, Cunningham-Rundles C, Pollack M S, Good R A & Dupont B (1978a) Response to wheat antigen in in vitro lymphocyte transformation among HLA-B8-positive normal donors. *Transplantation Proceedings* **10**: 977–979.

Cunningham-Rundles C, Brandeis W E, Good R A & Day N K (1978b) Milk precipitins, circulating immune complexes and IgA deficiency. *Proceedings of the National Academy of Sciences* **75**: 3387–3389.

Dausset J, Degos L & Hors J (1974) The association of the HL-A antigens with diseases. *Clinical Immunology and Immunopathology* **3**: 127–149.

De Marchi M, Carbonara A, Ansaldi N et al (1983) HLA-DR3 and DR7 in coeliac disease: immunogenetic and clinical aspects. *Gut* **24**: 706–712.

Dicke W K (1950) Coeliac disease: A study of the damaging effect of some cereals (especially wheat), caused by a factor outside of their starch, on the fat absorption of children with coeliac disease. *Transactions of the 6th International Congress of Paediatrics, Zurich*, p 117.

Dobberstein B, Kvist S & Roberts L (1982) Structure and biosynthesis of histocompatibility antigens (H-2, HLA). *Philosophical Transactions of the Royal Society of London* **B300**: 161–172.

Doherty M & Barry R E (1981) Gluten-induced mucosal changes in subjects without overt small-bowel disease. *Lancet* **1**: 517–520.

Dossetor J F B, Gibson A A M & McNeish A S (1981) Childhood coeliac disease is disappearing. *Lancet* **1**: 322–323.

Douglas A P (1976) The binding of a glycopeptide component of wheat gluten to intestinal mucosa of normal and coeliac human subjects. *Clinica Chimica Acta* **73**: 357–361.

Douglas A P & Booth C C (1970) Digestion of gluten peptides by normal human jejunal mucosa and by mucosa from patients with adult coeliac disease. *Clinical Science* **38**: 11–25.

Ecknauer R, Sircar B & Johnson L R (1981) Effect of dietary bulk on small intestinal morphology and cell renewal in the rat. *Gastroenterology* **81**: 781–786.

Egan-Mitchell B, Fottrell P F & McNicholl B (1981) Early or pre-coeliac mucosa: development of gluten enteropathy. *Gut* **22**: 65–69.

Ek J, Albrechtsen D, Solheim B G & Thorsby E (1978) Strong association between the HLA-DW3 related B cell alloantigen-DRW3 and coeliac disease. *Scandinavian Journal of Gastroenterology* **13**: 229–233.

Elson C O, Reilly R W & Rosenberg I H (1977) Small intestinal injury in the GvHR: an innocent bystander phenomenon. *Gastroenterology* **72**: 886–889.

Etzler M E (1979) Lectins as probes in studies of intestinal glycoproteins and glycolipids. *American Journal of Clinical Nutrition* **32**: 133–138.

Fairweather-Tait S J, Gee J M & Johnson I T (1983) The influence of cooked kidney beans (*Phaseolus vulgaris*) on intestinal cell turnover and faecal nitrogen excretion in the rat. *British Journal of Nutrition* **49**: 303–312.

Falchuk Z M (1983) Gluten-sensitive enteropathy. *Clinics in Gastroenterology* **12**: 475–494.

Falchuk Z M & Strober W (1974) Gluten sensitive enteropathy: Synthesis of antigliadin antibody in vitro. *Gut* **15**: 947–952.

Falchuk Z M, Rogentine G N & Strober W (1972) Predominance of histocompatibility antigen HL-A8 in patients with gluten-sensitive enteropathy. *Journal of Clinical Investigation* **51**: 1602–1605.

Falchuk Z M, Gebhard R L, Sessoms C & Strober W (1974a) An in vitro model of gluten-sensitive enteropathy. Effect of gliadin on intestinal epithelial cells of patients with gluten-sensitive enteropathy in organ culture. *Journal of Clinical Investigation* **53**: 487–500.

Falchuk Z M, Gebhard R L & Strober W (1974b) The pathogenesis of gluten sensitive enteropathy (celiac sprue): organ culture studies. In Hekkens W Th J M & Pena A S (eds) *Coeliac Disease*, pp 107–117. Leiden: Stenfert Kroese.

Falchuk Z M, Nelson D A, Katz A G et al (1980) Gluten sensitive enteropathy. Influence of histocompatibility type on gluten sensitivity in vitro. *Journal of Clinical Investigation* **66**: 227–233.

Ferguson A & Carswell F (1972) Precipitins to dietary proteins in serum and upper intestinal secretions of coeliac children. *British Medical Journal* **1**: 75–77.

Ferguson A & Jarrett E E E (1975) Hypersensitivity reactions in the small intestine. I. Thymus dependence of experimental 'partial villous atrophy'. *Gut* **16**: 114–117.

Ferguson A & McDonald T T (1977) Effects of local delayed hypersensitivity on the small intestine. In Porter R & Knight J (eds) *Immunology of the Gut, Ciba Foundation Symposium 46*, pp 305–327. Amsterdam: Excerpta Medica.

Ferguson A, MacDonald T T, McClure J P & Holden R J (1975) Cell-mediated immunity to gliadin within the small intestinal mucosa in coeliac disease. *Lancet* 1: 895–897.

Fox R A (1979) Membrane glycoproteins shed in defence of the cells of the gastrointestinal trac *Medical Hypotheses* 5: 669–682.

Franklin R H (1970) Post-vagotomy diarrhoea? *British Medical Journal* 1: 412.

Frazer A C (1956) Discussion of some problems of steatorrhoea and reduced stature. *Proceedings of th Royal Society of Medicine* 49: 1009–1013.

Frazer A C, Fletcher R F, Ross C A C et al (1959) Gluten-induced enteropathy. The effect of partiall digested gluten. *Lancet* 2: 252–255.

Galbraith R M, Eddleston A L W F, Williams R et al (1976) Enhanced antibody responses in activ chronic hepatitis: relation to HLA-B8 and HLA-B12 and porto-systemic shunting. *Lancet* 1 930–934.

Gardner M L G (1983) Evidence for, and implications of, passage of intact peptides across the intestina mucosa. *Biochemical Society Transactions* II: 810–813.

Gardner M L G, Lindblad B S, Burston D & Matthews D M (1983) Trans-mucosal passage of intac peptides in the guinea-pig small intestine in vivo: a re-appraisal. *Clinical Science* 64: 433–439.

Gee, S. (1888) On the coeliac affection. *St. Bartholomew's Hospital Reports* 24: 17–20.

Goda T, Yamada K, Bustamante S & Koldovsky O (1983) Dietary induced rapid decrease of microvilla carbohydrase activity in rat jejunoileum. *American Journal of Physiology* 245: G418–423.

Greenberg D A & Rotter J I (1981) Investigations of a two-locus model for coeliac disease. I McConnell R B (ed) *The Genetics of Coeliac Disease*, pp 251–262. Lancaster: MTP Press.

Hamilton I, Cobden I Rothwell J & Axon A T R (1982) Intestinal permeability in coeliac disease: th response to gluten withdrawal and single-dose gluten challenge. *Gut* 23: 202–210.

Holmes G K T, Asquith P & Cooke W T (1976) Cell mediated immunity to gluten fraction III in adul coeliac disease. *Clinical and Experimental Immunology* 24: 259–265.

How J, Row V V & Volpe R (1984) Antigen-specific suppressor cell function and autoimmune diseases *Lancet* 2: 463.

Howdle P D, Corazza G R, Bullen A W & Losowsky M S (1981) Gluten sensitivity of small intestina mucosa in vitro: Quantitative assessment of histological change. *Gastroenterology* 80: 442–450.

Howdle P D, Bullen A W & Losowsky M S (1982) Cell mediated immunity to gluten within the smal intestinal mucosa in coeliac disease. *Gut* 23: 115–122.

Howdle P D, Ciclitira P J, Simpson F G & Losowsky M S (1984) Are all gliadins toxic in coeliac disease' An in vitro study of α, β, γ and ω gliadins. *Scandinavian Journal of Gastroenterology* 19: 41–47.

Hudson D A, Purdham D R, Cornell H J & Rolles C J (1976) Non-specific cytotoxicity of wheat gliadir components towards cultured human cells. *Lancet* 1: 339–341.

Jackson D, Walker-Smith J A & Phillips A D (1983) Macromolecular absorption by histologicall normal and abnormal small intestinal mucosa in childhood: an in vitro study using organ culture *Journal of Pediatric Gastroenterology and Nutrition* 2: 235–247.

Jos J, Charbonnier L, Mosse J et al (1982) The toxic fraction of gliadin digests in coeliac disease Isolation by chromatography on Biogel P-10. *Clinica Chimica Acta* 119: 263–274.

Kagnoff M F (1982) Two genetic loci control the murine immune response to A-gliadin, a wheat protei that activates coeliac sprue. *Nature, London* 296: 158–160.

Kagnoff M F, Weiss J B, Brown R J, Lee T & Schanfield M S (1983) Immunoglobulin allotype marker in gluten-sensitive enteropathy. *Lancet* 1: 952–953.

Kay R A & Ferguson A (1984) Intestinal T cells, mucosal cell-mediated immunity and their relevance t food allergic disease. *Clinical Reviews in Allergy* 2: 55–68.

Keuning J J, Pena A S, van Leeuwen A, van Hooff J P & van Rood J J (1976) HLA-DW3 associatec with coeliac disease. *Lancet* 1: 506–508.

Kilshaw P J & Slade H (1982) Villus atrophy and crypt elongation in the small intestine of preruminan calves fed with heated soya bean flour or wheat gluten. *Research in Veterinary Science* 33: 305–308

Kimura A & Ersson B (1981) Activation of T lymphocytes by lectins and carbohydrate-oxidizing reagents viewed as an immunological recognition of cell-surface modifications seen in the context o 'self' major histocompatibility complex antigens. *European Journal of Immunology* II: 475–483.

Kosnai I, Kuitunen P, Savilahti E, Rapola J & Kohegyi J (1980) Cell kinetics in the jejunal cryp epithelium in malabsorption syndrome with cow's milk protein intolerance and in coeliac disease o childhood. *Gut* 21: 1041–1046.

Kottgen E, Kluge F, Volk B & Gerok W (1983) The lectin properties of gluten as the basis of the pathomechanism of gluten-sensitive enteropathy. *Klinische Wochenschrift* 61: 111–112.

Leading Article (1984) T cell receptors. *Lancet* 1: 776.

Levine R A, Briggs G W, Harding R S & Nolte L B (1966) Prolonged gluten administration in norma subjects. *New England Journal of Medicine* 274: 1109–1114.

Li E & Kornfeld S (1977) Effects of wheat germ agglutinin on membrane transport. *Biochimica et Biophysica Acta* **469**: 202–210.

Littlewood J M, Crollick A & Richards I D G (1980) Childhood coeliac disease is disappearing. *Lancet* **2**: 1359.

Logan R F A, Ferguson A, Cole S et al (1984) Is childhood coeliac disease declining? *Gut* **25**: A551.

Lorenzsonn V & Olsen W A (1982) In vivo responses of rat intestinal epithelium to intraluminal dietary lectins. *Gastroenterology* **82**: 838–848.

Losowsky M S, Walker B E & Kelleher J (1974) *Malabsorption in Clinical Practice*, pp 193–194. Edinburgh: Churchill Livingstone.

Madara J L & Trier J S (1980) Structural abnormalities of jejunal epithelial cell membranes in celiac sprue. *Laboratory Investigation* **43**: 254–261.

Mann D L, Katz S I, Nelson D L, Abelson L D & Strober W (1976) Specific B-cell antigen associated with gluten-sensitve enteropathy and dermatitis herpetiformis. *Lancet* **1**: 110–111.

Marsh M N (1983) Immunocytes, enterocytes and the lamina propria: an immunopathological framework of coeliac disease. *Journal of the Royal College of Physicians of London* **17**: 205–212.

Matsudaira P T (1983) Structural and functional relationship between the membrane and the cytoskeleton in brush border microvilli. In Porter R & Collins G M (eds) *Brush Border Membranes. Ciba Foundation Symposium 95*, pp 233–242. London: Pitman Books.

McCarthy D M, Nicholson J A & Kim Y S (1980) Intestinal enzyme adaptation to normal diets of different composition. *American Journal of Physiology* **239**: G445–451.

McConnell R B (1981) Membership of the Coeliac Society of the United Kingdom. In McConnell R B (ed) *The Genetics of Coeliac Diseases*. pp 65–69. Lancaster: MTP Press.

McKenna R, Stevens F M, Bourke M et al (1981) B-cell alloantigens associated with coeliac disease in the West of Ireland. In McConnell R B (ed) *The Genetics of Coeliac Disease*, pp 153–158. Lancaster: MTP Press.

McNeish A S (1980). Coeliac disease: duration of gluten-free diet. *Archives of Disease in Childhood* **55**: 110–111.

Mearin M L, Biemond I, Pena A S et al (1983) HLA-DR phenotypes in Spanish coeliac children: their contribution to the understanding of the genetics of the disease. *Gut* **24**: 532–537.

Morris P J (1973) In Discussion. In McDevitt H O & Landy M (eds) *Genetic Control of Immune Responsiveness*, pp 354–355. New York: Academic Press.

Mowat A M & Ferguson A (1981) Hypersensitivity in the small intestinal mucosa. V. Induction of cell-mediated immunity to a dietary antigen. *Clinical and Experimental Immunology* **43**: 574–582.

Nachbar M S & Oppenheim J D (1980) Lectins in the United States diet: a survey of lectins in commonly consumed foods and a review of the literature. *American Journal of Clinical Nutrition* **33**: 2338–2345.

Offord R E, Anand B S, Piris J & Truelove S C (1978) Further subfractionation of digests of gluten. In McNicholl B, McCarthy C F & Fottrell P F (eds) *Perspectives in Coeliac Disease*, pp 25–29. Lancaster: MTP Press.

O'Grady J G, Stevens F M, Keane R et al (1984) Intestinal lactase, sucrase and alkaline phosphatase in 373 patients with coeliac disease. *Journal of Clinical Pathology* **37**: 298–301.

Osoba D & Falk J (1978) HLA-B8 phenotype associated with an increased mixed leukocyte reaction. *Immunogenetics* **6**: 425–432.

Pang K-Y, Walker W A & Bloch K J (1981) Intestinal uptake of macromolecules. Differences in distribution and degradation of protein antigen in control and immunised rats. *Gut* **22**: 1018–1024.

Pang K-Y, Bresson J L & Walker W A (1983) Development of the gastrointestinal mucosal barrier. Evidence for structural differences in microvillus membranes from newborn and adult rabbits. *Biochimica et Biophysica Acta* **727**: 201–208.

Paulley J W (1954) Observations on the aetiology of idiopathic steatorrhoea. Jejunal and lymph node biopsies. *British Medical Journal* **2**: 1318–1321.

Pena A S, Mann D L, Hague N E et al (1978) Genetic basis of gluten-sensitive enteropathy. *Gastroenterology* **75**: 230–235.

Peters T J & Bjarnason I (1984) Coeliac syndrome: biochemical mechanisms and the missing peptidase hypothesis revisited. *Gut* **25**: 913–918.

Peters T J, Jones P E & Wells G (1978) Analytical subcellular fractionation of jejunal biopsy specimens: enzyme activities, organelle pathology and response to gluten withdrawal in patients with coeliac disease. *Clinical Science and Molecular Medicine* **55**: 285–292.

Phelan J J, Stevens F M, Cleere W F et al (1978) The detoxificaton of gliadin by the enzymic cleavage of a side-chain substituent. In McNicholl B, McCarthy C F & Fottrell P F (eds) *Perspectives in Coeliac Disease*, pp 33–39. Lancaster: MTP Press.

Polanco I, Biemond I, van Leeuwen A et al (1981) Gluten sensitive enteropathy in Spain: genetic an environmental factors. In McConnell R B (ed) *The Genetics of Coeliac Disease*, pp 211–231 Lancaster: MTP Press.

Poley J R & Klein A W (1983) Scanning electron microscopy of soy protein-induced damage of sma bowel mucosa in infants. *Journal of Pediatric Gastroenterology and Nutrition* 2: 271–287.

Price H, Zownir J & Prokipchuk E (1975) Coeliac disease. *Lancet* 2: 920–921.

Robertson D A F, Bullen A W, Field H, Simpson F G & Losowsky M S (1982) Suppressor cell activity splenic function and HLA-B8 status in man. *Journal of Clinical and Laboratory Immunology* 9 133–138.

Rolles C J, Kyaw-Myint T B, Sin W-K & Anderson C M (1974) Family study of coeliac disease. *Gut* 15 827.

Rolles C J, Kyaw-Myint T B, Sin W-K & Anderson M (1981) The familial incidence of asymptomati coeliac disease. In McConnell R B (ed) *The Genetics of Coeliac Disease*, pp 235–243. Lancaster MTP Press.

Ross I N & Asquith P (1979) Primary immune deficiency. In Asquith P (ed) *Immunology of the Gastrointestinal Tract*, pp 162–166. Edinburgh: Churchill Livingstone.

Rubin C E, Brandborg L L, Flick A L et al (1962) Studies of celiac sprue. III. The effect of repeate wheat instillation into the proximal ileum of patients on a gluten free diet. *Gastroenterology* 43 621–641.

Rubin W, Fauci A S, Sleisenger M H & Jeffries G H (1965) Immunofluorescent studies in adult celia disease. *Journal of Clinical Investigation* 44: 475–485.

Sandhu J S & Fraser D R (1983) Effect of dietary cereals on intestinal permeability in experiment enteropathy in rats. *Gut* 24: 825–830.

Savilahti E (1972) Immunoglobulin containing cells in the intestinal mucosa and immunoglobulins in th intestinal juice in children. *Clinical and Experimental Immunology* 11: 415–425.

Scholz S, Rossipal E, Brautbar Ch et al (1981) HLA-DR antigens in coeliac disease. A population an multiple case family study. In McConnell R B (ed) *The Genetics of Coeliac Disease*, pp 143–149 Lancaster: MTP Press.

Scott B B, Swinburne M L, Rajah S M & Losowsky M S (1974) HL-A8 and the immune response t gluten. *Lancet* 2: 374–377.

Scott H, Brandtzaeg P, Solheim, B G & Thorsby E (1981) Relation between HLA-DR-like antigens an secretory component (SC) in jejunal epithelium of patients with coeliac disease or dermatiti herpetiformis. *Clinical and Experimental Immunology* 44: 233–238.

Scott H, Brandtzaeg P, Thorsby E et al (1983a) Mucosal and systemic immune response patterns i celiac disease. *Annals of Allergy* 51: 233–239.

Scott H, Fausa O & Thorsby E (1983b) T-lymphocyte activation by a gluten fraction, glyc-gli. Studies adult coeliac patients and healthy controls. *Scandinavian Journal of Immunology* 18: 185–191.

Scott H, Hirschberg H & Thorsby E (1983c) HLA-DR3- and HLA-DR7-restricted T cell hyporespor siveness to gluten antigen: A clue to the aetiology of coeliac disease? *Scandinavian Journal c Immunology* 18: 163–167.

Sharon N (1977) Lectins. *Scientific American* 236: 108–119.

Shiner M (1956) Duodenal biopsy. *Lancet* 1: 17–19.

Shmerling D H, Rolles C J, Strober W et al (1981) Ethics and biopsy of relatives. In Discussion. I McConnell R B (ed) *The Genetics of Coeliac Disease*, pp 247–248. Lancaster: MTP Press.

Simpson F G, Bullen A W, Robertson D A F & Losowsky M S (1981) HLA-B8 and cell-mediate immunity to gluten. *Gut* 22: 633–636.

Simpson F G, Howdle P D, Robertson D A F & Losowsky M S (1983) Jejunal biopsy and lymphocyt co-culture in coeliac disease. *Scandinavian Journal of Gastroenterology* 18: 749–754.

Stern M & Dietrich R (1982) Gliadin- and immunoglobulin-containing cells of small intestinal lamin propria in childhood coeliac disease. *European Journal of Pediatrics* 139: 13–17.

Stern M, Fischer K & Gruttner R (1978) Immunofluorescent gliadin antibodies in childhood coelia disease. In McNicholl B, McCarthy C F & Fottrell P F (eds) *Perspectives in Coeliac Disease*, p 207–215. Lancaster: MTP Press.

Stevens F M, Phelan J J, McNicholl B et al (1978) Clinical demonstration of the reduction of gliadi toxicity by enzymic cleavage of a side-chain substitutent. In McNicholl B, McCarthy C F & Fottre P F (eds) *Perspectives in Coeliac Disease*, pp 41–50. Lancaster: MTP Press.

Stevens F M, Egan-Mitchell B, McCarthy C F & McNicholl B (1981) Factors in the epidemiology coeliac disease in the West of Ireland. In McConnell R B (ed) *The Genetics of Coeliac Disease*, p 7–14. Lancaster: MTP Press.

Stokes P L, Asquith P & Cokke W T (1973) Genetics of coeliac disease. *Clinics in Gastroenterology* **2** (3): 547–556.

Stokes P L, Asquith P, Holmes G K T, Mackintosh P & Cooke W T (1972) Histocompatibility antigens associated with adult coeliac disease. *Lancet* **2**: 162–164.

Stokes P L, Ferguson R, Holmes G K T & Cooke W T (1976) Familial aspects of coeliac disease. *Quarterly Journal of Medicine* **45**: 567–582.

Strober W (1978) An immunological theory of gluten-sensitive enteropathy. In McNicholl B, McCarthy C F & Fottrell P F (eds) *Perspectives in Coeliac Disease*, pp 169–182. Lancaster: MTP Press.

Strober W (1981). In Discussion. In McConnell R B (ed) *The Genetics of Coeliac Disease*, p 234. Lancaster: MTP Press.

Strober W (1982) The regulation of mucosal immune system. *Journal of Allergy and Clinical Immunology* **70**: 225–230.

Svejgaard A, Platz P, Ryder L P, Nielsen L S & Thomsen M (1975) HLA and disease associations – a survey. *Transplantation Reviews* **22**: 3–43.

Taylor K B, Truelove S C & Wright R (1964) Serologic reactions to gluten and cow's milk proteins in gastrointestinal disease. *Gastroenterology* **46**: 99–108.

Thomas H C & Parrot D M V (1974) The induction of tolerance to a soluble protein antigen by oral administration. *Immunology* **27**: 631–639.

Tosi R, Vismara D, Tanigaki N et al (1983) Evidence that coeliac disease is primarily associated with a DC locus allelic specificity. *Clinical Immunology and Immunopathology* **28**: 395–404.

Udall J N, Pang K, Fritze L, Kleinman R & Walker W A (1981) Development of gastrointestinal mucosal barrier. I The effect of age on intestinal permeability to macromolecules. *Pediatric Research* **15**: 241–244.

Van de Kamer J H & Weijers H A (1955) Coeliac disease: some experiments on the cause of the harmful effect of wheat gliadin. *Acta Paediatrica* **44**: 465–469.

Vasmant D, Feldmann G & Fontaine J-L (1982) Ultrastructural localization of concanavalin A surface receptors on brush-border enterocytes in normal children and during coeliac disease. *Pediatric Research* **16**: 441–445.

Vento S, Hegarty J E, Bottazzo G et al (1984) Antigen specific suppressor cell function in autoimmune chronic active hepatitis. *Lancet* **1**: 1200–1204.

Verkasalo M A (1982) Adherence of gliadin fractions to lymphocytes in coeliac disease. *Lancet* **1**: 1384–1386.

Vladutiu A O & Rose N R (1974) HL-A antigens: Association with disease. *Immunogenetics* **1**: 305–328.

Walker W A (1981) Intestinal transport of macromolecules. In Johnson L R (ed) *Physiology of the Gastrointestinal Tract* Vol. 2, pp 1271–1289. New York: Raven Press.

Walker W A (1984) Immunoregulation of small intestinal function. *Gastroenterology* **86**: 577–579.

Weinstein W M (1974) Latent celiac sprue. *Gastroenterology* **66**: 489–493.

Weiser M M (1983) Is gluten a plant lectin and if so does this property relate to coeliac disease? *Gastroenterology* **85**: 206–207.

Weiser M M & Douglas A P (1976) An alternative mechanism for gluten toxicity in coeliac disease. *Lancet* **1**: 567–569.

Weiser M M & Douglas A P (1978) Cell surface glycosyl transferases of the enterocyte in coeliac disease. In McNicholl B, McCarthy C F & Fottrell P F (eds) *Perspectives in Coeliac Disease*, pp 451–458. Lancaster: MTP Press.

Weiss J B, Austin R K, Schanfield M S & Kagnoff M F (1983) Gluten sensitive enteropathy. Immunoglobulin G heavy-chain (Gm) allotypes and the immune response to wheat gliadin. *Journal of Clinical Investigation* **72**: 96–101.

Welsh K (1981) HLA genes, immunoglobulin genes and human disease. *Nature, London* **292**: 673–674.

Woodrow J C (1981) The HLA system. In McConnell R B (ed) *The Genetics of Coeliac Disease*, pp 111–121. Lancaster: MTP Press.

Chapter 14
Irritable Bowel Syndrome

V. Alun Jones

Irritable bowel syndrome (IBS) is a common condition which accounts for between 33% and 70% of gastro-intestinal consultations in Britain (Drossman et al 1977; Harvey et al 1983). It occurs approximately twice as frequently in women as in men. The point at which people choose to seek advice about gut symptoms varies; Thompson and Heaton (1980) found that 30% of uncomplaining and apparently healthy British adults admitted to bowel disturbances. Those who seek medical attention have been suggested to be the more anxious. Affected patients complain of diarrhoea, constipation, or an alternation between the two, and abdominal pain. These may persist for many years but never lead to serious complications. There are no abnormalities to be found radiologically (Heaton 1983), and biochemical tests and mucosal biopsies are normal. Although IBS may follow bouts of gastro-enteritis, pathogenic bacteria are not present in the stools (Silverberg and Daum 1979).

The differential diganosis of IBS is wide, encompassing inflammatory bowel disease, colonic carcinoma, coeliac disease, alactasia, ulcer diathesis, biliary pathology and musculo-skeletal pain. As no specific diagnostic tests are available, IBS remains a diagnosis of exclusion and thus is probably a collection of conditions rather than a definite entity. This causes great difficulty in assessing clinical studies, as patient selection may vary from one centre to another. However, many gastro-enterologists reserve the label 'IBS' for those patients who clearly have an abnormality of gut motility, which can often be appreciated from spasm of the bowel at sigmoidoscopy. The abnormality of motility can be demonstrated in the small bowel and oesophagus as well as in the colon (Almy and Tulin 1947; Burns 1980; Corbett et al 1981; Whorwell et al 1981), but despite initial optimism (Snape et al 1976; Taylor et al 1978) no characteristic motility pattern specific to IBS can be demonstrated. The cause of the spasm remains unclear; antispasmodic drugs such as merbeverine and peppermint oil sometimes give temporary relief.

IBS is still considered by many to be a psychosomatic disorder (Almy and Tulin 1947; Young et al 1976), but other workers have found no higher level of anxiety in patients with IBS than in sufferers from other gut disease causing similar symptoms (Raymer et al 1984). Treatment by psychotherapy is often prolonged, and even when successful only provides a marginal improvement in the symptoms which the patients suffer (Svedlund et al 1983).

The possible role of diet in the pathogenesis of what modern gastroenterologists recognise as 'IBS' was first considered after reports that some patients suffered from alactasia (Weser et al 1965; Fung and Kho 1971). A recent study however, suggested that the incidence of alactasia in white gentiles with IBS was no higher than symptom-free controls from a similar background (Newcomer and McGill 1983). Furthermore many patients who may clearly be shown by biochemical tests to have alactasia remain symptom free (see Chapter 12). Alactasia, therefore, is usually considered a separate condition.

CLINICAL EXPERIENCE OF DIETARY MANAGEMENT

Numerous reports exist in the older literature of patients with abdominal symptoms finding relief by modification of their diets. As early as 1771, the King's physician Sir George Baker presented to the Royal College of Physicians a patient, Thomas Wood, 'A Miller of Billericay' whose abdominal symptoms were improved by a diet of 'sea biscuits and salt meat' (Drummond and Wilbraham 1959). Although many reports of abdominal pain and diarrhoea responding to dietary modification were made in the United States in the first half of the twentieth century (e.g. Duke 1921, 1923; Rowe 1928), this work was largely ignored by mainstream gastro-enterologists on both sides of the Atlantic, perhaps because the patients so treated were not dignified by the diagnostic label 'IBS'.

High fibre diets (in which the fibre was usually derived from wheat bran) were advocated for IBS in the late 1970s (Manning et al 1977), and were taken up with enthusiasm. Wheat fibre however, did not prove to be the answer to every patient's problems (Soltoff et al 1976; Longstreth et al 1982) and is now usually reserved for those with constipation.

During the past five years, considerable evidence has accumulated to support the suggestion that specific food intolerance may be responsible for some cases of IBS, especially those associated with diarrhoea. Cooper et al (1980) described seven cases of idiopathic diarrhoea which improved on a gluten-free diet, but in which the jejunal mucosa was normal when biopsied. Lessof et al (1980) reported a number of patients with diarrhoea which was shown by objective challenge to be caused by specific food intolerances.

Our initial study (Alun Jones et al 1982) was a search for food intolerance in 25 successive patients diagnosed on clinical grounds as having IBS: 21 agreed to follow a highly restricted diet of lamb, pears and water for one week before reintroducing other foods singly; 14 found subjective evidence of food intolerances, and were able to control their symptoms by avoiding the foods in question; 11 agreed to undergo objective challenges. In six of the latter, challenged by double blind trial on four occasions, using naso-gastric tubes with two test and two control foods, 21 out of 24 challenges were correctly identified. The other five patients received test soups, flavoured to disguise their constituents, given for four successive days on two occasions a month apart, and all were correctly identified (Alun Jones et al 1982).

We have since extended our experience of food intolerant IBS greatly (Hunter et al 1985). The foods concerned in producing symptoms in 122 patients are listed in Table 14.1. The number of foods affecting each patient varies from very few to more than 20 (Table 14.2), and those patients with multiple food intolerances are difficult to manage. However, the benefits of the successful identification of food intolerance in patients is considerable, for

Table 14.1. Percentage of patients intolerant to particular foods.

Food	%	Food	%	Food	%
Cereals		*Fruit*		Mushrooms	12
Wheat	60	Citrus	24	Parsnips	12
Corn	44	Apples	12	Tomatoes	11
Oats	34	Rhubarb	12	Cauliflower	11
Rye	30	Banana	11	Celery	11
Barley	24	Strawberries	8	Green Beans	10
Rice	15	Pineapples	8	Cucumber	10
		Pears	8	Turnip/swede	10
Dairy products		Grapes	7	Marrow	8
Milk	44	Melon	5	Beetroot	8
Cheese	39	Avocado pear	5	Peppers	6
Butter	25	Raspberries	4		
Yoghurt	24			*Miscellaneous*	
		Vegetables		Coffee	33
Fish		Onions	22	Eggs	26
White fish	10	Potatoes	20	Tea	25
Shell fish	10	Cabbage	19	Chocolate	22
Smoked fish	7	Sprouts	18	Nuts	22
		Peas	17	Preservatives	20
Meat		Carrots	15	Yeast	12
Beef	16	Lettuce	15	Sugar-beet	12
Pork	14	Leeks	15	Sugar-cane	12
Chicken	13	Broccoli	14	Alcohol	12
Lamb	11	Soya beans	13	Tap water	10
Turkey	8	Spinach	13	Saccharin	9
				Honey	2

From Hunter et al (1985), with kind permission of the authors and the publisher, Blackwell Scientific.

Table 14.2.

Intolerance of one food alone	5%
2–5 foods	28%
6–10 foods	35%
11–20 foods	17%
More than 20 foods	15%

From Hunter et al (1985), with kind permission of the authors and the publisher, Blackwell Scientific.

follow up reveals that the great majority remain well for long periods of time (Table 14.3).

There is still considerable dispute over the proportion of patients with IBS who have food intolerance. Our experience suggests that approximately 70% of those with abdominal pain and diarrhoea may be successfully managed by diet, but Bentley et al (1983) found only three patients out of a total of 19 to have food intolerances which could be objectively confirmed. This anomaly is probably related to differences in selection from a very heterogeneous group

Table 14.3. Questionnaires.

	May 1981	July 1982	December 1982
Date sent	May 1981	July 1982	December 1982
Date patients started diet	October 1979– March 1981	April 1981– May 1982	October 1979– March 1981
Length of follow-up	2–20 months	2–16 months	22–39 months
Nö. of patients	80	42	71
Replies	71 (89%)	41 (98%)	61 (86%)
No. of patients still on diet and improved	71 (100%)	41 (100%)	53 (87%)
Intolerance changed			
More foods	8 (11%)	2 (5%)	13 (25%)
Fewer foods	14 (20%)	10 (24%)	11 (21%)
Disappeared	0	0	3

From Hunter et al (1985), with kind permission of the authors and the publisher, Blackwell Scientific.

of patients. Furthermore, we consider that the diets used in their study were less than ideal, as some patients continued to eat wheat, which we have found to be the food most frequently implicated. Capsules were used to administer food in double blind trials, thus limiting challenges to a very small quantity. It seems possible that their protocol revealed subjects with immunologically mediated food allergies, but failed to identify non-atopic patients with food intolerance. These differenes between their experience and ours should not be allowed to cloud the major point at issue which is that Bentley et al (1983), like Cooper et al (1980), Lessof et al (1980), Gerrard (1984) and ourselves, confirmed objectively that patients exist whose abdominal symptoms may be reliably ascribed to food intolerance. With increasing experience, the true prevalence of food intolerance amongst patients with IBS will be determined, and it is to be hoped that this process will be aided by the development of diagnostic tests which allow an objective identification of patients suffering from this problem, and will avoid the inappropriate use of diet in patients who will not respond.

The detection of food intolerances

Many physicians develop scepticism on the subject of food intolerance because patients seize on 'food allergy' as the possible cause of all manner of persistent and unlikely symptoms. The patient may modify his own diet and it is not uncommon to encounter patients who claim to have 'food allergy' and whose symptoms are in no way alleviated by the bizarre and inadequate diets of their own devising. Nevertheless there exist patients with genuine food intolerances, and in the absence of any positive diagnostic marker for the condition it behoves the physician to recognise a complex of symptoms which suggests this possibility, and to have available a dietetic regime which will enable their accurate identification. It is well to remember that the inconveniences of diets are only justified when symptoms are both frequent and unpleasant. Patients who are mild cases of IBS do well with simple reassurance.

The patient with IBS may complain of a variety of symptoms, but those listed in Table 14.4 give a good idea of the sort of problem which is related to food intolerance. Patients suffering from abdominal pain of colonic origin, and/or diarrhoea, often associated with tiredness and headache, are most likely to be treated successfully by diet. Those with constipation do less well, and are probably best managed by increasing their intake of dietary fibre to at least 30 g per day.

The basic principle of studies of food intolerance is to provide a diet on which the patient's symptoms are relieved. When he feels *well*, and not before, foods may be tested by reintroduction one at a time. As food intolerances vary from patient to patient, the theoretical solution would be for nothing at all to be eaten, and for nutrition to be maintained parenterally. However, this is clearly too expensive and too dangerous to justify. Early studies were performed by confining patients to water alone, or to severely

Table 14.4. Analysis of presenting symptoms suffered by 122 patients subsequently found to be due to food intolerance.

Abdominal pain	73%
Diarrhoea	60%
Tiredness	42%
Headaches	38%
Constipation	22.5%
Abdominal distension	21.5%
Fluid retention	20%
Related conditions	
Migraine	11%
Atopy	10%

From Hunter et al (1985), with kind permission of the authors and the publisher, Blackwell Scientific.

limited diets such as the classic 'lamb and pears' — one meat, one fruit and spring water. These diets are unsatisfactory because they are nutritionally inadequate and because of the large number of foods which must subsequently be tested. Both these factors mean that food reintroduction must be rapid — at least two foods daily — which frequently leads to confusion and disillusionment, especially when reactions to foods are slow. If, as sometimes happens, symptoms come on only after 24–48 hours, the blame may be placed on the wrong food item.

With increasing experience of managing patients with IBS by dietary means we have established the frequency with which various foods are likely to cause problems (Table 14.1). Although any food seems to be able to cause problems in a small number of patients, the most important are cereals, dairy products, citrus fruits, beverages and food additives. Our standard exclusion diet avoids these, but permits the patient to have a nutritionally adequate diet of meat, fish, fruit and vegetables. The smaller number of foods to be reintroduced means that testing can be done slowly, which leads to greater accuracy.

If the IBS patient is not considerably improved after two weeks on the exclusion diet, it is best to tell him firmly that food intolerance is *not* the cause of his difficulties, and to forbid any further dietary manœuvres. Of course some patients with multiple intolerances may be missed in this way, but those patients are very difficult indeed to manage, and are probably better off not knowing of their condition. It is important to recheck all foods believed to provoke symptoms when testing has been completed. Some food reactions may have been coincidence (as for example when diarrhoea occurs at the time of a menstrual period) and some intolerances are very short-lived. The final diet should be checked for nutritional adequacy by a dietitian. Vitamin and calcium supplements are occasionally needed. Once the diet is established, the offending foods should be avoided as conscientiously as possible, but should be retested at six-monthly intervals to confirm that they still provoke symptoms.

A full account of the exclusion diet, for use by patients, has been published by Workman et al (1984).

It cannot be denied that an exclusion diet presents a stern challenge to the perseverence and self-discipline of most patients, who take 8–10 weeks to complete it sucessfully. However, our data on long term follow up of these patients confirm that the vast majority consider the effort well worth while (Hunter et al 1985).

MECHANISMS OF FOOD INTOLERANCE

Immunological studies

The objective demonstration of food intolerance in many patients with IBS has led to increased interest in the mechanisms by which the symptoms are provoked. In popular parlance this is clearly an example of 'food allergy' but we have yet to succeed in demonstrating a convincing immunological abnormality. Although all three of Bentley et al's (1983) patients with IBS caused by foods also suffered from atopic disease, our experience in a much larger series (Hunter et al 1985) has been that this is true of only 10% of our food-intolerant patients with IBS, which is similar to the incidence in the general population. Furthermore, skin tests (whether prick or intra-dermal) are unreliable in diagnosing food intolerances in these patients (Lehmann 1980).

Immunological studies in the laboratory have also been largely negative. In contrast to patients with asthma, eczema and urticaria, most patients with diarrhoea caused by food intolerances have normal levels of IgE (Lessof et al 1980; Alun Jones et al 1982). In double blind challenge studies we found no difference between test and control days in the circulating eosinophil count, plasma histamine, or in immune complexes in the serum. Incubation of basophils with food antigens, including milk proteins and gliadin, led to no increased release of histamine (Alun Jones et al 1982; McLaughlan et al 1983a).

In contrast, we found that the incubation with gliadin of jejunal biopsies from patients with wheat intolerance and coeliac disease led to an increased release of histamine when compared with biopsies taken from normal subjects and treated similarly. The controls had been biopsied because they were either relatives of coeliac patients, or were suffering from steatorrhoea, later shown to be of pancreatic origin (Figure 14.1) (McLaughlan et al 1983b). In view of the absence of any similar response the basophils from the same patients were treated in the same way (McLaughlan et al 1983a); these results raise the possibility of the existence of a local immune response in the jejunum of patients with food intolerant IBS. However, it could also represent a pseudo-allergic reaction (see Chapter 8). Molecules other than

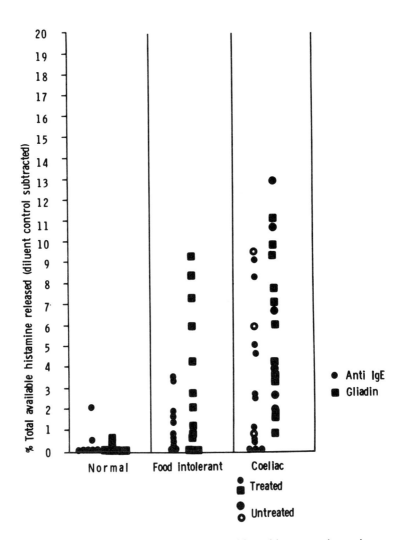

Figure 14.1. Percentage of total histamine released from biopsy specimens in response to incubation with gliadin or anti-IgE. From McLaughlan et al (1983b), with kind permission of the authors and the publisher, Medicine Publishing Foundation.

those recognised as messengers of the immune system may occupy the receptor sites on immune effector cells, causing them to release the mediators of the immune response, such as histamine. Plant lectins have been shown to be capable of this effect (Helm and Froese 1981), and it is possible that this is the role of gliadin in jejunal biopsies. This possibility requires further investigation.

Gut hormones

In view of the abnormalities of gut motility observed in IBS, the possible role of gut hormones in its pathogenesis has been examined. Many gut hormones are related to gut motility in physiological concentrations. Besterman et al (1981) performed a study in the hope that there might be characteristic hormone profile for IBS as there is for other conditions such as coeliac disease (see Chapter 13), but no significant abnormality of gut hormone release was detected. We have attempted to refine the study of gut hormones in IBS by selecting patients with food intolerant IBS and measuring gut hormone release before and after both challenge and control meals. No difference was found in the release of motilin, cholecystokinin, gastrin, secretin, insulin, GIP, enteroglucagon or neurotensin (Alun Jones et al 1984a).

Prostaglandins

The role of prostaglandins in food intolerant IBS has attracted attention. Buisseret et al (1978) reported the case of a woman who suffered diarrhoea after eating mussels but who found that she could prevent this reaction by taking the prostaglandin synthetase inhibitor ibuprofen. Objective challenge confirmed that the ingestion of mussels produced both diarrhoea and an increase in the prostaglandins (PGE_2 and $PGF_{2\alpha}$) measurable in both blood and faeces, and that ibuprofen could block these effects. A number of similar patients were also described.

In the light of this report we studied PGE_2 production in the rectum in patients with food intolerant IBS (Alun Jones et al 1982). A dialysis bag made of Visking tubing and mounted on a catheter was passed into the rectum of patients undergoing objective double blind food challenges; the bag was replaced at hourly intervals. PGE_2 was measured by radioimmunoassay. A significant increase in PGE_2 production was seen after food challenge (Figure 14.2) and in another study PGE_2 production was shown to correlate significantly wtih faecal weight (Figure 14.3). Control studies indicated that the rise in prostaglandins was not a consequence of the insertion of the dialysis bags (Alun Jones et al 1983). However, although increased PGE_2 production is the rule in patients with diarrhoea, it is not universal amongst patients, and those with the symptom of abdominal pain alone frequently show very little change in PGE_2 after food challenges. What is more, it is our experience that many patients derive little benefit from prostaglandin inhibitors. Thus we believe that the release of prostaglandins is likely to be a secondary phenomenon, rather than the true cause of the condition.

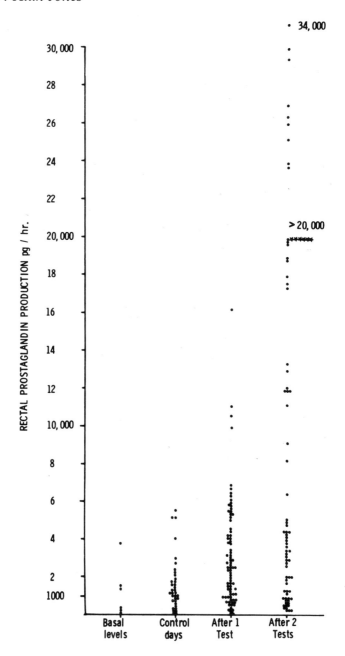

Figure 14.2. Individual levels of rectal prostaglandin production in response to food challenge. From Alun Jones et al (1982), with kind permission of the authors and the editor of *Lancet*.

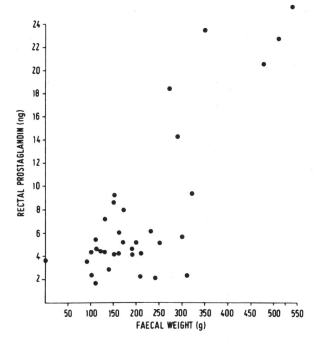

Figure 14.3. Relation between prostaglandin level and wet faecal weight. From Alun Jones et al (1982), with kind permission of the authors and the editor of *Lancet*.

Role of antibiotics

Many women with IBS report that their problems begin after gynaecological operations (Fielding 1977) and we performed a study to assess prospectively the importance of hysterectomy in the pathogenesis of IBS (Alun Jones et al 1984b). In an initial study, the course of 113 patients who underwent hysterectomy with or without prophylactic metronidazole was followed. All had been free of gut symptoms pre-operatively, but 13 had developed the symptoms of IBS when reviewed 6–8 weeks later; 12 of these were from the 74 who had received prophylactic metronidazole, while only one was from the 39 who had not.

A double blind trial was then set up using metronidazole or placebo suppositories as prophylaxis at the time of hysterectomy. If infection occurred it was treated appropriately by other antibiotics. An analysis of 100 patients (Table 14.5) again supported the aetiological role of antibiotic usage in the development of IBS. Seven out of the 62 patients who had received antibiotics developed the syndrome, but none of the 20 who did not receive antibiotics developed IBS.

Faecal flora

In view of the relationship between antibiotics and surgery, we have undertaken studies on the faecal flora of patients with IBS (Bayliss et al

Table 14.5. Post-operative IBS in previously asymptomatic patients having metronidazole prophylaxis or placebo with hysterectomy, and those having other antibiotics in addition.

	Patients	Irritable bowel syndrome
Metronidazole alone	26	2
Placebo alone	20	0
Metronidazole + other antibiotics	14	1
Placebo + other antibiotics	22	4

From Alun Jones et al (1984b), with kind permission of the authors and the editor of *Journal of Obstetrics and Gynaecology*.

Table 14.6. Excretion of aerobic bacteria in faeces (viable bacteria/g dry weight faeces).

	n	Samples	Mean	Range
Patients	6	30	2.2×10^9	2.9×10^7 to 1.1×10^{10}
Controls	6	6	9.8×10^7	3.9×10^6 to 2.7×10^8

From Bayliss et al (1984), with kind permission of the authors and the editor of *Proceedings of the Nutrition Society*.

1984). Six patients, well on a wheat free diet, were found to have high faecal counts of aerobic bacteria compared to age and sex matched controls (Table 14.6). In two patients increases of two orders of magnitude in the count of aerobic bacteria were seen after food challenge (Figure 14.4), although counts of anaerobic bacteria did not change and were comparable to those of the controls. Further studies on faecal bacteria are in progress.

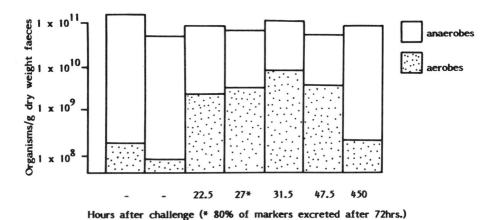

Figure 14.4. Effect of wheat challenge on faecal flora.

CONCLUSION

Objective food intolerances have been demonstrated by a number of independent workers to occur in some patients with IBS, and at present the trial of an exclusion diet should be considered in all patients with unexplained colonic pain or diarrhoea. The mechanisms of this food intolerance remain obscure, but it seems probable that with their further clarification a new condition will be defined, which, like alactasia, may be regarded as a separate entity, distinguishable from the Irritable Bowel Syndrome.

REFERENCES

Almy T P & Tulin M (1947) Alterations in colonic function in man under stress: experimental production of changes simulating irritable bowel colon. *Gastroenterology* **8**: 616–626.

Alun Jones V, McLaughlan P, Shorthouse M, Workman E & Hunter J O (1982) Food intolerance: a major factor in the pathogenesis of irritable bowel syndrome. *Lancet* **2**: 1115–1117.

Alun Jones V, McLaughlan P, Shorthouse M, Workman E & Hunter J O (1983) Food intolerance, prostaglandins, and irritable bowel syndrome. *Lancet* **1**: 124.

Alun Jones V, Hunter J O, Adrian T E & Bloom S R (1984a). Gut hormones in food intolerant irritable bowel syndrome. *Abstracts of the 12th International Congress of Gastroenterology*, 526.

Alun Jones V, Wilson A J, Hunter J O & Robinson R E (1984b). The aetiological role of antibiotic prophylaxis with hysterectomy in irritable bowel syndrome. *Journal of Obstetrics and Gynaecology* **5** (Suppl. 1): s22–s23.

Bayliss C E, Houston A P, Alun Jones V, Hishon S & Hunter J O (1984) Microbiological studies on food intolerance. *Proceedings of the Nutrition Society* **43**: 16a.

Bentley S J, Pearson D J & Rix K J B (1983) Food hypersensitivity in irritable bowel syndrome *Lancet* **2**: 295–297.

Besterman H S, Sarson D L, Rambaud J C et al (1981). Gut hormone responses in the irritable bowel syndrome. *Digestion* **21**: 219–224.

Buisseret P D, Youlten L J F, Heinzelman D I & Lessof M H (1978) Prostaglandin-synthesis inhibitors in prophylaxis of food intolerance. *Lancet* **1**: 906–908.

Burns T W (1980) Colonic motility in the irritable bowel syndrome. *Archives of Internal Medicine* **140**: 247–251.

Cooper B T, Holmes G K T, Ferguson R et al (1980) Gluten-sensitive diarrhoea without evidence of coeliac disease. *Gastroenterology* **79**: 801–806.

Corbett C L, Thomas S, Read N W et al (1981) Electrochemical detector for breath hydrogen determination. Measurement of small bowel transit time in normal subjects and patients with irritable bowel syndrome. *Gut* **22**: 836–840.

Drossman D A, Powell D W & Sessions J T (1977) The irritable bowel syndrome. *Gastroenterology* **73**: 811–822.

Drummond J C & Wilbraham A (1959) *The Englishman's Food*. London: Jonathan Cape.

Duke W D (1921) Food allergy as a cause of abdominal pain. *Archives of Internal Medicine* **28**: 151–165.

Duke W D (1923) Food allergy as a cause of illness. *Journal of the American Medical Association* **81**: 886–889.

Fielding J F (1977) The irritable bowel syndrome part 1; clinical spectrum. *Clinics in Gastroenterology* **6**: 607–622.

Fung W-P & Kho K M (1971) The importance of milk intolerance in patients presenting with chronic (nervous) diarrhoea. *Australian and New Zealand Journal of Medicine* **1**: 374–376.

Gerrard J W (1984) Food intolerance. *Lancet* **2**: 413.

Harvey R F, Salih S Y & Read A E (1983) Organic and functional disorders in 2000 gastroenterology out-patients. *Lancet* **1**: 632–634.

Heaton K W (1983). IBS; still in search of its identity. *British Medical Journal* **287**: 852–853.

Helm R M & Froese A (1981) Binding of the receptors for IgE by various lectins. *International Archives of Allergy and Applied Immunology* **65**: 81–84.

Hunter J O, Workman E & Alun Jones V (1985) The role of diet of the management of irritable bowel syndrome. In Gibson P R & Jewell D P (eds) *Topics in Gastroenterology*, Vol. 12 Oxford: Blackwell Scientific. (In press.)

Lehman C W (1980) A double blind study of sub-lingual provocation food testing: a study of its efficacy. The leukocytic food allergy test: a study of its reliability and reproducibility. Effect of diet and sub-lingual food drops on this test. *Annals of Allergy* **45**: 144–158.

Lessof M H, Wraight D G, Merrett T G, Merrett J & Buisseret P D (1980) Food allergy and intolerance in 100 patients. *Quarterly Journal of Medicine* **195**: 259–271.

Longstreth G F, Fox D D, Youkeles L, Forsythe A B & Wolochon A (1981) Psyllium therapy in the irritable bowel syndrome: a double blind trial. *Annals of Internal Medicine* **95**: 53–56.

McLaughlan P, Easter G B, Hunter J O & Coombs R R A (1983a) Histamine release from blood basophils. In *The Second Fisons Food Allergy Workshop*, pp 52–53. Oxford: Medicine Publishing Foundation.

McLaughlan P, Hunter J O, Easter G B et al (1983b) Histamine release in vitro from the jejunal mucosa following challenge with gliadin and also anti-IgE. In *The Second Fisons Food Allergy Workshop*, pp 7–9. Oxford: Medicine Publishing Foundation.

Manning A P, Heaton K W, Uglow P & Harvey R F (1977) Wheat fibre and the irritable bowel syndrome: a controlled trial. *Lancet* **2**: 417–418.

Newcomer A D & McGill D B (1983) Irritable bowel syndrome. Role of lactose deficiency. *Mayo Clinic Proceedings* **58**: 339–341.

Raymer D, Weininger O & Hamilton J R (1984) Psychological problems in children with abdominal pain. *Lancet* **2**: 439–440.

Rowe A H (1928) Food allergy. Its manifestations, diagnosis and treatment. *JAMA* **91**: 1623–1631.

Silverberg M & Daum F (1979). IBS in children and adolescents. *Practical Gastroenterology* **2**: 25.

Snape W J L Jr, Carlson G N & Cohen S (1976) Colonic myoelectric activity in IBS. *Gastroenterology* **70**: 326–330.

Scoltoff J, Krag B, Gudmand-Hoyer E, Kristensen E, Wulff H R (1976) A double blind trial of the effect of wheat bran on symptoms of irritable bowel syndrome. *Lancet* **1**: 270–272.

Svedlund J, Sjodin I, Ottosson J-O & Dotevall G (1983) Controlled study of psychotherapy in irritable bowel syndrome. *Lancet* **2**: 589–591.

Taylor I, Darby C & Hammond P (1978) Comparison of recto-sigmoid myoelectrical activity in the irritable colon syndrome during relapses and remissions. *Gut* **19**: 923–929.

Thompson W G & Heaton K W (1980) Functional bowel disorders of apparently healthy people. *Gastroenterology* **79**: 283–288.

Weser E, Rubin W, Ross L & Sleisenger M H (1965) Lactose deficiency in patients with the 'irritable bowel syndrome'. *New England Journal of Medicine* **273**: 1070–1075.

Whorwell P J, Clouter C & Smith C L (1981) Oesophageal motility in the irritable bowel syndrome. *British Medical Journal* **282**: 1101–1102.

Workman E, Hunter J O & Alun Jones V (1984) *The Allergy Diet*. London: Dunitz.

Young S J, Alpers D H, Norlan C C & Woodruff R A (1976) Psychiatric illness and the irritable bowel syndrome. *Gastroenterology* **70**: 162–166.

Chapter 15
The Dietary Management of Crohn's Disease

J. O. Hunter

Crohn's disease is an unpleasant chronic granulomatous inflammation, which may affect any part of the gut from mouth to anus, but which predominantly involves the terminal ileum and the colon. Extra-intestinal manifestations such as anaemia, arthritis, uveitis and abscesses are common, and medical treatment involving corticosteroids, immunosuppressive drugs and antibiotics is often ineffective. Many patients require extensive gastro-intestinal surgery. Although it may affect any age group, Crohn's disease is commonest in young adults; its cause is unknown (Sachar et al 1980).

Early reports of links between Crohn's disease and diet (e.g. Rowe and Uyeyama 1953) have been regarded by gastro-enterologists as curiosities rather than as a basis for the rational management of the disease (Korelitz 1980), despite reports published in the 1970s of improvement of patients with Crohn's disease following total parenteral nutrition (TPN) (Fischer et al 1973; Reilly et al 1976; Driscoll and Rosenberg 1978; Mullen et al 1978; Dickinson et al 1980). The mechanism for this improvement was unknown and was generally ascribed to 'total bowel rest', rather than to any beneficial effect of avoiding specific foods.

Our interest in the role of diet arose with the case of a girl of 18 who presented with persistent diarrhoea and who was in good general health. Examination, including sigmoidoscopy, was normal and as it was thought that she had irritable bowel syndrome she was started on the elimination diet which was then our standard management (Alun Jones et al 1982). A routine rectal biopsy, however, showed characteristic changes of Crohn's disease. She was unwilling then to start corticosteroid therapy as her diarrhoea had abated and she wished to continue to explore diet as a means of controlling her symptoms. She discovered that wheat provoked her symptoms, and has now been well on a wheat-free diet for over four years. A further biopsy confirmed the diagnosis of Crohn's disease, which was limited to her rectum as radiological studies were normal. An objective challenge was made with wheat; this confirmed the association of this food with her diarrhoea and a subsequent jejunal biopsy showed that she did not have coeliac disease.

In the light of this woman's improvement, and in view of the known effects of food in other gastro-intestinal diseases such as coeliac disease (Chapter 13), cow's milk intolerance (Chapter 12) and the irritable bowel syndrome (Chapter 14), it seemed quite likely that food intolerance might underlie the success of TPN in Crohn's disease, and this led to a determined evaluation of dietary therapy for the condition.

METHODS OF INDUCING REMISSION

In some patients with fairly mild Crohn's disease it may be possible to achieve remission of symptoms by means of exclusion diets based on those used in the management of irritable bowel syndrome (Chapter 14). Most patients with Crohn's disease, however, are severely undernourished, and restricted oral diets are not suitable.

TPN is of proven value in the management of active Crohn's disease (Fischer et al 1973; Reilly et al 1976; Driscoll and Rosenberg 1978; Mullen et al 1978; Dickinson et al 1980) (see also Chapter 16) but has the disadvantages that it is invasive and highly expensive, not least because of the need for supervision by a specialised nutrition team to ensure the meticulous care which is required to prevent complications such as infection. Elemental diets have the advantage of being simple, safe and comparatively cheap (currently at £15 per patient per day, against £50 for TPN). A number of reports have now appeared claiming excellent results for elemental diets in gaining remission in active Crohn's disease (Morin et al 1982; O'Morain et al 1980, 1983, 1984).

Randomised trial of elemental diet and TPN

To decide whether TPN or elemental diet (ED) was the treatment of choice for achieving remission in our patients, we set up a randomised study. Successive patients admitted to Addenbrooke's Hospital, Cambridge, with active Crohn's disease were eligible for inclusion if the Crohn's Disease Activity Index (CDAI) (National Co-operative Crohn's Disease Study 1979) was greater than 150, and if there was no evidence to suggest a surgical complication of the disease, such as intestinal obstruction, abscess, or major fistula.

Patients were randomly allocated to receive either TPN or elemental diet. TPN was given by tunnelled line into the subclavian vein by an infra-clavicular approach. The calorie requirement of the patients was calculated in relation to body weight, modified to take account of the presence of Crohn's disease (basal metabolic rate [BMR]$+0$–10%) and of starvation if present (BMR-0–10%) and of activity about the ward (BMR$+40\%$). Most patients received between 1.4 and 2.1 times the estimated resting energy expenditure depending on the desired repletion of energy stores. Between 0.17 and 0.3 g of nitrogen per kg were given depending on the extent of nitrogen depletion. Electrolytes given were: sodium 90 mmol, potassium 80 mmol, calcium 7.5 mmol, magnesium 7.5 mmol, phosphorus 30 mmol with additional sodium and potassium if required, and trace elements according to the American Medical Association recommendations (American Medical Association 1979). All vitamins were included except B_{12}, K and D (the two former being given by intra-muscular injection). The total comprised a volume of 2.5 – 3.5 l per day, and was prepared under sterile conditions by the pharmacy at Addenbrooke's Hosptial, or by Travenol Ltd., Thetford.

The elemental diet used was E028, manufactured by Scientific Hospital Supplies Ltd., Liverpool. Each 100 g box was given with 650 ml of distilled or spring water. The mixture was pleasantly palatable and naso-gastric tubes were not necessary. The recommended daily intake of E028 for an adult is 500 g, but many patients are unable to tolerate this quantity at first. Patients were therefore started on 300 g daily, building up to 500 g after 2–3 days.

Patients allocated to either regime were allowed to drink spring or distilled water freely, but took nothing else by mouth. All medication for Crohn's disease was tailed off and stopped during the first week. Patients were not confined to bed.

From day seven the CDAI was recalculated daily. When the CDAI fell below 150 the patient was considered to be in remission. If the CDAI remained above 150 on day 14 the treatment was considered to have failed.

Details of patients admitted to the trial are given in Table 15.1. Two (1TPN, 1E028) were found to have previously unsuspected surgical complica-

Table 15.1. Clinical details of patients (*n*=36) in controlled trial of TPN and ED.

Age (years)	<20	21–30	31–40	41–50	>50
TPN	6	6	4	1	2
ED	2	5	5	4	1

Sex	Male	Female
TPN	4	15
ED	5	12

Length of history (months)	<12	13–24	25–36	37–48	49–60	>61
TPN	9	2	3	1	0	4
ED	3	3	0	1	0	10

Area of disease	Ileal	Colonic	Ileo-colonic	Old colectomy
TPN	6	5	8	3
ED	7	5	5	1

Table 15.2. Results of controlled trial of TPN and ED. No significant difference was discovered between the two groups. However the fall in CDAI in both groups is significant (*p*<0.01, paired student's *t* test).

	TPN ($\bar{x}$ ± s.d.)	ED ($\bar{x}$ ± s.d.)
No. recruited	19	17
Withdrawals	3	1
Unable to comply	0	3
Failure of method to induce remission in 14 days	2	2(NS)
Days to remission	9.0 ± 3.08	8.8 ± 2.56 (NS)
	(*n*=16)	(*n*=13)
Mean pre-trial CDAI	267.2 ± 94.2	247.7 ± 59.0 (NS)
Mean pre-trial albumin (g/L)	28.3 ± 6.99	29.3 ± 6.25 (NS)
Mean pre-trial orosomucoid (%)	213 ± 79	180 ± 68 (NS)
Mean post-trial CDAI	114.9 ± 84.9	118.7 ± 82.7 (NS)
Mean post-trial albumin (g/L)	28.5 ± 6.93	31.2 ± 4.85 (NS)
Mean post-trial orosomucoid (%)	205 ± 74	162 ± 50 (NS)

CDAI = Crohn's Disease Activity Index; NS = not significant

tions; one woman was found to be suffering from an enteropathy produced by oral gold salts for rheumatoid arthritis (TPN) and another, with severe uveitis, was also being managed by the opthalmologists who were unwilling for her steroids to be withdrawn (TPN). Although the majority of patients found no difficulty in drinking E028, three declared that it was unpalatable and refused to continue. Of the patients who persisted with E028 for 14 days, only two failed to go into remission but both subsequently settled for TPN. It was interesting that as the trial proceeded, and as nurses on the ward realised the improvement that could be achieved with elemental diet, patients ceased to find E028 unpalatable. It seems probable that earlier patients might also have persevered if the same degree of support offered to later patients had been available.

The results of TPN were very similar. Only two patients failed to go into remission after 14 days. No difference was detected between the two groups in the number of days required to reach remission, the change of CDAI, erythrocyte sedimentation rate (ESR) and serum albumin levels (Table 15.2).

Thus no significant difference was found between the two treatments, both of which were highly successful. In view of the greater simplicity, safety and cheapness of elemental diet we now consider this to be the treatment of choice, although patients who fail to go into remission may still be considered for subsequent TPN (Alun Jones et al 1985b).

Food reintroduction: identification of specific food intolerances

During the period of artificial feeding all medication for Crohn's disease is tailed off. This is to ensure that any remission is indeed related to food withdrawal and to prevent the masking of subsequent reaction when food testing begins.

When the patients are symptom-free they are instructed to reintroduce one new food into their diets each day following the order shown in Table 15.3, which withholds those foods most likely to cause difficulty until later, in the hope of avoiding reactions when the diet is very limited. The elemental diet is used as a nutritional supplement during the early days of this phase.

Patients are asked to keep a diary record of all foods eaten and the time at which any symptoms, such as abdominal pain and diarrhoea, occur. If a reaction is provoked the process of reintroduction is interrupted and only foods known to be safe are eaten until symptoms clear. Once a food has been tested and found not to provoke symptoms it may be eaten freely thereafter. Foods which cause symptoms were avoided and tested again some weeks later to confirm the reaction. When food testing is complete the resulting diet is analysed for nutritional adequacy (Workman et al 1984).

MAINTENANCE OF REMISSION

Controlled trial of diets

Although most reports have suggested that the majority of patients in remission on TPN or ED relapse promptly when they restart normal eating

Table 15.3. Order of food reintroduction of foods for patients with Crohn's disease. The list is based on the frequency with which foods provoke symptoms.

1. Chicken	21. Potatoes	41. White bread
2. Pears	22. Butter	42. Courgettes or marrow
3. Rice	23. Eggs	43. Soya beans
4. Carrots	24. Coffee beans	44. Cabbage
5. White fish	25. Leeks	45. Oats
6. Runner beans	26. Cane sugar	46. Rhubarb
7. Beef	27. White wine	47. Instant coffee
8. Peas	28. Oranges	48. Honey
9. Turkey	29. Brussel sprouts	49. Melon
10. Tap water	30. Beet sugar	50. Celery
11. Banana	31. Wheat	51. Lemon
12. Milk	32. Onion	52. Olive oil
13. Tomatoes	33. Parsnips	53. Turnip or swede
14. Tea	34. Cheddar cheese	54. Yoghurt
15. Cauliflower	35. Mushrooms	55. Broccoli
16. Apple	36. Corn	56. Rye bread
17. Lamb	37. Spinach	57. Monosodium glutamate
18. Lettuce	38. Grapefruit	58. Prawns or shrimps
19. Pork	39. Plain chocolate	59. Saccharin tablets
20. Yeast tablets	40. Grapes	

and require continuing corticosteroids (Hanauer et al 1984; Ostro et al 1984), a number of patients with Crohn's disease are known to enjoy spontaneous remissions (National Co-operative Crohn's Disease Study 1979). We were concerned that the benefit apparent in our patients might possibly be a long term effect of the previous artificial feeding, and not necessarily the consequence of the search for food intolerances. A controlled trial was therefore set up in patients who had settled satisfactorily after either TPN or ED. They were randomly assigned to follow the regime for the detection of food intolerances which has been outlined above (FI), or the unrefined carbohydrate, fibre-rich diet (UCFR) which has been suggested as an adjunct to conventional medical management of patients with Crohn's disease, who have undergone gastro-intestinal surgery (Heaton et al 1979). Patients were followed up in the out-patients clinic for six months, and were seen by the dietitian as often as was thought necessary to provide adequate guidance and encouragement in following their diets. They were also seen each month by a physician who objectively assessed the activity of their disease without knowing which dietary regime they were following. Patients whose CDAI rose above 150 were considered treatment failures.

It was planned to include 40 patients in this study but because those on the fibre-rich diet relapsed so rapidly it was considered unethical to continue after the time when 20 patients had been enrolled. Their clinical details are given in Table 15.4. Eight patients on the fibre-rich diet relapsed within the first two months — some within a few days of restarting normal eating (Figure 15.1).

Table 15.4. Clinical details of 20 patients in out-patient trial of diet in the prolongation of remission.

Age (years)	<19	20–29	30–39	40–49	>50
UCFR	1	3	3	3	0
FI	2	4	2	2	0

Length of history (months)	<12	13–24	25–26	37–48	49–60	>60
UCFR	2	2	2	0	1	3
FI	3	0	3	1	2	1

Area of disease	Ileum	Terminal ileum	Colon	Rectum
UCFR	2	10	4	0
FI	4	7	10	2

Previous management	New patient	Steroids	Sulphasalazine	Surgery	Azathioprine	Antibiotics
UCFR	1	9	7	3	2	2
FI	4	5	4	1	0	1

Sex: 9 women and 1 man in both groups. Method of achieving remission: TPN 13, ED 7.

Table 15.5. Results of controlled trial of diet in prolongation of remission.

	UCFR ($\bar{x} \pm$ s.d.)	FI ($\bar{x} \pm$ s.d.)
No. recruited	10	10
Withdrawals	0	0
Relapsing before six months	10	3
	($p < 0.05$, Fisher's exact test)	
Mean pre-trial ESR	26 ± 24.0	37.9 ± 21.7 (NS)
Mean pre-trial orosomucoid (%)	232.5 ± 68.2	236.1 ± 89.9 (NS)
Mean time to relapse (months)	1.375 ± 1.74	2.75 ± 1.98
Mean ESR at relapse	30.8 ± 25.7	41.3 ± 28.04
Mean orosomucoid at relapse (%)	220.5 ± 66.9	230 ± 124.89

FI patients in remission for 6 months

	Initial	3 months	6 months
ESR	37.9 ± 21.7	16.1 ± 8.8*	16.2 ± 12.5*
Orosomucoid (%)	232.5 ± 68.2	138.3 ± 36.6*	140 ± 41.5*

*$p < 0.05$, Student's t test.

Two remained well for longer, but all had relapsed by six months. Although two patients in the other group failed to grasp the principles of the search for food intolerances and never achieved a diet on which they were symptom free, seven remained well after six months. The difference between the two groups is significant ($p < 0.05$, Fisher's Exact Test). Detailed results are given in Table 15.5.

Thus the prolonged remission seen in these patients is a consequence of the discovery and avoidance of foods of which the patient is intolerant and not merely a prolonged benefit of artificial feeding (Alun Jones et al 1984).

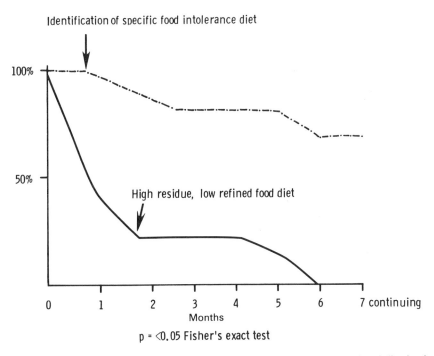

Figure 15.1. Percentage of patients remaining well in randomised study of diet in the prolongation of remission in Crohn's disease.

Overall clinical experience

These dietary manipulations form the basis of a therapeutic strategy for the long term management of Crohn's disease. Remission is at first achieved by elemental diet or occasionally TPN; it is then prolonged by the avoidance of specific foods which vary from patient to patient. This technique has become the standard management of patients with active Crohn's disease presenting at our clinic. Only those in whom the disease is inactive or those who suffer surgical complications are considered unsuitable for dietary treatment, although it is clearly necessary that patients should be able and willing to co-operate with the regime.

Up to the end of September 1984 a total of 77 patients had been started on this management. These represented a broad spectrum of Crohn's disease whose clinical features, including the duration of the disease and the extent of involvement of the gut, are well representative of the condition (Table 15.6).

Thirteen patients have been unable satisfactorily to complete the regime for the detection of food intolerances and were thus unable to establish a diet on which they remained symptom free. This was not only because they were

Table 15.6. Clinical details of patients with Crohn's disease undergoing dietary management.

No. of patients	24 male
	53 female
Age range	16–65 years
	(mean 35.5)
Length of history	0–20 years
	(mean 6 years)
Extent of disease	
Oral	1
Jejunal	6
Ileal	20
Terminal ileal	53
Colonic	48
Rectum	11
Previous treatment	
Corticosteroids	47
Sulphasalazine	31
Azathioprine	10
Long-term antibiotics	10
Surgery	29
New patient	17

unable or unwilling to persevere with diet, although seven patients did come into that category, usually because of pressure from sceptical members of their families. Three patients found so many foods to provoke symptoms that the resulting diet was nutritionally inadequate. Despite a return to conventional medical management all three have since undergone major colonic surgery. Finally, three men relapsed dramatically in the early stages of food reintroduction and all underwent emergency surgery. Because of this we now ask patients with severe Crohn's disease to reintroduce the first few foods under close observation in the hospital, and delay the introduction of foods known to cause difficulty until late in the food reintroduction phase.

Sixty-four patients have successfully completed the food testing and have remained well on diet alone. The numbers of foods to which they were

Table 15.7. Subjective food intolerances reported by patients who established a diet on which they remained symptom free.

No. of foods	No. of patients
Nil	5
1	11
2	6
3	10
4	8
5	3
6	5
7	5
8	3
9	3
>10	5

intolerant, and the foods involved are shown in Tables 15.7 and 15.8. These include patients with extensive Crohn's disease of the colon and the small intestine, including the terminal ileum, but we have had little experience of patients with severe anal disease. Extra-intestinal problems such as arthritis, uveitis and aphthous oral ulceration have cleared in a highly satisfactory manner. As perhaps might be foreseen, the diet has had no effect on pre-existing recto-vaginal and enteric fistulae, nor on fibrous intestinal strictures, although narrowing of the terminal ileum produced by inflamma-

Table 15.8. Foods reported by patients to have been responsible for provoking their symptoms.

Wheat	28	Beef ⎫ Rice ⎬	5
Dairy products	24	Tea	4
Brassicas	16	Fish	3
Maize (corn)	12	Onions	2
Yeast ⎫ Tomatoes ⎬	11	Chicken ⎫ Barley	
Citrus fruits ⎫ Eggs ⎬	10	Rye Turkey	
Tap water ⎫ Coffee ⎬ Banana	8	Additives ⎬ Alcohol Chocolate	1
Potatoes ⎫ Lamb ⎬ Pork	7	Shellfish Swede ⎭	

Table 15.9. Changes in ESR and serum orosomucoid concentrations over 24 months in 64 patients successfully establishing a diet.

	ESR		Orosomucoid	
	Mean ± s.d.	No. of patients*	Mean ± s.d. (%)	No. of patients*
Before start of dietary management	34.8±25.6	43	215.7±86.0	41
After induction of remission	31.6±24.6	33	185±77.2	35
0 – 6 months	24.8±18.7¶	52	156.3±55.7†	51
7 – 12 months	19.1±13.1†	29	147±62.8†	25
13 – 18 months	14.4±12.6†	15	135±39.9†	15
19 – 24 months	15.9±15.8‡	12	139±44.4†	12

*Refers to those patients for whom data were available.
†$p < 0.01$, ‡$p < 0.02$, ¶$p < 0.05$, compared to value before start of dietary management (Student's t test).

tion and oedema has been seen to resolve on radiographs (Figure 15.2). In all cases an adequate state of nutrition has been achieved. Indicators of systemic inflammation such as the ESR and serum orosomucoid level have returned to normal in most patients (Table 15.9) and repeat radiographs have often shown striking improvements (Figures 15.2, 15.3).

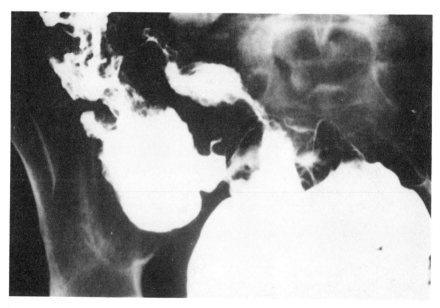

Figure 15.2. (a) CW: A barium follow through examination on 28.7.82 shows a narrowed irregular and ulcerated terminal ileum.

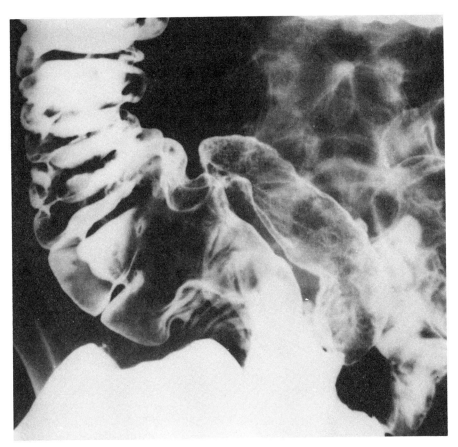

Figure 15.2. (b) A pneumocolon on 11.2.83 demonstrates normal distension of the terminal ileum with some fibrotic lines, but no active ulceration.

Nine of the 64 patients have since relapsed. In two, pre-existing terminal ileal strictures caused subacute obstruction and were resected. In retrospect, early surgery might have been a more appropiate treatment than diet. A further two patients found the restrictions of the diet irksome and asked to restart corticosteroids in order to eat freely. One patient with wheat intolerance suffered a severe relapse after remaining well for 36 months and it was later discovered that his bakery had started to include wheat flour in its rye bread. Although he previously had terminal ileal disease, he developed a total Crohn's colitis and a rectal abscess which only settled with prolonged TPN, corticosteroids and surgical drainage. Three patients relapsed for no obvious reason, although in two of them this followed a bout of gastro-enteritis. One man developed cardiac arrhythmias and proved to have myocardial sarcoidosis requiring treatment with corticosteroids.

Four patients have been lost to follow up (they were well up to 9, 11, 19 and 22 months respectively); fifty-one remain in remission on diet alone (15 for

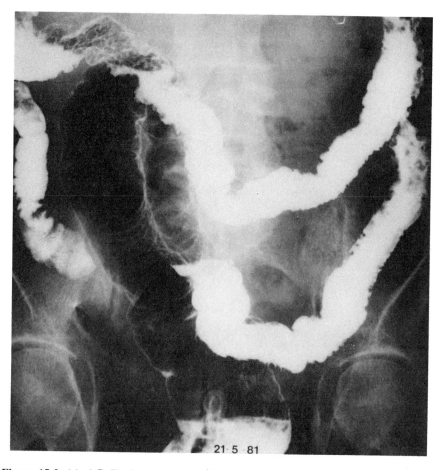

Figure 15.3. (a) AC: Barium enema on 21.5.81 demonstrates widespread ulceration, particularly in the descending and transverse colon. The recto-sigmoid is relatively spared.

more than 2 years, the longest for 51 months); three have succeeded in becoming pregnant, and numerous patients with long experience of the orthodox management of Crohn's disease and its side effects have emphasised how well they feel on diet (Alun Jones et al 1985a).

The most informative assessment of the value of diet in these patients is provided by the overall relapse rates (Table 15.10). Patients who are successful in establishing a satisfactory diet have an average relapse rate of less than 10% per annum over the next three years. This is comparable with the recurrence rate after successful surgery (Fielding et al 1972; Lee and

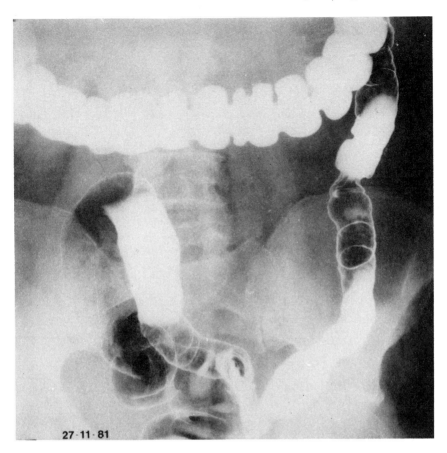

27-11-81

Figure 15.3. (b) Repeat enema on 27.11.81 shows a normal colon with no ulceration and return to normal of the haustral pattern.

Papaiannou 1980). It would be wrong to draw firm conclusions from a comparison between this work and other reports of the treatment of Crohn's disease as patient selection may vary and the enthusiasm with which they are treated may influence their progress. However, it helps to put results of dietary management into perspective to realise that in the European Co-operative Crohn's Study (Malchow et al 1984), the percentage of patients with acute Crohn's disease, who remained in remission after two years treatment with corticosteroids, was less than 40%. The equivalent figure for our patients is nearly 65%. If we consider only patients who were successful in

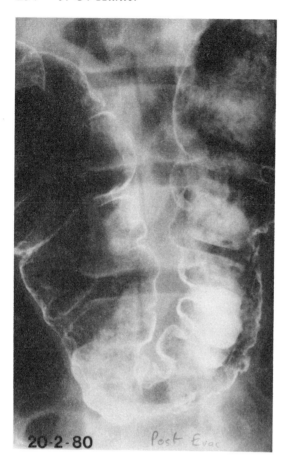

20-2-80   *Post Evac*

Figure 15.3. (c) CC: Barium enema on 20.2.80 shows an abnormal segment of distal transverse colon with obliteration of haustral markings and ulceration.

establishing a satisfactory diet, the percentage still in remission at two years is much higher, at 80%. It is possible, of course, that patients who are successful in dietary studies suffer a less severe form of the disease and certainly the overall figures for subsequent surgery in our series (10 out of 13 in those who failed to establish a diet; three out of 64 in those who succeeded) would fit with such an interpretation. However, it could equally be argued that the benefits of diet are such that they are the cause of the reduction in the need for surgery. Clearly a controlled trial of diet and orthodox management is necessary to establish the true place of dietary management amongst the various options available.

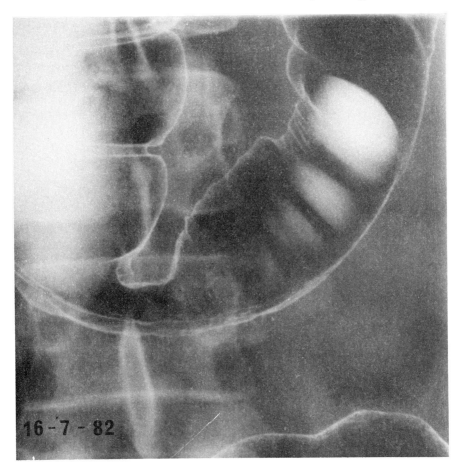

Figure 15.3. (d) Repeat enema on 16.7.82 shows a normal mucosa in this area.

CONCLUSION

Dietary manipulation represents a therapeutic strategy for the long-term management of Crohn's disease, whose results would seem to compare favourably with orthodox treatment without carrying the same risk of side effects. Further controlled trials are necessary finally to establish its value in relationship to other established lines of treatment. Food intolerance may be a factor in the aetiology of Crohn's disease or could be a consequence of it. Research into the mechanisms which link foods to symptoms may eventually allow successful treatment involving neither drugs, surgery nor restrictive diets.

Table 15.10. Overall relapse rates (Bradford Hill 1977) in patients successfully establishing a diet.

Time span after treatment (months)	Number well at beginning of time span	Number lost to follow up during time span	Number well observed for only part of time span	Number exposed to risk of relapse during time span	Number relapsing during time span	Proportion relapsing during time span	Proportion remaining well during time span	Proportion remaining well from start of treatment to end of each time span
0 – 6	64 (77)	–	19	54.5 (67.5)	2 (15)	0.036 (0.222)	0.964 (0.778)	0.964 (0.778)
7 – 12	43	1	10	37.5	5	0.135	0.865	0.834 (0.673)
13 – 18	27	–	5	24.5	1	0.041	0.959	0.800 (0.645)
19 – 24	21	2	6	17	–	0.00	1.0	0.800 (0.645)
25 – 30	13	–	2	12	–	0.00	1.0	0.800 (0.645)
31 – 36	11	–	2	10	1	0.1	0.9	0.720 (0.581)
27 – 42	8	–	4	6	–	0.00	1.0	0.720 (0.581)
43 – 48	4	–	3	2.5	–	0.00	1.0	0.720 (0.581)
49 – 54	1	–	–	1	–	0.00	1.0	0.720 (0.581)

Figures in parentheses give values corrected to include patients unable to establish dietary control.

REFERENCES

Alun Jones V, McLaughlan P, Shorthouse M, Workman E & Hunter J O (1982) Food intolerance: A major factor in the pathogenesis of irritable bowel syndrome. *Lancet* **2**: 1115–1117.

Alun Jones V, Dickinson R J, Workman E, Freeman A H & Hunter J O (1984) Controlled trial of diet in the management of Crohn's disease. *Abstracts of the 12th International Congress of Gastroenterology*: 943.

Alun Jones V, Dickinson R J, Workman E et al (1985a) The management of Crohn's disease by diet. Submitted for publication.

Alun Jones V, Dickinson R J & Hunter J O (1985b) Controlled trial of elemental diet and total parenteral nutrition in the induction of remission in Crohn's disease. In preparation.

American Medical Association Department of Food and Nutrition (1979) Guidelines for essential trace element preparations for parenteral use. *JAMA* **241**: 2051–2053.

Bradford Hill A (1977) *A Short Textbook of Medical Statistics*, pp 205–213. London: Hodder and Stoughton.

Dickinson R J, Ashton M G, Axon A T et al (1980) Controlled trial of intravenous hyperalimentation and total bowel rest as an adjunct to the routine therapy of acute colitis. *Gastroenterology* **79**: 1199–1204.

Driscoll R H Jr & Rosenberg I H (1978) Total parenteral nutrition in inflammatory bowel disease. *Medical Clinics of North America* **62**: 185–201.

Fielding J F, Cooke W T & Williams J A (1972) The incidence of recurrence in Crohn's disease. *Surgery, Gynecology and Obstetrics* **134**: 467.

Fischer J E, Foster J S, Abel R M, Abbott W M & Ryan J A (1973) Hyperalimentation as primary therapy for inflammatory bowel disease. *American Journal of Surgery* **125**: 165–173.

Hanauer S B, Sitrin M D, Bengoa J M, Newcomb S A & Kirsner J B (1984). Long term follow up of patients with Crohn's disease treated by supportive total parenteral nutrition. *Gastroenterology* **86**: 1106.

Heaton K W, Thornton J R & Emmett P M (1979) Treatment of Crohn's disease with an unrefined-carbohydrate, fibre-rich diet. *British Medicial Journal* **2**: 764–766.

Korelitz B I (1980) Therapy of inflammatory bowel disease, including use of immunosuppressive agents. *Clinics in Gastroenterology* **9**: 331–349.

Lee E C G & Papaioannou N (1980) Recurrences following surgery for Crohn's disease. *Clinics in Gastroenterology* **9**: 419–438.

Malchow H, Ewe K, Brandes J W et al (1984) European Co-operative Crohn's Disease Study (ECCDS): Results of drug treatment. *Gastroenterology* **86**: 249–266.

Morin C L, Roulet M, Roy C C, Weber A & Lapointe N (1982) Continuous elemental enteral alimentation in the treatment of children and adolescents with Crohn's disease. *Journal of Parenteral Nutrition* **6**: 194–199.

Mullen J L, Clark Hargrove W, Dudrick S J, Fitts W T & Rosato E F (1978) Ten years experience with intravenous hyperalimentation and inflammatory bowel disease. *Annals of Surgery* **187**: 523–529.

National Co-operative Crohn's Disease Study (1979) *Gastroenterology* **77**: 825–944.

O'Morain C, Segal A W & Levi A J (1980) Elemental diets in the treatment of acute Crohn's disease. *British Medical Journal* **281**: 1173–1175.

O'Morain C, Segal A W, Levi A J & Valman H B (1983) Elemental diet in acute Crohn's disease *Archives of Disease in Childhood* **53**: 44–47.

O'Morain C, Segal A W & Levi A J (1984) Elemental diet as primary therapy of acute Crohn's disease; a controlled trial. *British Medical Journal* **288**: 1859–1862.

Ostro M J, Greenberg G R & Jeejeebhoy K N (1984) TPN and complete bowel rest in the management of Crohn's disease. *Gastroenterology* **86**: 1203.

Reilly J, Ryan J A, Strole W & Fischer J E (1976) Hyperalimentation in inflammatory bowel disease. *American Journal of Surgery* **131**: 192–200.

Rowe A Jr & Uyeyama K (1953) Regional enteritis — its allergic aspects. *Gastroenterology* **23**: 554–571.

Sachar D B, Auslander M O & Walfish J S (1980) Aetiological theories of inflammatory bowel disease. *Clinics in Gastroenterology* **9**: 231–257.

Workman E, Alun Jones V, Wilson A J & Hunter J O (1984) Diet in the management of Crohn's disease. *Applied Nutrition: Human Nutrition* **38**A: 469–473.

Chapter 16
Parenteral Nutrition

Graham Neale

The concept of parenteral nutrition has a long history (Lee 1980). Early experiments were undertaken with opium (Oldenburg 1665), fat (Courten 1712), blood (Blundell 1828; Levenson et al 1949), milk (Hodder 1873), glucose (Landerer 1887), protein hydrolysates (Neumeister 1889), and amino acids (van Slyke and Meyer 1913). The effective use of saline infusions to correct dehydration dates from the cholera epidemics of 150 years ago, following the abnormalities in blood chemistry reported by O'Shaughnessy (1832). Nevertheless the modern era of intravenous nutrition did not really begin until this century when Woodyatt et al (1915) quantified the rate of utilisation of glucose infused intravenously and claimed that 'the way is open for experiments with amino acids, polypeptides, etc'. These did not come until 20 years later when Elman (1937), in a series of classical experiments, showed that serum proteins regenerated more rapidly with infusions of a solution of 5% amino acids and 5% glucose than with 10% glucose. A complete mixture of amino acids was first used by Shohl and Blackfan (1940).

The use of large veins for the infusion of hypertonic solutions was the next important advance (Zimmerman, 1945) and this allowed experiments on the use of 20% glucose supplemented with vitamins, electrolytes and plasma (Dennis and Karlson 1952). Japanese chemists made an invaluable contribution by developing methods for the large scale synthesis of L-amino acids which had clear advantages over protein hydrolysates. Not only did the use of L-amino acids overcome the loss of poorly metabolised peptides in urine, it also paved the way for the formulation of amino acid mixtures for specific nutrition purposes, such as the requirements of uraemic patients (Freund et al 1978; Blackburn et al 1979; Eriksson 1981). Finally, after a long struggle starting in the 1920s a safe and effective fat emulsion was developed for intravenous use by Wretlind et al (1978) (see also Yamakawa et al 1929; Hallberg et al 1966).

Thus parenteral feeding progressed from regimens of saline and dextrose, with or without a source of nitrogen, to one which encompassed all essential nutrients (Geyer 1960). Total parenteral nutrition was used primarily for the short term support of malnourished patients who had undergone major surgery for severe abdominal disease. Over the next decade reports on its longer term use in medical disorders, such as Crohn's disease (Hallberg et al 1966) and unresponsive coeliac disease (Neale 1968), began to appear. Subsequently the full potential of parenteral feeding to meet total nutritional needs for growth, development and positive nitrogen balance was recognised in a key paper by Dudrick et al (1968). Today, most of the practical problems appear to have been solved and intestinal failure is no longer a sentence of death (Shils 1975). Patients may be kept alive for years without using their gastro-intestinal tract. Although total parenteral nutrition (TPN) is expensive and the list of potential complications is long, it is a form of treatment which seems to have come of age (Leading article, *British Medical Journal* 1979).

THE PROVISION OF TPN

Parenteral nutrition is now used in all large hospitals but, like all invasive technical procedures, it carries a moderately high risk of technical complications (Table 16.1), as well as the metabolic side-effects of feeding nutrients at a constant rate directly into the circulation (see Table 16.5). The technical problems may be minimised by using a nutrition team (Ryan 1976), and this service should be established in any large hospital using parenteral nutrition regularly for nutritional support or as a mode of therapy. The organisation of the nutrition service must depend on local circumstances and staffing. Some centres (e.g. Hope Hospital, Manchester) have a small ward for surgical patients requiring prolonged nutritional support. The staff of the ward also provide an advisory service for the whole hospital. In other centres, one clinical unit takes a special interest in parenteral nutrition and information diffuses throughout the hospital.

Nutrition service at a teaching hospital

At Addenbrooke's Hospital (Cambridge), the pharmacy and diet kitchen have been established as the means of providing a centralised service. The

Table 16.1. Total parenteral nutrition: technical complications.

(1) Damage caused by insertion of the line
    Bleeding
    Pneumothorax
    Air embolism

(2) Line incorrectly placed
    Jugular vein
    Right heart

(3) Blocking of line
    Fibrin clot
    Local thrombosis
    Pulmonary embolism

(4) Line damaged
    Cut by insertion needle
    Snap at hub
    Loss of line into circulation

(5) Infection
    Contaminated tip (10–30% after 1 month)
    With bacteraemia (2–5% after 1 month)

team consists of the following: a senior clinician in charge, a senior registrar/ research fellow with training in clinical biochemistry, and a part-time specialist nurse (20 hours a week), who provide day to day management; an anaesthetist with an interest in intensive care who is responsible for the maintenance of expertise in the placing of central venous lines; a pharmacist with special skills in the provision of sterile solutions; and a dietitian who is primarily concerned with enteral feeding and who covers the transition from parenteral to enteral nutrition. Patients remain under the care of the admitting team who can obtain formula feeds only through the pharmacy or diet kitchen.

In practice, ward doctors contact a member of the nutrition team and ask for advice. The patient is assessed with respect to nutritional well-being, likely requirements and the means of providing these. Often ward staff and members of the nutrition team find it necessary to discuss in some detail how best to proceed before they reach an agreed decision regarding optimal care for the patient and the most efficient use of an expensive resource. About one in four requests for total parenteral nutrition are modified to supplementary feeding for the short term, either via a peripheral vein or via a fine bore enteral tube. Occasionally it may be agreed that artificial feeding is unnecessary. Discussion is invaluable, not only for providing the best solution to clinical problems, but also as an effective means of education. Good-will is maintained by ensuring that the management of patients remains firmly in the hands of clinical teams.

The nutrition team gives a whole hospital service (excluding the neonatal ward). Its role has been accepted because the team provides cover for 24 hours a day, has a central source of equipment and materials, deals with problems promptly, and has demonstrated its efficiency in reducing complications. In the nutrition team at Addenbrooke's Hospital, the nurse specialist acts as the pivot. She is known in every ward of the hospital, she runs classes and seminars for pupil nurses and trained staff and she maintains the records of the work of the nutrition team (Table 16.2). The team meets as a whole

Table 16.2. Total parenteral nutrition: demand for service at Addenbrooke's and related hospitals (approximately 900 acute beds) 1981–1984.

Year	No. of patients	Patient days of TPN	Average days of TPN per patient	Catheter problems	Catheter sepsis
1980 (data incomplete)	20	240	12.0	14	2
1981	69	1083	15.7	10	4
1982	72	1103	15.3	7	2
1983	86	1469	17.1	4	4*
1984 (first 9 months)	72	1384†	16.4‡	0	2*

*Sepsis only in patients undergoing TPN for more than six weeks.
†Includes 201 days home TPN.
‡Average applies only to hospital patients.

only once or twice a year. The system evolves as new developments are worked out by individual members (e.g. changes in the method of line insertion — anaesthetist; changes in formulation of nutrients — research pharmacist; agreement on standardised regimens — clinicians/intensive care specialists; and development of the cheapest form of enteral nutrition — dietitian).

Home parenteral nutrition

The system has been simplified to enable patients with appropriate conditions to live at home. This may take the form of weekend leave or short term feeding to rest the bowel. Long term parenteral nutrition has also been used successfully in three female patients with total intestinal failure: one, aged 47, with severe Crohn's disease; one, aged 40, with mesenteric fibromatosis and massive intestinal resection; and one aged 35, with severe systemic sclerosis. Over a period of four years these are the only patients who were considered suitable for long term parenteral nutrition in a catchment area of approximately half a million people. There seems little danger of a massive increase in demand for home parenteral nutrition.

THE NEED FOR TOTAL PARENTERAL NUTRITION (TPN)

TPN is required when the patient has reached the point of requiring nutritional support and the gastro-intestinal tract is unavailable. After an era of over-use the statement above summarises generally accepted dogma. Nevertheless, it is one which leaves room for major disagreement. When is the patient seriously malnourished? How long should one maintain a patient solely on sugar, salt and water? How does one decide that the gut has failed?

Moreover clinicians have begun to extend TPN to patients for whom enteral feeding is possible but increasing the contents of the intestine may be harmful, at least in the short term. Again, there are no absolute indications. A great deal more information is required regarding the mechanisms by which food may damage the gut and the effect of TPN on gastro-intestinal inflammation.

BIOCHEMICAL CONSIDERATIONS

The requirements for nutritional support of the healthy adult have been established (American Medical Association 1979) but there are still many imponderables. For example, there are few hard data on the need for trace elements or vitamins in patients fed parenterally. This is almost certainly of no importance in short term feeding (e.g. up to six weeks) but may be of considerable significance for the occasional patient requiring maintenance TPN for months. The metabolic requirements may be different when nutrients are fed directly into the systemic circulation, thus by-passing the portal circulation and thereby over-riding control mechanisms for the maintenance of optimal metabolic status. This may be particularly true for the divalent cations. Body iron status is largely controlled by absorptive mechanisms and the infusion of large quantities of iron could readily cause iron overload. In practice this should not occur. Changes in the metabolism of other divalent cations are more subtle. In the case of calcium, hypercalcuria, hypercalcaemia and an unusual form of metabolic bone disease have all been described. In addition, electrolyte disorders secondary to magnesium deficiency are not uncommon.

The absolute nutritional requirements for healthy body function include salt and water to preserve intra- and extra-cellular hydration; fuels of respiration (principally carbodydrate and fat) to provide energy-rich phosphate bonds for external work and the energy required for the maintenance of cellular integrity; amino acids for protein synthesis; essential fatty acids, vitamins, co-factors, minerals and trace elements for cell structure and function. A simple set of regimens is shown in Table 16.3.

Sources of energy

Cellular energy is derived principally from glucose, fatty acids and some amino acids via 2-carbon fragments and the tri-carboxylic acid pathway. Although subject to metabolic control this vital biochemical pathway is readily primed by intermediates which are not rate limiting.

Table 16.3. Total parenteral nutrition (Addenbrooke's Hospital).

Basic daily regimen	
Volume	2.5 litres
Energy	1600, 2000, 2500 kcal
Nitrogen	12.8 g
Sodium	90 mmol
Potassium	80 mmol
Calcium	7.5 mmol
Magnesium	7.5 mmol
Phosphate	30 mmol
Cu, Zn, Mn, Cr, I, Fe	Adequate trace amounts* (Addenbrooke's solution)
Vitamins A, B complex, C and E, folic acid	As in Multibionta*

Variants of basic regimen	Fat	CHO : fat	Indications
(1) Standard (2000 kcal)	550 kcal	2 : 1	Most sick adult patients
(2) Standard high fat	1100 kcal	0.7 : 1	Hyperglycaemia†
(3) 1600 kcal	550 kcal	1.4 : 1	Small subjects; those with excess body fat
(4) 2500 kcal	1100 kcal	1 : 1	Hypercatabolic underweight adults

*Solutions given alternate days.
†These patients may be managed on standard regimen with added insulin.

Carbohydrates

In patients fed by the parenteral route, glucose is now established as the carbohydrate of choice. Glucose is cheap and readily assimilated, blood levels are easily monitored and, when necessary, can be controlled by the judicious use of insulin. Fructose, sorbitol and xylitol offer no metabolic advantages and are prone to cause lactic acidosis, hyperuricaemia and liver dysfunction.

Acetyl-CoA is formed from glucose by the glycolytic pathway. This pathway offers a maximum rate of oxidation of approximately 5 mg of glucose per kg body weight per minute, or approximately 1 750 kcal per day for a 70 kg man. Thus, in the short term, it is possible to cover energy requirements of the hospitalised patient using glucose alone. Nevertheless there are disadvantages. Glucose is irritant to peripheral veins and when large quantities are given, there is always a risk of exceeding the maximum rate of oxidation, thereby causing hyperosmolar dehydration. Thus monitoring the patient is more important when glucose is used as the principal source of energy.

Lipids

Lipids are given as fat emulsions which consist mainly of triglycerides. These are metabolised to glycerol and free fatty acids. The glycerol is converted to glucose or enters the glycolytic pathway. Free fatty acids are oxidised after crossing the mitochondrial membranes, bound to carnitine. Alternatively, fatty acids may be converted to ketone bodies which themselves are important fuels of respiration. In addition to calories, intravenous lipid preparations contain essential fatty acids (linoleic, linolenic and arachidonic acids) which are needed for the synthesis of cell membranes. Requirements for essential fatty acids are small, but a deficiency syndrome is well recognised in man (Press et al 1974). Lipid preparations are non-irritant to veins and provide a high energy yield in a small volume. But they are expensive and, in patients with impaired clearance mechanisms, hyperlipidaemia may be a troublesome complication. Alternative fuels of lipid origin have been suggested: medium chain triglycerides, short chain fatty acids and glycerol aceto-acetate. At present they do not seem to offer significant advantages.

Choice of fuels

A 50:50 contribution to energy requirements by carbohydrate and fat would probably be the easiest to manage. In practice, however, it is usual to give rather more energy in the form of carbohydrate because lipid preparations are so expensive. It is particularly wasteful not to use complete bottles of lipid emulsion which contain either 550 kcal or 1 100 kcal.

Amino acids

Much of the controversy regarding the optimum means of providing energy appears to have subsided. With nitrogen, however, the arguments are far from being resolved.

In patients with major trauma or severe illnesses, wasting of body protein is universal. Much work has been undertaken to devise ways of maintaining nitrogen balance. Unfortunately, easy methods of monitoring the effect of short term feeding do not provide clear-cut answers. The excretion of nitrogen in urine is a good marker of body losses (assuming a fixed loss in faeces and from the skin), but this nitrogen represents a combination of catabolised tissue protein and deaminated dietary nitrogen. Augmenting the amount of amino acids infused may do no more than increase urinary nitrogen.

All solutions contain adequate amounts of essential amino acids (Table 16.4). The branched chain amino acids appear to have a specific effect on protein synthesis (Odessy and Goldberg 1972) and may be as effective as a full mixture of amino acids in reversing the increase in nitrogen excretion after mild surgical trauma (Freund et al 1979).

Table 16.4. Essential amino acids.

Phenylalanine
Tryptophan
Histidine
Arginine
Lysine
Threonine
Methionine
Valine*
Leucine*
Isoleucine*

*Branched-chain amino acids.

The optimal amount and the most appropriate mix of non-essential amino acids is unresolved. They are metabolised by: (1) incorporation into protein molecules (with or without transamination); (2) deamination with (a) conversion of ammonia to urea, (b) conversion of the carbon chain to glucose or keto acids, or total metabolism to CO_2 and water with formation of ATP. Deamination is wasteful. It is better to provide energy as carbohydrate or lipid, both of which have a protein sparing effect. It is often stated that 200 kcal of energy should be given for each gram of amino acid nitrogen. In practice it is probably better to take protein and energy requirements as independent variables.

There is some evidence that transamination is impaired in sick subjects. Thus amino acid solutions with a high proportion of certain cheap, non-essential amino acids (such as glutamate, alanine or glycine) may be less than ideal for patients requiring TPN. At present, however, there is insufficient evidence to favour one preparation over another. The effect of by-passing the gut may be especially important with respect to the nitrogen economy of the body. With enteral feeding, glutamate is converted to glutamine and alanine is released from the gut. Normally there is little glutamate in the systemic circulation. The situation is different during parenteral feeding but the implications, particularly with respect to hormones mediating intermediary metabolism, are not well understood.

Finally, it is clear that changes in nitrogen metabolism in response to trauma and disease do not constitute a simple, graded response. Patients with renal or hepatic insufficiency behave quite differently from those with intact mechanisms of intermediary metabolism in these two key organs. Moreover some severely ill patients do not become ketotic during fasting; their body protein stores waste rapidly and their nitrogen requirements may be both quantitatively and qualitatively different from those who are less sick (Williamson et al 1977).

THE PHYSIOLOGICAL EFFECTS OF PARENTERAL NUTRITION

Long term TPN has important physiological and metabolic effects (Table 16.5), most of which are far from being fully understood.

Table 16.5. Total parenteral nutrition: metabolic side-effects.

Disturbance	Precipitating factors
Extra-cellular fluid	
Overload	Excess volume in patient with renal insufficiency
Hyperosmolar dehydration	Excess glucose
Acidoses	
Lactic acidosis	Especially with fructose, ethanol
Hypochloraemic acidosis	Excess chloride
Hyperuricaemia	Occasional especially with fructose, sorbitol (? xylitol)
Carbohydrate	
Hyperglycaemia	Excess glucose; unmasked diabetes
Hypoglycaemia	Post-infusion rebound
Fat	
Hyperlipidaemia	Excess fat emulsion (especially septicaemia)
Fatty liver	Mechanism uncertain
Essential fatty acid deficiency	Fat-free regimen
Nitrogen	
Azotaemia	Excess nitrogen (renal insufficiency)
Hyperammonaemia	Use of protein hydrolysates (hepatic insufficiency)
Altered cerebration (headache)	Amino acid induced
Cholestatic hepatitis	Amino acid induced (especially children)
Mineral disturbances	
Calcium, magnesium deficiency	Inadequate provision (especially with gastro-intestinal disease)
Hypophosphataemia	Carbohydrate with inadequate phosphate
Metabolic bone disease	Cause uncertain

Small intestine

Intra-luminal nutrition is vital for the maintenance of normal mucosal growth and adaptive hyperplasia after extensive resection fo the small intestine. All of the following participate in the regulation of mucosal growth: the absorption of nutrients (Dowling et al 1974; Feldman et al 1976; Spector et al 1977); the stimulus of work (Richter et al 1983); pancreatico-biliary secretions (Williamson et al 1978a; Weser et al 1981); circulating enteric hormones (Dworkin et al 1976; Hughes and Dowling 1978; Williamson et al 1978b; Weser et al 1981); neurovascular responses (Touloukian and Spencer 1972; Tutton 1977).

In the broadest terms, parenteral nutrition is most frequently indicated when the patient requires prolonged nutritional support and the gut is not available, nor likely to be available, for many days or weeks. These indications are met most frequently on surgical wards (Table 16.6) and in neonatal units (Dudrick et al 1969). The clinician should always seek to use the gastro-intestinal tract if at all possible (see Chapter 1). Fine-bore nasogastric or nasoduodenal tubes can be used to by-pass upper gastro-intestinal obstruction (oro-pharyngeal and oesophageal) and fine needle catheter jejunostomy is useful in some post-operative patients (Ryan and Page 1984). Stasis of intestinal contents, with or without vomiting, is an important contra-indication to enteral nutrition. Aspiration of the regurgitated contents of the stomach may readily cause a life-threatening pneumonia.

The clinical importance of the many physiological studies is far from certain. Nevertheless it is clear that nutrients in the lumen of the small intestine are vital for normal structure and function. Parenteral nutrition should be total for as short a time as possible. This is particularly important in the care of patients with the short bowel syndrome. Adaptation will be delayed without some form of enteral nutrition. A formula diet is often useful during the recovery phase (Young et al 1975).

Pancreas and biliary tree

Pancreatic secretory responses fall dramatically during periods of intravenous nutrition (Stabile et al 1984). The long term effects are uncertain. There is also a slowing in the entero-hepatic circulations of bile salts. Stasis in the gall bladder may lead to the formation of sludge and gall-stone formation is enhanced. Intra-hepatic cholestasis also occurs in some patients undergoing parenteral feeding.

Metabolic complications of parenteral nutrition

Disorders as a result of deficiency or excess of nutrients are now well recognised (Table 16.5). It is important to avoid overfeeding sick patients. Obsessional concern with increasing or maintaining body weight may lead to excess deposition of fat and a high respiratory quotient. Excess nitrogen may exacerbate renal failure and disturb cerebration.

Conversely the requirements for minerals, vitamins and trace elements are still not fully understood. Deficiency syndromes may occur in patients undergoing prolonged intravenous feeding (Table 16.7).

Table 16.6. Total parenteral nutrition: Addenbrooke's Hospital, 1981–1984.

Surgical wards		
Pre-operative management		
Nutritional rehabilitation	13	
Intestinal obstruction or stasis	11	
		24
Post-operative management		
Intestine not available	35	
Intestinal leaks	17	
Intestinal resection	10	
Nutritional rehabilitation	7	
		69
Intensive care		
Multiple organ failure	10	
Pancreatitis	5	
Road traffic accidents	5	
Hepatic failure	4	
		28
		121
Medical wards		
'Resting' intestine		
Crohn's disease*	53	
Food intolerance	3	
Malabsorption	2	
		58
Nutritional support		
Leukaemia (cytotoxic drugs)	12	
Colitis (with malnutrition)	8	
Subacute obstruction	4	
Neoplasia (cytotoxic drugs)	4	
Pregnancy (hyperemesis)	2	
Anorexia	1	
Starvation	1	
		32
		90

*The high number of patients with Crohn's disease reflects in part the work of a specialist unit in a regional hospital caring for patients with peculiarly difficult problems; and in part the management of patients in a controlled trial of TPN versus formula feeding in inducing remission (see Chapter 15).

Table 16.7. Total parental nutrition: deficiency syndromes.

Nutrient	Major signs	Reference
Chromium	Glucose intolerance, neuropathy	Jeejeebhoy et al (1977)
Copper	Anaemia, neutropaenia	Dunlop et al (1974)
Magnesium	Tetany, hypocalcaemia, hypokalaemia	Main et al (1981)
Selenium	Cardiomyopathy, myalgia	van Rij et al (1979) Fleming et al (1984)
Zinc	Peri-stomal and acral dermatitis	Kay et al (1976)
Phosphate	Anaemia, cardio-respiratory dysfunction	Thompson and Hodges (1984)
Essential fatty acids	Dermatitis	Press et al (1974) O'Neill et al (1977)
Carnitine	Fatty liver, myopathy and reactive hypoglycaemia	Worthley et al (1983)
Folic acid	Pancytopaenia	Woods (1980)
Biotin	Hair loss, eczematous dermatitis, depression	Mock et al (1981) Khaladi et al (1984)

More complex disturbances occur with respect to calcium, magnesium and phosphate metabolism, as well as carnitine and the use of lipids (Meguid and Borum 1984), methionine and folate metabolism (Wardrop et al 1977) and disturbances of acid–base balance.

PARENTERAL NUTRITION: MEETING BODY REQUIREMENTS

There is no simple method of determining exact body requirements for parenteral nutrition. In practice this is unimportant because patients rarely need this form of nutritional support for more than a month. A standard regimen may be used without apparent untoward effect for most patients (Occasional review, *British Medical Journal* 1983).

At Addenbrooke's Hospital, independent estimates of requirements for nitrogen and calories are made from a knowledge of body weight, ideal body weight, a crude estimate of body composition and metabolic state. This is a useful teaching exercise as well as providing a guideline for the nutrition team. Analysis of data obtained from 200 patients showed that almost all could be fitted reasonably closely to a standard regimen, but that it is worth having low and high calorie preparations also available (Table 16.3).

Nutrients are best delivered from a big bag filled aseptically in the pharmacy (Giovanni 1976). Many centres include all nutrients together. We prefer to infuse lipid emulsion separately over a period of eight hours. This allows nursing staff to check the clarity of the electrolyte–carboydrate solution and clinicians to ensure that the infused lipid is adequately cleared from the circulation.

Delivery of infusions

In most large centres with considerable experience of TPN, nutrients are delivered to the superior vena cava via a silastic catheter which is inserted below the clavicle and tunnelled onto the anterior chest wall (Powell-Tuck 1980). Mechanical complications and the risk of sepsis are minimised by following a standardised procedure under the supervision of a nurse specialist (Table 16.8).

Table 16.8. Care of central venous line.

(1) Used solely for intravenous feeding.
(2) Full aseptic precautions for all manipulations of line.
(3) Line disconnected only once a day for change of solution.
(4) Skin puncture site cleaned and dressed regularly.

If a patient becomes pyrexial, venous blood samples should be taken and the puncture site swabbed for bacteriological culture. It is then necessary to examine the patient for evidence of focal infection, unrelated to the feeding line. In practice, a central venous line carefully inserted and cared for is usually not the cause of pyrexia (especially during the first two weeks).

If a specific cause for the pyrexia is not found, it is not unreasonable to clear the line of fibrin with urokinase followed by a short course of antibiotics. Some authorities however prefer to remove all 'probably infected' lines and to culture the tips of catheters. Certainly it is safer to remove the line if the skin tunnel becomes inflamed or if there is not a rapid response to antibiotics. Following the removal of an infected line the pyrexia should settle promptly. A new line can be safely established within 24 hours.

A different approach to the problem of sepsis associated with central venous catheters has been developed in Italy (Bozzetti et al 1983). The subclavian catheter is secured without making a subcutaneous tunnel (von Meyenfeldt et al 1980) and the catheter is changed weekly over a guide-wire irrespective of suspected sepsis. This method is described as having limited value in the prevention of sepsis but appears to be useful in treatment (Bozzetti et al 1984). Against these claims one has to weigh the risk of pulmonary thrombo-embolism (Scarpa et al 1982) and further studies are needed to determine the value of this technique.

TOTAL PARENTERAL NUTRITION : INDICATIONS AND CONTRAINDICATIONS

A treatment which currently costs nearly £50 per day for materials alone carries important economic implications. Nevertheless TPN is now established as a safe and effective treatment which decreases morbidity in a wide range of conditions (Table 16.9).

Parenteral nutrition may also be indicated to 'rest' the gastro-intestinal tract, especially when there is pathology of the small intestine which is

Table 16.9. Indications for TPN.

---

(1) *Small intestine unavailable*
    Neonatal conditions
        Congenital structural disorders
        Enterocolitis
    Surgical conditions
        Intestinal obstruction
        Prolonged post-operative ileus
        Severe abdominal trauma
        Peritonitis
        Massive intestinal resection
    Medical conditions
        Severe malabsorption
        Recurrent vomiting
          (e.g. severe anorexia,
            prolonged hyperemesis)

(2) *To allow healing of gastro-intestinal pathology*
    Fistulae
        Gastro-intestinal
        Pancreatic
    Diffuse inflammatory disease
        Crohn's disease
        Radiation enteritis
        Pancreatitis
    Diffuse mucosal enteropathy
        Jejuno-ileitis (primary or secondary)
        Cytotoxic drugs
        Protein-calorie malnutrition

(3) *To improve or maintain nutritional status (in some cases in preparation for surgery)*
    Ulcerative colitis
    Intra-abdominal sepsis
    Multiple organ pathology (including some cases of renal or hepatic failure)
    Severe trauma including burns
    Unconscious patients for whom tube feeding contra-indicated

(4) *Intestinal failure*
    Massive resection of small intestine
    Intestinal pseudo-obstruction
        Idiopathic
        Systemic sclerosis
        Diffuse amyloidosis
        Fibrosing conditions of the mesentery
    Irreversible damage
        Crohn's disease
        Irradiation

---

expected to heal with time. Thus such treatment has been shown to be helpful in the treatment of diffuse Crohn's disease (Driscoll and Rosenberg 1978; Meryn et al 1983) and some remarkable recoveries from life-threatening states have been described (Greenberg et al 1976). The results of a controlled trial to test the beneficial effects of TPN against those of formula feeding in Crohn's disease are described in Chapter 15. Resting the small intestine is also useful in the management of patients with acute radiation enteritis, and in those suffering the severe side-effects (stomatitis, dysphagia, nausea and diarrhoea) of treatment with cytotoxic drugs (Copeland et al 1975).

Parenteral nutrition is of considerable benefit to patients with gastro-intestinal (Towne et al 1973) or pancreatic fistulae (Bivins et al 1984) and may speed healing (MacFadyen et al 1973). It is important to note that external fistulae from a segment of diseased small intestine (Crohn's disease, irradi-ated bowel) rarely heal without surgical intervention. In such cases TPN may be used to buy time and to improve the nutritional condition of the patient (Leading article, *Lancet* 1979). This is also the case in the care of severely malnourished patients with ulcerative colitis, those with prolonged pancreati-tis and in some cases of intra-abdominal sepsis.

Intestinal failure

Finally, total parenteral nutrition may be indicated in patients with small intestinal failure. The decision to give TPN to a patient in whom the small intestine is irreparably damaged places a great burden on the patient, the attending clinician and health services. To date in the UK fewer than 200 patients have been admitted to programmes for home TPN. Approximately one-third have been able to return to normal feeding but several have died of their disease. Our experience in East Anglia suggests that at any one time, not more than 1–2 patients per million of the population should be taking long-term TPN. Thus such treatment should be offered only by regional centres. Patients undergoing home parenteral nutrition require considerable help from specialised services. Nevertheless, feeding may be restricted to the sleeping hours, permitting near-normal activities during the day (Ladefogen and Jarnum 1978). The cost for each patient is approximately £20 000 per annum.

It is impossible to give clear guidelines regarding the contra-indications for long-term parenteral nutrition. The clinician has the responsibility of deter-mining the quality of life and in individual cases taking a decision may be extremely difficult. Home parenteral nutrition will be particularly difficult to manage in patients with continuing sepsis, in the elderly and infirm and in patients with cardiovascular disease.

CONCLUSION

Parenteral nutrition is a major therapeutic advance but it is expensive and likely to remain so. Further studies are necessary to define its value in 'resting the bowel' in inflammatory disorders and food related diseases.

Acknowledgements

I am grateful to all members of the nutrition team at Addenbrooke's Hospital for their help in developing the ideas expressed in this chapter. Dr Marinos Elia has been my mentor in intermediary metabolism as well as providing clinical care for patients; Dr Michael Lindop initiated the service and has ensured a very high standard of operative care in the insertion of lines; Mr Donald McHutchison and Shirley Shipton have developed a practical and highly efficient pharmaceutical service with research support from Dr Michael Allwood. Diane Talbot and Karen Horgan have provided skill and expertise in enteral nutrition. But the key role has been played by Sylvia Cottee as nurse specialist. She has been responsible for the day-to-day management of patients, has kept meticulous records and has demonstrated extraordinary skill in keeping the team together and building up goodwill throughout the hospital.

REFERENCES

Allwood M C, McHutchison D & Elia M (1984) *A Guide to the Operation of a TPN Service.* Thetford Travenol.

American Medical Association Department of Food and Nutrition (1979) Guidelines for essential trace element preparations for parenteral use. *JAMA* **241**: 2051–2053.

Bivins B A, Bell R M, Rapp R P & Toedebusch W H (1984) Pancreatic exocrine response to parenteral nutrition. *Journal of Parenteral and Enteral Nutrition* **8**: 34–36.

Blackburn G L, Moldawer L L, Usmi S, O'Keefe S J D & Bistrian B R (1979) Branched chain amino acid administration and metabolism during starvation, injury and infection. *Surgery* **86**: 307–315.

Blundell J (1828) The after management of floodings and on transfusion. *Lancet* **1**: 673.

Bozzetti F, Terno G, Bonfanti G et al (1983) Prevention and treatment of central venous catheter sepsis by exchange via a guidewire. A prospective controlled trial. *Annals of Surgery* **198**: 48–52.

Bozzetti F, Terno G, Bonfanti G & Gallus G (1984) Blood culture as a guide for the diagnosis of central venous catheter sepsis. *Journal of Parenteral and Enteral Nutrition* **8**: 386–398.

Copeland E M, MacFadyen B V, Lanzott V J & Dudrick S J (1975) Intravenous hyperalimentation as an adjunct to cancer chemotherapy. *American Journal of Surgery* **129**: 167–173.

Courten W (1712) Experiments and observations of the effects of several sorts of poisons upon animals made at Montpelier in the years 1678 and 1679 by the late William Courten. *Philosophical Transactions of the Royal Society of London* **27**: 485–500.

Dennis C & Karlson K E (1952) Surgical measures as supplements to the management of idiopathic ulcerative colitis; cancer, cirrhosis and arthritis as frequent complications. *Surgery* **32**: 892–912.

Dowling R H, Feldman E J & McNaughton J (1974) Importance of luminal nutrition for intestinal adaptation following small bowel resection. *Digestion* **10**: 216–217.

Driscoll R H & Rosenberg I H (1978) Total parenteral nutrition in inflammatory bowel disease. *Medical Clinics of North America* **62**: 185–201.

Dudrick S J, Wilmore D W, Vars H M & Rhoads J E (1968) Long-term total parenteral nutrition with growth, development and positive nitrogen balance. *Surgery* **64**: 134–142.

Dudrick S J, Wilmore D W, Vars H M & Rhoads J E (1969) Can intravenous feeding as the sole means of nutrition support growth in the child and restore weight loss in an adult? An affirmative answer *Annals of Surgery* **169**: 974–984.

Dunlop W M, James G W (III) & Hume D M (1974) Anaemia and neutropaenia caused by copper deficiency. *Annals of Internal Medicine* **80**: 470–476.

Dworkin L D, Levine G M, Farber N J & Spector M H (1976) Small intestinal mass of the rat is partially determined by indirect effects of intraluminal nutrition. *Gastroenterology* **71**: 626–630.

Elman R (1937) Amino acid content of the blood following intravenous injection of hydrolysed casein *Proceedings of the Society for Experimental Biology and Medicine* **37**: 437–440.

Eriksson L L (1981) Metabolic effects of branched-chain amino acids in patients with liver cirrhosis Thesis Karolinska Institute, Huddinge University Hospital, pp 1–55. Stockholm: Dahlberg.

Feldman E J, Dowling R H, Mcnaughton J & Peters T J (1976) Effects of oral versus intravenous nutrition on intestinal adaptation after small bowel resection in the dog. *Gastroenterology* **70**: 712–719.

Fleming C R, McCall J T, O'Brien J F et al (1984) Selenium status in patients receiving home parenteral nutrition. *Journal of Parenteral and Enteral Nutrition* **8**: 258–262.

Freund H, Yoshimura N, Lunetta L & Fischer J E (1978) Infusion of the branched-chain amino acids in decreasing muscle catabolism in vivo. *Surgery* **83**: 611–616.

Freund H, Hoover H C, Atamain S & Fishcher J E (1979) Infusion of the branched-chain amino acids in post-operative patients: anti-catabolic properties. *Annals of Surgery* **190**: 18–23.

Geyer R (1960) Parenteral nutrition. *Physiological Reviews* **40**: 150–186.

Giovanni, R (1976) The manufacturing pharmacy; solutions and incompatabilities. In Fischer J E (ed) *Total Parenteral Nutrition*, Ch 3, pp 27–53. Boston: Little, Brown.

Greenberg E R, Haber G B & Jeejeebhoy K N (1976) Total parenteral nutrition (TPN) and bowel rest in the management of Crohn's disease. *Gut* **17**: 828.

Hallberg D, Schuberth O & Wretlind A (1966) Experimental and clinical studies with fat emulsion for intravenous nutrition. *Nutritio et Dieta* **8**: 245–281.

Hodder E M (1873) Transfusion of milk in cholera. *Practitioner* **10**: 14–16.

Hughes C A & Dowling R H (1978) Cholecystokinin and secretin prevent the intestinal mucosal hypoplasia of total parenteral nutrition in the dog. *Gastroenterology* **75**: 34–41.

Jeejeebhoy K N, Chu R C, Marliss E B, Greenberg G R & Bruce-Robertson A (1977) Chromium deficiency glucose intolerance and neuropathy reversed by chromium supplementation in a patient receiving long-term total parenteral nutrition. *American Journal of Clinical Nutrition* **30**: 531–538.

Kay R G, Tasman-Jones C, Pybus J, Whitin R & Black H (1976) A syndrome of acute zinc deficiency during total parenteral nutrition in man. *Annals of Surgery* **183**: 331–340.

Khaladi N, Wesley J R, Thoene J G, Whitehouse W M (Jr) & Baker W L (1984) Biotin deficiency in a patient with short bowel syndrome during home parenteral nutrition. *Journal of Parenteral and Enteral Nutrition* **8**: 311–314.

Ladefogen K & Jarnum S (1978) Long-term parenteral nutrition. *British Medical Journal* **2**: 262–266.

Landerer S A (1887) Uber Transfusion und Infusion. *Archiv fuer Klinische Chirurgie* **34**: 807–812.

Leading article (1979) Parenteral nutrition before surgery? *British Medical Journal* **2**: 1529–1530.

Leading article (1979) Nutritional management of entero-cutaneous fistulae. *Lancet* **2**: 507–508.

Lee H A (1980) The development of parenteral nutrition. In Truelove S C & Kennedy H J (eds) *Topics in Gastroenterology*, pp 3–14. Oxford: Blackwell Scientific.

Levenson S M, Birkhill F R, Maloney M A & Bell J A (1949) The metabolic fate of the infused erythrocyte. *Annals of Surgery* **30**: 723–746.

MacFadyen B V, Dudrick S J & Ruberg R L (1973) Management of gastro-intestinal fistulae with parenteral hyperalimentation. *Surgery* **74**: 100–105.

Main A N H, Morgan R J, Russell R I et al (1981) Mg deficiency in chronic inflammatory bowel disease and requirements during intravenous nutrition. *Journal of Parenteral and Enteral Nutrition* **5**: 15–19.

Meguid M M & Borum P (1984) Carnitine deficiency with hyperbilirubinemia, generalised skeletal muscle weakness and reactive hypoglycaemia in a patient on long term total parenteral nutrition. *Journal of Parenteral and Enteral Nutrition* **8**: 51–52.

Meryn S, Lochs H, Pamperl H, Kletter K & Mulac K (1983) Influence of parenteral nutrition on serum levels of proteins in patients with Crohn's disease. *Journal of Parenteral and Enteral Nutrition* **7**: 553–556.

Mock D M, Lorimer A A de, Liebman W M Sweetman L & Baker H (1981) Biotin deficiency: an unusual complication of parenteral nutrition. *New England Journal of Medicine* **304**: 820–823.

Neale G (1968) Clinico-pathological Conference: Adult coeliac disease resistant to treatment. *British Medical Journal* **2**: 678–683.

Neumeister R (1889) Ueber die nächste Einwerkung gespannter Wasserdämpfe auf Proteïne und über eine Gruppe eigenthümlicher Eiweisskörper und Albumosen. *Zeitschrift für Biologie* **8**: 57–83.

Occasional review (1983) Total parenteral nutrition: value of a standard feeding regimen. *British Medical Journal* **286**: 1323–1327.

Odessey R & Goldberg A L (1972) Oxidation of leucine by rat skeletal muscle. *American Journal of Physiology* **223**: 1376–1378.

Oldenburg H (1665) An account of the rise and attempts of a way to convey liquors immediately into the mass of blood. *Philosphical Transactions of the Royal Society of London* **7**: 128–130.

O'Neill J A Jr, Caldwell M D & Meng H C (1977) Essential fatty acid deficiency in surgical patients. *Annals of Surgery* **185**: 535–542.

O'Shaughnessy W B (1832) Report on the clinical pathology of the malignant cholera. *Lancet* **1**: 929–936.

Powell-Tuck J (1980) Long term intravenous feeding. In Karran S J & Alberti K G M M (eds) *Practical Nutrition Support*. Ch 28, pp 300–311. Tunbridge Wells: Pitman Medical.

Press M, Kikuchi H, Shimoyama T & Thompson G R (1974) Diagnosis and treatment of essential fatty acid deficiency in man. *British Medical Journal* 2: 247–250.

Richter G C, Levine G M & Shiau Y F (1983) The effects of luminal glucose versus non-nutritive infusates on jejunal mass and absorption in the rat. *Gastroenterology* 85: 1105–1112.

Ryan J A (1976) Complications of total parenteral nutrition. In Fischer J E (ed) *Total Parenteral Nutrition*, Ch 4, pp 55–100. Boston: Little, Brown.

Ryan J A Jr & Page C P (1984) Intrajejunal feeding: development and current status. *Journal of Parenteral and Enteral Nutrition* 8: 187–198.

Scarpa D, Terno G, Bozzetti F et al (1982) Subclavian venous thrombosis due to indwelling catheters: a prospective study on 52 patients. *Journal of Parenteral and Enteral Nutrition* 6: 336–337.

Shils M E (1975) A programme for total parenteral nutrition at home. *American Journal of Clinical Nutrition* 28: 1429–1435.

Shohl A T & Blackfan K D (1940) The intravenous administration of crystalline amino acids to infants. *Journal of Nutrition* 20: 305–316.

Spector M H, Levine G M & Deren J J (1977) Direct and indirect effects of dextrose and amino acids on gut mass. *Gastroenterology* 72: 706–710.

Stabile B E, Borzatta M & Stubbs R S (1984) Pancreatic secretory responses to intravenous hyperalimentation and intraduodenal elemental and full liquid diets *Journal of Parenteral and Enteral Nutrition* 8: 377–380.

Thompson J S & Hodges R E (1984) Preventing hypophosphataemia during total parenteral nutrition. *Journal of Parenteral and Enteral Nutrition* 8: 137–139.

Touloukian R J & Spencer R P (1972) Ileal blood flow preceding compensatory intestinal hypertrophy. *Annals of Surgery* 175: 320–325.

Towne J B, Hamilton R F & Stephenson D V (1973) Mechanism of hyperalimentation in the suppression of upper gastro-intestinal secretions. *American Journal of Surgery* 126: 714–721.

Tutton P J M (1977) Neural and endocrine control systems acting on the population kinetics of the intestinal epithelium. *Medical Biology* 55: 201–208.

van Rij A M, Thomson C D, McKenzie J M & Robinson M F (1979). Selenium deficiency in total parenteral nutrition. *American Journal of Clinical Nutrition* 32: 2076–2085.

van Slyke D D & Meyer G M (1913) The fate of protein digestion products in the body. *Journal of Biological Chemistry* 16: 197–229.

von Meyenfeldt M M F, Stapert J, Jong P C M de et al (1980) TPN catheter sepsis: lack of effect of subclavian tunnelling of PVC catheters on sepsis rate. *Journal of Parenteral and Enteral Nutrition* 4: 514–517.

Wardrop C A J, Lewis M H, Tennant G B, Williams R H P & Hughes L E (1977) Acute folate deficiency associated with intravenous nutrition with amino acid–sorbitol–ethanol: prophylaxis with intravenous folic acid. *British Journal of Haematology* 37: 521–526.

Weser E, Bell D & Tawil T (1981) Effects of octapeptide-cholecystokinin, secretin, and glucagon on intestinal mucosal growth in parenterally nourished rats. *Digestive Diseases and Sciences* 26: 409–416.

Williamson D H, Farrell R, Kerr A & Smith R (1977) Muscle protein catabolism after injury in man as measured by urinary excretion of 3-methyl-histidine. *Clinical Science and Molecular Medicine* 52: 527–532.

Williamson R C N, Bauer F L R, Ross J S & Malt R A (1978a) Contribution of bile and pancreatic juice to cell proliferation in ileal mucosa. *Surgery* 83: 570–576.

Williamson R C N, Bucholz T W & Malt R A (1978b) Humoral stimulation of cell proliferation in small bowel after transection and resection. *Gastroenterology* 75: 249–254.

Woods H F (1980) Metabolic complications with special reference to folate deficiency. In Truelove S C & Kennedy H J (eds) *Topics in Gastroenterology*, pp 51–62. Oxford: Blackwell Scientific.

Woodyatt R T, Sansum W D & Wilder R M (1915) Prolonged and accurately timed injection of sugar. *Journal of the American Medical Association* 65: 2067–2070.

Worthley L I G, Fishlock R C & Snoswell A M (1983) Carnitine deficiency with hyperbilirubinaemia, generalised skeletal muscle weakness and reactive hypoglycaemia in a patient on long term total parenteral nutrition. *Journal of Parenteral and Enteral Nutrition*. 7: 176–180.

Wretlind, A (1978). Parenteral nutrition. *Surgical Clinics of North America* 58: 1055–1070.

Yamakawa S, Nomura T & Fujinaga I (1929) Zur Frage der emulgierten Fets vom Dickdarm aus. *Tohuku Journal of Experimental Medicine* 14: 265.

Young E A, Heuler N, Russell P & Weser E (1975) Comparative nutritional analysis of chemically defined diets. *Gastroenterology* 69: 1338.

Zimmerman B (1945) Intravenous tubing for parenteral therapy. *Science* 101: 567–568.

Chapter 17
Gall-stones

K. W. Heaton

The traditional classification of gall-stones into cholesterol, mixed, and pigment stones, is obsolete. All gall-stones are mixed in composition and there is a continuum from almost pure cholesterol stones to almost pure calcium salt stones. Of the calcium-rich stones, a small minority are composed mainly of calcium bilirubinate and can reasonably be called pigment stones, but the majority are made up of the inorganic calcium salts, carbonate and phosphate, or of calcium palmitate. Remarkably little is known of the aetiology or pathogenesis of calcium-rich stones except that calcium bilirubinate stones form in the gall-bladder in haemolytic states and in the bile ducts when these ducts are infested or infected. Pigment-rich stones are the main variety found in the peoples of the Orient, and probably in those of other developing countries, at least in rural areas. In Western and other urbanised communities, the majority of gall-stones (70–80%) are composed chiefly of cholesterol as crystalline cholesterol monohydrate. They are almost always radiolucent. Calcium-rich stones are often, but not necessarily, radio-opaque.

This review will be concerned essentially with cholesterol-rich gall-stones. In practice this will cover most of the problem, since gall-stones are much more prevalent in Western-type communities than in rural, developing areas of the world (Brett and Barker 1976; Heaton 1981). Stones in the gall-bladder can reasonably be considered a 'Western disease' (Trowell and Burkitt 1981).

CHOLESTEROL-RICH GALL-STONES

Pathogenesis

The steps in the formation of a gall-stone are: (1) secretion by the liver of bile supersaturated with cholesterol; (2) precipitation of microcrystals of cholesterol monohydrate; (3) growth of crystals and/or their entrapment in a mucous gel in the gall-bladder, leading to the formation of macroscopic stones. Many factors influence this process which has been the subject of intensive research for nearly 20 years but is still only partially understood (Bouchier 1983; Heaton 1985).

Supersaturation of gall-bladder bile with cholesterol is the prerequisite of this process. Cholesterol is a highly insoluble lipid. The detergent system which holds it in solution in the gall-bladder consists of micelles of bile salts and lecithin. The system breaks down when it is called upon to solubilise too much cholesterol; that is, when there is increased secretion of cholesterol by the liver into bile. It also breaks down if there is a deficiency of bile salts, that is, a small circulating pool of bile salts. Normally the body contains about 3 g of bile salts (roughly 40% cholate, 40% chenodeoxycholate and 20% deoxycholate) which are efficiently conserved by active absorption from the terminal ileum. Reabsorbed bile salts are avidly extracted from the portal blood and returned to the biliary tree, so completing the enterohepatic circulation. Patients with gall-stones, at least those who are non-obese, tend to have a small bile salt pool, usually 1.5–2.0 g. This may provide insufficient micelles to solubilise a normal amount of cholesterol.

Thus there are two defects of hepatic metabolism which can lead to supersaturated bile, increased secretion of cholesterol and decreased production of bile salts. Characteristics associated with increased secretion of cholesterol are adiposity, raised serum triglycerides and a high level of deoxycholate in the bile salt pool. Cholesterol secretion is decreased when the bile is enriched with chenodeoxycholate or the trace bile salt ursodeoxycholate by oral administration of these compounds. The balance of chenodeoxycholate and deoxycholate may be an important determinant of supersaturated bile.

The cholesterol saturation index (CSI) of fasting gall-bladder bile (which can easily be obtained by duodenal intubation) is a valuable indicator of the risk of gall-stones. However, it has one important limitation. In Western countries many people, especially the obese and the aged, have supersaturated bile (CSI>1.0) but fail to develop gall-stones. Such people have no crystals of cholesterol monohydrate in their bile, whereas in people with cholesterol-rich gall-stones, the bile either contains such crystals or develops them rapidly when the bile is incubated in vitro. Recent research has shown that the bile of patients with gall-stones contains a potent nucleating factor which promotes the crystallisation of cholesterol (Burnstein et al 1983). It is probably a protein or a mixture of proteins.

The role of the gall-bladder in gall-stone formation is that of providing a quiet backwater in which crystals can form and grow, a role which is enhanced if gall-bladder contraction is impaired; the gall-bladder also provides the nucleating factor or factors and, if it is inflamed or infected, it may contribute to supersaturation by inappropriately absorbing bile salts.

Risk factors for cholesterol gall-stones

The old saw about 'fair, fat, fertile and forty' has some truth in it in that there is certainly increased prevalence of stones in females over males and in multigravidae over nullipara (Table 17.1). However, the link with ageing carries on well past the forties, indeed until death. Such basic facts have been elucidated from autopsy surveys, but they tell us more about personal traits which confer susceptibility to the disease than about its aetiology.

Obesity

The link with obesity is obviously important. It was discovered by simple clinical observation and confirmed by autopsy surveys (Newman and Northup 1959; Burnett 1971; Záhoř et al 1974) but a recent large case-control study suggests it may be a significant risk factor only in women and may operate

Table 17.1. Risk factors for cholesterol-rich gall-stones.

Definite	Putative
Age	Lowered plasma HDL cholesterol
Female sex	Raised plasma insulin (fasting)
Obesity (? young only)	Raised biliary deoxycholic acid
Multiparity	
Hypertriglyceridaemia	
Clofibrate treatment	

N.B. Oestrogens only accelerate. Diabetes probably acts via obesity.

only under the age of 50 years (Scragg et al 1984a). In a population where most people are obese, as in the Pima Indians of Arizona, there may be no excess of obesity amongst those in whom gall-stones are formed (Sampliner et al 1970).

Obesity probably favours gall-stones through its effects on cholesterol metabolism. Total daily synthesis of cholesterol is directly proportional to body fat (Nestel et al 1973). Biliary secretion is the main pathway for the excretion of cholesterol from the body, so it is hardly surprising that the rate at which cholesterol is secreted into bile is proportional to body weight as a percentage of ideal (Bennion and Grundy 1978). Fat Americans and Europeans almost always have bile supersaturated with cholesterol. However, not all patients with cholesterol gall-stones are fat and, in primitive communities like rural Zimbabwe and Tonga, fat women generally have bile which is unsaturated with cholesterol (Heaton et al 1977; Stace et al 1981). Clearly, other factors are important.

Hypertriglyceridaemia

The link between gall-stones and raised fasting serum triglycerides is even closer than that with obesity. Patients with this type of hyperlipoproteinaemia have a very high incidence of gall-stones (Ahlberg et al 1979) and secrete bile which is supersaturated with cholesterol (Ahlberg et al 1980). Even when levels of plasma triglycerides are in the normal range, there is a significant correlation between the plasma triglyceride concentration and the cholesterol saturation index of bile (Thornton et al 1981). Conversely, patients with gall-stones have higher plasma triglycerides than controls of equal weight (Kadziolka et al 1977). In their big case-control study Scragg et al (1984b) found hypertriglyceridaemia to be a risk factor for gall-stones in those aged under 50 years, even when they controlled for obesity by multivariate analysis.

Hyperinsulinaemia

In the Adelaide case-control study, a raised plasma insulin in the fasting state was a risk factor for gall-stones and this finding was independent of levels of plasma triglycerides (Scragg et al 1984b). However, when we compared the cholesterol saturation index of bile with the fasting (and post-glucose) insulin levels in the plasma of 25 non-obese middle-aged women, we found no correlation (Thornton et al 1980).

Low plasma high density lipoprotein cholesterol

Three lines of evidence incriminate low levels of plasma high density lipoprotein (HDL) cholesterol as a risk factor for gall-stones. First, the levels have been found to be low in women who give a history of gall-bladder disease (Petitti et al 1981). Second, in the Adelaide case-control study, HDL cholesterol was negatively associated with the risk of gall-stones (Scragg et al 1984b). Third, in our study of middle-aged women we found a negative correlation between plasma HDL cholesterol and the cholesterol saturation index of bile (Thornton et al 1981). The nature of this link is debatable, but one possibility is that HDL cholesterol is the main source of cholesterol for the synthesis of bile salts by the liver.

Diverticular disease and hiatus hernia

In Amiens, gall-stones were found twice as often as expected in patients with diverticular disease of the colon and in patients with sliding hiatus hernia (Capron et al 1978, 1981). Patients with hiatus hernia were found to have markedly supersaturated gall-bladder bile (Capron et al 1978). These provocative findings have not been confirmed (or disproved) by any other studies. Clinicians talk of Saint's triad when all three diseases are found in the same patient but, at present, there is no evidence that this concurrence is more than a chance event.

CURRENT DIETARY THEORIES

The theories concerning the effect of diet on the formation of gall-stones which carry any credence today implicate excess energy intake, high cholesterol intake, lack of dietary fibre and high sucrose intake. There is no evidence that dietary fat plays any part in the aetiology of gall-stones (except insofar as it contributes to excessive energy intake) though it is widely accepted that a low fat diet helps to reduce the frequency of biliary colic in patients who have gall-stones.

Excess or high energy intake

Excess energy intake over expenditure is not necessarily the same as high energy intake. Dietary surveys indicate that fatter people do not eat more than thinner ones — they may even eat less, presumably because of their greater energy efficiency (Keen et al 1979). Nevertheless, the theory that high energy intake predisposes to gall-stones has gained some credence. This theory arose from three case-control studies carried out in Marseilles between 1956 and 1968 (Sarles et al 1957, 1969; Hauton 1967), which all showed a higher energy intake in patients with gall-stones. However, these early examples of the case-control technique do not satisfy modern standards (Scragg 1984) and a difference in energy intake was not found in six later case-control studies (Wheeler et al 1970; Burnett 1971; Reid et al 1971; Sarles et al 1978a; Coste et al 1979; Smith and Gee 1979), including a later one from Marseilles (Sarles et al 1978a). In the Adelaide study (Scragg et al 1984a) a high energy intake increased the relative risk of gall-stones in young and middle-aged women and in young men, but not in older subjects of either sex (Figure 17.1). These variations with age and sex help to explain the contradictory data obtained in smaller studies.

The idea that high energy intake is a causative factor was strengthened by a comparison of the published autopsy prevalence of gall-stones in seven countries (France, Sweden, Portugal, South Africa, Uganda, India and Japan) and the estimated average intake of calories in these countries (Sarles et al 1978b). There appeared to be a good correlation, at any rate up to 3000 kcal (12.6 MJ) per day. However, no statistical testing was carried out and the prevalence rates were not age-standardised. Also correlations were present with animal fat and protein and, no doubt, they could have been found with many other indicators of affluence.

For an individual, a long term increase in energy intake certainly increases the risk of gall-stones if it results in increased body fat. Studies on T-tube bile have suggested that, in the short term too, changes in energy intake may affect the cholesterol concentration of bile (Sarles et al 1968, 1971) but the setting of these experiments was unphysiological and the changes in energy were drastic. In a more physiological study, a 24% change in energy intake (induced by changing sucrose intake) did not affect the cholesterol saturation of duodenal bile over a six-week period (Werner et al 1984).

If excess (or high) energy intake is a risk factor, it follows that any dietary item or any eating habit which inflates energy intake will itself be a risk factor.

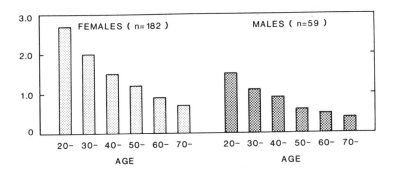

Figure 17.1. Relative risk (after controlling for alcohol, sugar in drinks and sweets, and cholesterol) of gall-stones at different ages associated with an increase in calorie intake of 500 kcal/day. From Heaton (1984). Copyright (1984), reprinted by permission of John Wiley & Sons. Data from the Adelaide case-control study (Scragg et al 1984a).

The two dietary items which are most often blamed for inflating energy intake are refined carbohydrate, especially sugar, and fat. There is no evidence from epidemiology, case-control studies or human experiments to incriminate dietary fat in causing gall-stones. There is, however, considerable evidence to incriminate refined sugars.

High cholesterol intake

Western populations with a high incidence of gall-stones tend to eat more cholesterol than people in developing countries, but no statistical correlations have been demonstrated between cholesterol intake and gall-stone prevalence. Case-control studies provide little support. In the Adelaide study (Scragg et al 1984a) cholesterol intake was similar in male cases and their matched community controls. In female cases aged under 50 years, intake was 40 mg/day higher than in controls, but in women over 50 intake was 52 mg/day lower. On multiple regression analysis, cholesterol was *negatively* associated with gall-stones (but only in females and when included in a statistical model with fat or calories).

Human experiments have also given conflicting results. Two American studies (DenBesten et al 1973; Lee et al 1983) found that adding cholesterol to the diet for three weeks raised the cholesterol content of bile. The first study is hard to interpret because it involved adding egg yolks to a liquid formula diet and it is unsafe to extrapolate findings to a normal solid diet. Also, there was a significant rise in serum cholesterol during the experiment, whereas patients with gall-stones do not have raised serum cholesterol levels — they may even be reduced (van der Linden 1961) — and, other things being equal, there is no correlation between serum cholesterol and bile cholesterol saturation (Thornton et al 1981). The second study (Lee et al 1983) is also hard to interpret because as yet it has been published only as an abstract. However, it purports to show that the saturation index of duodenal bile in seven healthy women rose from 0.89 ± 0.04 to 1.06 ± 0.04 ($p<0.05$) when eggs were added to their diet to raise its cholesterol content from 500 to 1 000 mg/day for three weeks. Also, in six women with radiolucent gall-stones, the saturation index rose from 1.28 ± 0.06 to 1.48 ± 0.05 ($p<0.01$).

In total opposition are the results of Dam et al (1971). They fed 5–10 eggs a day to young volunteers for six weeks and, despite a rise in the serum cholesterol, there was no tendency for the cholesterol content of bile to rise; in fact, in most subjects the bile salts/cholesterol ratio improved. Similarly, Andersén and Hellström (1979) found no change in bile cholesterol saturation when 5 eggs a day were fed for two weeks.

In animals, feeding cholesterol can induce supersaturated bile and cholesterol gallstones, at least in rodents, such as the mouse, prairie dog and gerbil, also in the squirrel monkey (van der Linden and Bergman 1977). However, it is doubtful if these experiments are relevant to the human disease. Animals on these regimes become saturated with cholesterol, which in no way resembles the situation in patients with gall-stones. For example, in gerbils the serum cholesterol rose from 104 to 867 mg/dl. At the same time, the liver became so stuffed with cholesterol, it swelled to three times its normal size and most of the animals died (Bergman and van der Linden 1971). Animal species vary greatly in how their bile responds to cholesterol feeding (Ho 1976); in hamsters, bile saturation actually decreases. In the author's view, animal models have not thrown any light on the dietary aetiology of human gall-stones. They may even be misleading.

Fibre-depleted diet and high sucrose intake

These two theories are so interconnected that the arguments and evidence for them will be considered together.

Cleave used the term 'refined carbohydrate' (Cleave and Campbell 1966; Cleave 1974) to encompass all of the carbohydrate-containing items in man's diet which have been processed so as to remove a fibre-rich fraction. The main examples in Western diets are sugars (white or brown) and syrups, which are fibre-free, and white flour from which the bran and germ have been removed. A better term is fibre-depleted foods since white flour and other 'refined' foods like white rice are not by any means pure carbohydrate. Dietary fibre is defined (Trowell et al 1976) as the plant polysaccharides and lignin which escape digestion by the alimentary enzymes of man. It is composed chiefly of plant cell walls, which are complex, highly organised structures. Wheat bran contains about 40% dietary fibre and is the richest source of fibre in the diet. Up to 50% of bran is fermented by anaerobic bacteria in the colon. Fibre from other sources is fermented more extensively and the resultant growth of bacteria is largely responsible for the greater bulk of the stools on a high-fibre diet (Stephen and Cummings 1980). The products of fermentation are the short-chain fatty acids, acetic, propionic and butyric, together with the gases hydrogen, carbon dioxide and, in some people, methane (see Chapters 5 and 6).

Cleave proposed that eating fibre-depleted foods in place of natural full-fibre foods damages health in two main ways. It provides insufficient fibre for the optimal function of the large intestine, and it disturbs energy balance and carbohydrate metabolism by making carbohydrate foods too easily ingested and digested. Amongst the diseases caused by eating fibre-depleted foods, Cleave included gall-stones (Cleave and Campbell 1966). I believed he was right but argued that the explanation for the link lay in disturbed hepatic metabolism (Heaton 1975) rather than, as he believed, in promotion of gall-bladder infection. Eventually he conceded that a metabolic link was likely (Cleave 1974).

In its current form the fibre-depletion theory has two parts: (1) fibre-depleted foods, especially sugars, lead to excessive energy intake and, possibly, to excessive insulin levels, both of which favour gall-stone formation, mainly by increasing cholesterol synthesis; (2) lack of indigestible material in the diet allows increased formation and/or absorption of deoxycholic acid in the colon; this in turn leads to increased cholesterol secretion into bile.

This unifying hypothesis is shown in Figure 17.2 in schematic form.

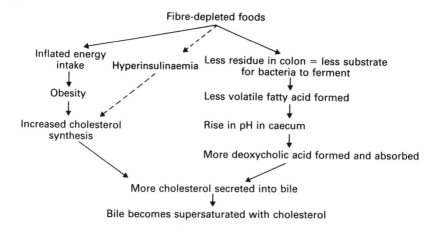

Figure 17.2.

Epidemiological evidence

Population comparisons. The fibre-depletion theory has not been formally tested by population comparisons and it would be difficult to do so, in view of the great heterogeneity of dietary fibre. Moreover, fibre is hard to analyse and measure chemically and data are not yet available for the fibre intakes of whole populations. However, the exchange of traditional, lightly processed staple foods for the modern Western diet almost always involves a reduction in fibre intake and it always includes a greater intake of fibre-free sugars. Hence, the fibre-depleted food theory could help to explain the marked geographical and historical variations in gall-stone prevalence.

Case-control studies. Only one case-control study has looked specifically at the intake of refined sugars. Workers in Rome and Milan (Alessandrini et al 1982) used a food frequency questionnaire to compare the sugar and fibre intake of 160 patients with radiolucent gall-stones and 160 hospital controls matched for age and sex, all with negative cholecystograms. The gall-stone patients ate significantly more refined sugar, about 23 g/day versus 19 g/day in the controls ($p < 0.05$). The intakes are surprisingly low in both groups.

The Adelaide case-control study (Scragg et al 1984a) looked at total sugar intake, which is mainly refined (fibre-depleted) sugar in most people, and also at sugar in drinks and sweets which is an important fraction of refined sugar intake. As shown in Table 17.2, total sugar intakes were considerably higher in both men and women with gall-stones under the age of 50 but were not significantly different over the age of 50 years. Sugar in drinks and sweets was higher in all groups with gall-stones except older men. These were the biggest and most consistent differences in any nutrient in this study. Dietary fibre intakes were looked at in both the foregoing studies. Alessandrini et al (1982) found slightly but significantly ($p < 0.05$) lower intakes of total dietary fibre

Table 17.2. Daily intake of sugars and dietary fibre in patients with gall-stones and matched community controls.

	Females				Males			
	Age<50		Age>50		Age<50		Age>50	
	Cases	Controls	Cases	Controls	Cases	Controls	Cases	Controls
Sugars: total (g)	‡147±7	113±4	128±8	126±7	*160±15	121±10	135±12	153±10
Sugars: drinks and sweets (g)	‡53±4	28±3	†36±4	23±2	*58±5	40±7	46±6	40±5
Dietary fibre (g)	19.2±0.8	17.7±0.7	18.1±0.9	21.9±1.2	17.4±2.1	18.3±1.6	18.5±2.2	22.6±1.9

*$p<0.05$, †$p<0.01$, ‡$p<0.001$.
From Heaton (1984), reprinted by permission of John Wiley & Sons. Copyright (1984). Data from the Adelaide case-control study (Scragg et al 1984a).

and of fruit and vegetable fibre in patients with gall-stones, but there was no difference in cereal fibre. As shown in Table 17.2, Scragg and colleagues found no difference in total dietary fibre intake in any age or sex group. However, on multivariate analysis, fibre was negatively associated with gall-stones in both sexes.

Hence, case-control studies support the theory that refined carbohydrate in the form of sugars is an aetiological factor in gall-stones. They give limited support to the idea that a low intake of dietary fibre is pathogenic. The power of case-control studies is limited if there is little variation in the intake of a nutrient within the population studied.

Experimental studies in man

The published experimental studies consist of one on the effects of refined carbohydrate in general, and one investigating refined sugar in particular, together with several studies using wheat bran. All studies have involved analysing duodenal bile for its lipid composition and for the relative proportions of bile salts.

The effects of wheat bran on the cholesterol saturation of bile are shown in Figure 17.3. In four groups of subjects whose bile was initially supersaturated, the bile became less saturated, whereas in three groups with initially unsaturated bile there was no change (Pomare et al 1976; McDougall et al 1978; Tarpila et al 1978; Watts et al 1978; Huijbregts et al 1980). Thus, bran appears to have a consistent normalising effect on bile. This effect is relatively weak, however, and in only a minority of subjects does bran convert supersaturated into unsaturated bile.

The mode of action of bran has not been proved. However, in all groups of subjects in whom bile has become less saturated there has also been a fall in the proportion of deoxycholate in the bile salt pool. It is relevant because, besides bran, there are several other measures which lower the deoxycholate content of bile and all of them also make the bile less saturated with cholesterol. These measures are treatment with metronidazole (Low-Beer and Nutter 1978), with ampicillin (Carulli et al 1981), with lactulose (Thornton and Heaton 1981), or with senna laxative (Marcus and Heaton 1984), also oral administration of *Streptococcus faecium* (Salvioli et al 1982) and the reversal of hypothyroidism with thyroxine treatment (Angelin et al 1983).

Deoxycholic acid is a secondary bile acid, i.e. a bacterial breakdown product of an original or primary bile acid. It is formed by the dehydroxylation of cholic acid.

Measures that increase the deoxycholic acid content of bile tend to raise the cholesterol saturation of bile, and people with gall-stones tend to have an increased proportion of deoxycholic acid in their bile (Low-Beer and Pomare 1975; Heaton 1985). Why deoxycholic acid should favour more saturated bile is unproven but there are two plausible explanations. First, being the most detergent of the major bile acids, deoxycholic acid may leach out excessive amounts of cholesterol as it is being secreted from the liver cell into the bile (Carulli et al 1984). Second, deoxycholic acid displaces chenodeoxycholic acid from the bile (either by competing with it for intestinal absorption or by

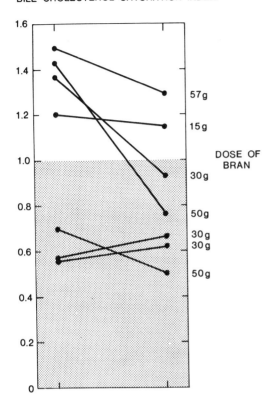

EFFECT OF WHEAT BRAN ON
BILE CHOLESTEROL SATURATION INDEX

DOSE OF
BRAN

Figure 17.3. Cholesterol saturation index of duodenal bile in seven groups of subjects before and during treatment with wheat bran in the daily dose stated. Each point represents mean values for a group (Pomare et al 1976; McDougall et al 1978; Tarpila et al 1978; Watts et al 1978; Huijbregts et al 1980). A saturation index of more than 1.0 indicates supersaturation with cholesterol. From Heaton (1984). Copyright (1984), reprinted by permission of John Wiley & Sons.

suppressing its synthesis) and this removes an agent which is known to lower cholesterol secretion. Whatever the mode of action of deoxycholic acid, bran may act by reducing it.

As to how bran reduces the amount of circulating deoxycholate, there are three possibilities. First, it provides solid matter in the colon to which bile acids and especially deoxycholic acid would tend to adsorb (Eastwood and Hamilton 1968; Story and Kritchevsky 1976). Second, it reduces the time available for deoxycholic acid to be absorbed by speeding up colonic transit; simply taking a senna laxative has the same effect as bran (Marcus and Heaton 1984). Third, up to 50% of bran is metabolised by bacteria to short-chain fatty acids which would lower the pH in the right colon. At low pH, deoxycholic acid is precipitated and so made unavailable for absorption. Also bacterial dehydroxylases become inactive, so less deoxycholic acid is formed — a mechanism which accounts for the actions of lactulose on bile (Thornton and Heaton 1981).

We have studied the effects on bile of replacing fibre-depleted carbohydrate in the diet with full-fibre foods (Thornton et al 1983). Thirteen women with asymptomatic, radiolucent gall-stones were studied after six weeks on a diet containing substantial amounts of fibre-depleted starch and sugar, and again after six weeks on a diet devoid of these products but with free access to all full-fibre foods. The cholesterol saturation index of bile averaged 1.50 on the fibre-depleted diet and 1.20 on the full-fibre diet. On the full-fibre diet, bile was less saturated in all but one person (who ate immoderately of nuts and, unlike the rest, gained weight). There was little change in the deoxycholate content of bile, so it was thought that the beneficial effect of full-fibre foods was not the same as the bran effect. It was speculated that benefit was due to the drastic reduction in the intake of refined sugars (from 106 to 6 g/day). However, we had to drop this idea when a subsequent six-week cross-over study comparing two diets, closely similar except for their sucrose contents (112 and 16 g/day, respectively), showed no difference in bile saturation index (Werner et al 1984). Thus, the short-term beneficial effect of a full-fibre diet is unexplained.

An important finding in both these studies was that mean energy intake was substantially higher on a sucrose-rich diet (23% and 24.5% higher respectively) without the subjects being aware of eating more. These findings give strong support to Cleave's hypothesis. They also help to explain the close association between gall-stones and obesity.

In the sucrose study, the high sucrose period caused an elevation of the plasma triglyceride levels and a fall in the HDL cholesterol concentrations (Werner et al 1984). This is further evidence incriminating sucrose in gall-stone formation since such changes in plasma are strongly linked with an increased risk of gall-stones (see above).

Animal experiments

No animal experiments have been reported which set out to test the fibre-depletion hypothesis. However, many lithogenic dietary regimes have been reported and, although the diets vary widely, they have one feature in common – they are all semi-synthetic or semi-purified (for references, see Heaton, 1975). In practice this means that the carbohydrate component of the diet is always in refined or fibre-depleted form, usually glucose or sucrose, but sometimes corn-starch. The idea that lack of fibre explains the lithogenicity of these diets is supported by two observations. First, in the hamster, the diet loses its lithogenic effect if it is supplemented with bulking agents such as agar and carboxymethyl cellulose, and even if the animal is allowed to eat the straw laid on the floor of its cage. Second, in the rabbit, stones dissolve rapidly if ordinary chow is fed.

CONCLUSION

Eating fibre-depleted rather than full-fibre foods inflates energy intake and depresses fibre intake. In the short term it makes bile more saturated with cholesterol, though the mechanism is unknown and seems not to be loss of a 'bran effect'. Bran seems to work by removing deoxycholic acid from the bile through its effects on colonic function.

In the long term, if obesity results from this or any eating habit the formation of gall-stones will be promoted. Patients with gall-stones tend to eat more sugar than other people in a Western community, but their fibre intake is similar (and low). Populations prone to cholesterol gall-stones tend to be on Western-style diets which are low in fibre and high in refined or fibre-depleted carbohydrate foods. A high intake of cholesterol may be an additional factor.

REFERENCES

Ahlberg J, Angelin B, Einarsson K, Hellström K & Leijd B (1979) Prevalence of gallbladder disease in hyperlipoproteinemia. *Digestive Diseases and Sciences* 24: 459–464.

Ahlberg J, Angelin B, Einarsson K, Hellström K & Leijd B (1980) Biliary lipid composition in normo- and hyperlipoproteinemia. *Gastroenterology* 79: 90–94.

Alessandrini A, Fusco M A, Gatti E & Rossi P A (1982) Dietary fibres and cholesterol gall-stones: a case control study. *Italian Journal of Gastroenterology* 14: 156–158.

Andersén E & Hellström K (1979) The effect of cholesterol feeding on bile acid kinetics and biliary lipids in normolipidemic and hypertriglyceridemic subjects. *Journal of Lipid Research* 20: 1020–1027.

Angelin B, Einarsson K & Leijd B (1983) Bile acid metabolism in hypothyroid subjects: response to substitution therapy. *European Journal of Clinical Investigation* 13: 99–106.

Bennion L J & Grundy S M (1978) Risk factors for the development of cholelithiasis in man. *New England Journal of Medicine* 299: 1161–1167 and 1221–1227.

Bergman F and van der Linden W (1971) Reaction of the mongolian gerbil to a cholesterol-cholic acid-containing gall-stone inducing diet. *Acta Pathologica et Microbiologica Scandinavica* 79: 476–486.

Bouchier I A D (1983) Biochemistry of gallbladder formation. *Clinics in Gastroenterology* 12: 25–48.

Brett M & Barker D J P (1976) The world distribution of gall-stones. *International Journal of Epidemiology* 5: 335–341.

Burnett W (1971) The epidemiology of gall-stones. *Tijdschrift voor Gastroenterologie* 14: 79–89.

Burnstein M J, Ilson R G, Petrunka C N, Taylor R D & Strasberg S M (1983) Evidence for a potent nucleating factor in the gallbladder bile of patients with cholesterol gallstones. *Gastroenterology* 85: 801–807.

Capron J-P, Payenneville H, Dumont M, Dupas J-L & Lorriaux, A (1978) Evidence for an association between cholelithiasis and hiatus hernia. *Lancet* 2: 329–331.

Capron J-P, Piperaud R, Dupas J-L, Delamarre J & Lorriaux A (1981) Evidence for an association between cholelithiasis and diverticular disease of the colon: a case-controlled study. *Digestive Diseases and Sciences* 26: 523–527.

Carulli N, Ponz de Leon M, Loria P et al (1981) Effect of the selective expansion of the cholic acid pool on bile lipid composition: possible mechanism of bile acid induced biliary cholesterol desaturation. *Gastroenterology* 81: 539–546.

Carulli N, Loria P, Bertolotti M et al (1984) Effects of acute changes of bile acid pool composition on biliary lipid secretion. *Journal of Clinical Investigation* 74: 614–624.

Cleave T L (1974) *The Saccharine Disease*. Bristol: Wright.

Cleave T L & Campbell G D (1966) *Diabetes, Coronary Thrombosis and The Saccharine Disease*. Bristol: Wright.

Coste T, Karsenti P, Berta J L, Cubeau J & Guilloud-Bataille M (1979) Facteurs diététiques de la lithiase biliare: comparaison de l'alimentation d'un groupe de lithiasiques à l'alimentation d'un group témoin. *Gastroenterologie, Clinique et Biologique* 3: 417–424.

Dam H, Prange I, Jensen M K, Kallehauge H E & Fenger H J (1971) Studies on human bile. IV. Influence of ingestion of cholesterol in the form of eggs on the composition of bile in healthy subjects. *Zeitschrift für Ernährungswissenschaft* 10: 178–187.

DenBesten L, Connor W E, Bell S (1973) The effect of dietary cholesterol on the composition of human bile. *Surgery* 73: 266–273.

Eastwood M A, Hamilton D (1968) Studies on the adsorption of bile salts to non-absorbed components of diet. *Biochimica et Biophysica Acta* 152: 165–173.

Hauton J (1967) Cholelithiasis. In *Proceedings of 3rd World Congress of Gastroenterology, Tokyo 1966* (vol 4) pp 109–116. Basel: Karger.

Heaton K W (1975) Gallstones and cholecystitis. In Burkitt D P & Trowell H C (eds) *Refined Carbohydrate Foods and Disease. Some Implications of Dietary Fibre*, pp 173–194. London: Academic Press.

Heaton K W (1981) Gallstones. In Trowell H C & Burkitt D P (eds) *Western Diseases: Their Emergence and Prevention*, pp 47–59. London: Edward Arnold.

Heaton K W (1984) The role of diet in the aetiology of cholelithiasis. *Nutrition Abstracts and Reviews: Reviews in Clinical Nutrition* 54: 549–560.

Heaton K W (1985) Bile salts. In Wright R, Millward-Sadler G H, Alberti K G M M & Karran S (eds) *Liver and Biliary Disease*, 2nd edn. London: Baillière Tindall. In press.

Heaton K W, Wicks A C B & Yeates J (1977) Bile composition in relation to race and diet: studies in Rhodesian Africans and in British subjects. In Paumgartner G & Stiehl A (eds) *Bile Acid Metabolism in Health and Disease*, pp 197–202. Lancaster: MTP Press.

Ho K-J (1976) Comparative studies on the effect of cholesterol feeding on biliary composition. *American Journal of Clinical Nutrition* 29: 698–704.

Huijbregts A W M, van Berge-Henegouwen G P, Hectors M P C, van Schaik A & van der Werf S D J (1980) Effects of a standardised wheat bran preparation on biliary lipid composition and bile acid metabolism in young healthy males. *European Journal of Clinical Investigation* 10: 451–458.

Kadziolka R, Nilsson S & Scherstén T (1977) Prevalence of hyperlipoproteinaemia in men with gallstone disease. *Scandinavian Journal of Gastroenterology* 12: 353–355.

Keen H, Thomas B J, Jarrett R J & Fuller J H (1979) Nutrient intake, adiposity, and diabetes. *British Medical Journal* 1: 655–658.

Lee D W, Gilmore C J, Bonorris G G et al (1983) Effect of dietary cholesterol on biliary lipids in women with and without gall-stones. In Paumgartner G, Stiehl A & Gerok W (eds) *Bile Acids and Cholesterol in Health and Disease (Falk Symposium 33)*, pp 237–238. Lancaster: MTP Press.

Low-Beer T S & Nutter S (1978) Colonic bacterial activity, biliary cholesterol saturation, and pathogenesis of gall-stones. *Lancet* 2: 1063–1065.

Low-Beer T S & Pomare E W (1975) Can colonic bacterial metabolites predispose to cholesterol gall-stones? *British Medical Journal* 1: 438–440.

McDougall R M, Yakymyshyn L, Walker K & Thurston O G (1978) The effect of wheat bran on serum lipoproteins and biliary lipids. *Canadian Journal of Surgery* 21: 433–435.

Marcus S N & Heaton K W (1984) Intestinal transit, deoxycholic acid and the cholesterol saturation of bile. *Gut* 25: A1141–A1142.

Nestel P J, Schreibman P H & Ahrens E H (1973) Cholesterol metabolism in human obesity. *Journal of Clinical Investigation* 52: 2389–2397.

Newman H F & Northup J D (1959) The autopsy incidence of gall-stones. *International Abstracts of Surgery* 109: 1–13.

Petitti D B, Friedman G D & Klatsky A L (1981) Association of a history of gallbladder disease with a reduced concentration of high-density-lipoprotein cholesterol. *New England Journal of Medicine* 304: 1396–1398.

Pomare E W, Heaton K W, Low-Beer T S & Espiner H J (1976) The effect of wheat bran upon bile salt metabolism and upon the lipid composition of bile in gallstone patients. *American Journal of Digestive Diseases* 21: 521–526.

Reid J M, Fullmer S D, Pettigrew K D et al (1971). Nutrient intake of Pima Indian women: relationships to diabetes mellitus and gallbladder disease. *American Journal of Clinical Nutrition* 24: 1281–1289.

Salvioli G, Salati R, Bondi M et al (1982) Bile acid transformation by the intestinal flora and cholesterol saturation in bile. Effects of *Streptococcus faecium* administration. *Digestion* 23: 80–88.

Sampliner R E, Bennett P H, Comess L J, Rose F A & Burch T A (1970) Gallbladder disease in Pima Indians. Demonstration of high prevalence and early onset by cholecystography. *New England Journal of Medicine* 283: 1358–1364.

Sarles H, Chalvet H, Ambrosi L & D'Ortoli G (1957) Étude statistique des facteurs dietetiques dans la pathogenie de la lithiase biliaire humaine. *Semaines des Hôpitaux de Paris* 58: 3424–3428.

Sarles H, Hauton J, Lafont H et al (1968) Role de l'alimentation sur la concentration du cholesterol biliaire chez l'homme lithiasique et non-lithiasique. *Clinica Chimica Acta* 19: 147–155.

Sarles H, Chabert C, Pommeau Y et al (1969) Diet and cholesterol gallstones. A study of 101 patients with cholelithiasis compared to 101 matched controls. *American Journal of Digestive Diseases* 14: 531–537.

Sarles H, Crotte C, Gerolami A et al (1971) The influence of calorie intake and of dietary protein on the bile lipids. *Scandinavian Journal of Gastroenterology* 6: 189–191.

Sarles H, Gerolami A & Bord A (1978a). Diet and cholesterol gallstones. A further study. *Digestion* 17: 128–134.

Sarles H, Gerolami A & Cros R C (1978b). Diet and cholesterol gallstones. A multicenter study. *Digestion* **17**: 121–127.

Scragg R K R (1984) Diet, obesity, plasma lipids and insulin in gallstone disease. PhD thesis, University of Adelaide.

Scragg R K R, McMichael A J & Baghurst P A (1984a) Diet, alcohol, and relative weight in gall stone disease: a case-control study. *British Medical Journal* **288**: 1113–1119.

Scragg R K R, Calvert G D & Oliver J R (1984b) Plasma lipids and insulin in gallstone disease: a case-control study. *British Medical Journal* **289**: 521–525.

Smith D A & Gee M I (1979) A dietary survey to determine the relationship between diet and cholelithiasis. *American Journal of Clinical Nutrition* **32**: 1519–1526.

Stace N H, Pomare E W, Peters S, Thomas L & Fisher A (1981) Biliary lipids and dietary intakes (including dietary fiber) in four different female populations. *Gastroenterology* **80**: 1291.

Stephen A M & Cummings J H (1980) Mechanism of action of dietary fibre in the human colon. *Nature*, London **284**: 283–284.

Story J A & Kritchevsky D (1976) Comparison of the binding of various bile acids and bile salts in vitro by several types of fiber. *Journal of Nutrition* **106**: 1292–1294.

Tarpila S, Miettinen T A & Metsäranta L (1978) Effects of bran on serum cholesterol, faecal mass, fat, bile acids and neutral sterols, and biliary lipids in patients with diverticular disease of the colon. *Gut* **19**: 137–145.

Thornton J R & Heaton K W (1981) Do colonic bacteria contribute to cholesterol gallstone formation? Effects of lactulose on bile. *British Medical Journal* **282**: 1018–1020.

Thornton J R, Heaton K W & MacFarlane D G (1980) Plasma lipids, insulin and gallstone risk. *Clinical Science* **59**: 9P.

Thornton J R, Heaton K W & MacFarlane D G (1981) A relation between high-density-lipoprotein cholesterol and bile cholesterol saturation. *British Medical Journal* **283**: 1352–1354.

Thornton J R, Emmett P M & Heaton K W (1983) Diet and gallstones: effects of refined and unrefined carbohydrate diets on bile cholesterol saturation and bile acid metabolism. *Gut* **24**: 2–6.

Trowell H C & Burkitt D P (1981) *Western Diseases: Their Emergence and Prevention*. London: Edward Arnold.

Trowell H C, Southgate D A T, Wolever T M S et al (1976) Dietary fibre redefined. *Lancet* **1**: 967.

Van der Linden W (1961) Some biological traits in female gallstone-disease patients. *Acta Chirurgica Scandinavica Supplementum* **269**.

Van der Linden W & Bergman F (1977) Formation and dissolution of gallstones in experimental animals. *International Reviews of Experimental Pathology* **17**: 173–233.

Watts J McK, Jablonski P & Toouli J (1978) The effect of added bran to the diet on the saturation of bile in people without gall-stones. *American Journal of Surgery* **135**: 321–324.

Werner D, Emmett P M & Heaton K W (1984) The effects of dietary sucrose on factors influencing cholesterol gallstone formation. *Gut* **25**: 269–274.

Wheeler M, Hills L L & Laby B (1970) Cholelithiasis: a clinical and dietary survey. *Gut* **11**: 430–437.

Záhoř Z, Sternby N H, Kagan A et al (1974). Frequency of cholelithiasis in Prague and Malmö. An autopsy study. *Scandinavian Journal of Gastroenterology* **9**: 3–7.

Chapter 18
Nutritional Fatty Liver

J. D. Maxwell

Among patients on the Continent of Europe 'crise de foie' is a common complaint in which the symptoms of malaise and upper abdominal pain are popularly attributed to liver dysfunction as a result of dietary indiscretion. Although European gastro-enterologists have now discarded this notion, the relationship between dietary factors and liver disease continues to attract attention.

The liver's position in relation to the portal circulation emphasises its crucial role in the storage, metabolism and transport of almost all nutrients absorbed from the gut, and via the hepatic artery of lipid and other substances from depots. The complex biochemical functions of the hepatocytes themselves require optimal nutrition. Thus it is not surprising that abnormalities of diet may be important in the pathogenesis of structural and/or functional disorders of the liver (Nayak 1979).

In this chapter I shall first discuss the development of the concept of nutritional liver injury from early experimental studies, and its subsequent reassessment. Then I shall attempt to redefine the role of diet in the pathogenesis of liver injury in a number of conditions in which nutritional factors have been implicated.

HISTORICAL BACKGROUND: CONCEPT OF NUTRITIONAL LIVER INJURY

Early animal experiments showed that two types of liver disease could be induced in rats fed nutritionally deficient diets. In animals given protein deficient diets, acute massive necrosis developed, followed by coarsely nodular and fibrotic liver. The other type of liver disease, produced by prolonged feeding of a lipotrope-deficient diet was a severe and progressive fatty change resulting in diffuse hepatic fibrosis and formation of micronodules (Himsworth and Glynn 1944).

Himsworth extrapolated from these observations in animals to suggest that all fatty liver and cirrhosis in man were caused by nutritional deficiency (Himsworth 1950). Clinical experience at that time seemed to support this view since most alcoholics who developed cirrhosis were obviously malnourished, and the fatty liver of chronic alcoholics preceding the development of cirrhosis was very similar to the sequence of events in the animal model. Moreover, among the malnourished populations of Africa and Asia both macronodular (portal) and micronodular (fatty) cirrhosis were frequently encountered. Severe protein-energy malnutrition (kwashiorkor) seen in children in these developing areas was characterised by grossly fatty liver, which was considered a fore-runner of cirrhosis (Trowell et al 1954).

The concept of nutritional liver disease was at first universally accepted, and indeed is still used as a euphemism for alcoholic liver disease. However this view was challenged by a more critical attitude to experimental studies, in particular by the realisation that different species vary greatly in their reactions to liver injury so that results in rodents may have little relevance to man. Protein and choline deficiency was found to induce fatty liver and cirrhosis only in certain animal species (notably the rat), but not in humans or non-human primates, who lack the enzyme choline oxidase (Sidransky and Farber 1960). Non-human primates were a more suitable model for investigating the effects of nutrition on the liver, but protein deficiency did not produce fatty liver or cirrhosis in baboons (Patrick 1973). Subsequently Rubin and Lieber (1974) showed that baboons fed a nutritionally adequate diet supplemented with alcohol developed all features of human alcoholic liver disease, including cirrhosis.

In many forms of chronic liver disease, multiple factors may be involved, so that it is difficult to define the contribution made by diet. At present it appears that malnutrition has only a very limited primary role, although there is some evidence that it may play a subsidiary part in the development of certain types of liver disease. However, there is increasing recognition that various dietary toxins can result in liver disease, and that under certain circumstances even normal dietary constituents may have deleterious effects on liver structure or function. These aspects will be discussed in subsequent sections of this and the following chapter.

RE-EVALUATION OF THE ROLE OF NUTRITION IN PATHOGENESIS OF CERTAIN FORMS OF LIVER DISEASE

Alcoholic liver disease

The progression of hepatic changes through steatosis to cirrhosis in chronic alcoholics has been recognised since the early nineteenth century. Thus when animal experiments demonstrated that rats fed protein and choline deficient diets consistently developed fatty changes leading to cirrhosis (Himsworth and Glynn 1944) it was readily accepted that human alcoholic liver disease was due to dietary deficiency. The failure of alcohol administered in the drinking water to cause significant hepatic changes (Klatskin et al 1954) in experimental animals seemed to support this view.

However, the failure of early animal experiments to demonstrate a direct hepatotoxic effect of alcohol has now been ascribed to methodological difficulties since animals are reluctant to consume drinking water containing alcohol, and when this was administered as part of a nutritionally adequate liquid diet to baboons the whole spectrum of human alcoholic liver disease from fatty change through hepatitis to cirrhosis was induced (Rubin and Lieber 1974). Studies on human volunteers given nutritionally adequate diets also showed that the addition of alcohol rapidly induced fatty change which could not be prevented by excess protein, but which regressed on withdrawal of alcohol (Rubin and Lieber 1968).

It is difficult to reconcile these findings with other reports indicating that moderately high alcohol intake (160 g/day) did not impede recovery in patients with alcoholic liver disease who were also given a nutritious diet (Patek 1979). Further evidence provided in favour of a nutritional basis for alcoholic liver disease has come from retrospective studies of alcohol intake and dietary habits in hospitalised alcoholic patients. The degree and duration of alcohol excess was not different between patients with and without cirrhosis, but cirrhotics had significantly lower calorie and protein intakes than non-cirrhotics (Patek 1979). However, retrospective studies such as this are complicated by the difficulty in differentiating cause and effect. Severe liver disease may result in anorexia, and it is not clear whether differences in dietary intake between cirrhotics and non-cirrhotics were the cause or consequence of the disease (Lieber et al 1979). Nevertheless, abstinence results in regression of precirrhotic hepatic abnormalities and improves life expectancy in patients with alcoholic liver disease (Brunt et al 1974). Moreover, epidemiological studies have shown excessive alcohol consumption to be the cause of most cirrhosis in developed Western countries, and that this is related to the severity and duration of alcohol excess, but not to dietary deficiency as judged by weight loss and economic status of the subjects (Lelbach 1975; Patek et al 1975).

The possibility that protein deficiency may potentiate the effect of alcohol remains under investigation, since such a phenomenon has been observed for fatty liver in the rat (Lieber et al 1969) and rhesus monkey (Nayak 1979) and appears to hold for some other hepatotoxins (Carey et al 1966). It is also of interest to speculate whether deficiency of micronutrients (such as zinc, which is a co-factor for various metallo-protein enzymes) might also potentiate the hepato-toxic effects of alcohol.

At present the evidence for a direct toxic effect of alcohol seems overwhelming, but the range of alcohol intake which can normally be tolerated without liver damage may be determined by the individual's nutritional status. However, above a certain threshold, no protection against alcohol toxicity is provided by dietary manipulation (Patek 1979; Morgan 1982).

Complex nutritional deficiencies may result from chronic alcoholism due to accompanying liver and pancreatic disease. It is also recognised that alcohol ingestion, as well as causing diminished food intake from anorexia, may result in malabsorption and intestinal injury (Morgan 1982). Thus, regardless of the continuing controversy concerning the place of nutrition in the pathogenesis of liver injury in the alcoholic, it seems rational to correct nutritional deficiencies when present, especially in view of the interaction of alcoholism and nutrition.

Overnutrition and liver disease

Histological abnormalities are found in the majority of greatly obese subjects. It is now well recognised that between 65% and 90% of morbidly obese patients have some degree of hepatic steatosis (Salmon and Reedyk 1975;

Baddeley 1976). Much of this hepatic lipid accumulation in obesity probably represents a local manifestation of a generalised increase in lipid stores. Although marked fatty change is most prevalent in the heaviest patients, the relationship between steatosis and degree of obesity is inexact (Figure 18.1).

This poor correlation may be partly explained by the fact that histological estimates provide only a rough guide to total hepatic lipid concentration (Holzbach et al 1974). In addition it seems likely that in a proportion of obese individuals, alcohol provides a significant contribution to total calories, and to hepatic steatosis (Juhl and Quaade 1970). It is interesting that other abnormalities occasionally reported in liver biopsies from grossly overweight subjects include focal necrosis, and established cirrhosis (Brown et al 1974) and that liver function tests may be unreliable in obese subjects in detecting these underlying histological findings (Galambos and Wills 1978) which can all be produced by alcohol excess. Such reports emphasise the importance of pre-operative assessment of liver morphology in grossly overweight individuals before embarking on surgery for obesity (Maxwell 1980).

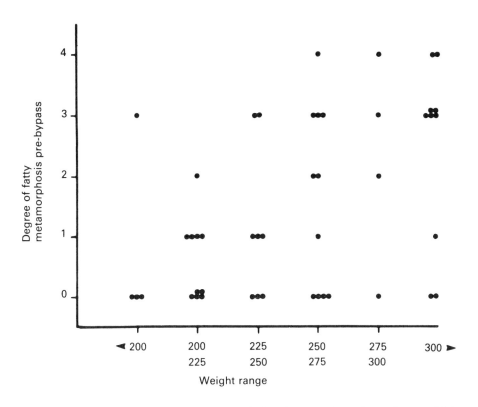

Figure 18.1. The extent of hepatic steatosis in obese patients in various weight categories before intestinal by-pass surgery. From Salmon and Reedyk (1975), with kind permission of the authors and the editor of *Surgery, Gynecology and Obstetrics*.

Malnutrition and liver disease

It has been estimated that over 100 million children throughout the developing world are affected by some form of malnutrition, varying from mild varieties, through non-oedematous wasting (marasmus), to severe oedematous malnutrition (kwashiorkor) with a high mortality. In these children, intermittent diarrhoea and anorexia are commonly seen in association with growth retardation. Hepatic abnormalities are also well recognised, particularly in kwashiorkor where the liver appears large, yellow, soft, and greasy. Microscopically severe fatty change is often associated with hepatocellular inflammation and necrosis. Fatty change initially and predominantly affects periportal liver cells, but with increasing duration and severity of disease the whole of every lobule may be involved so that morphologically the organ resembles adipose tissue and is only recognised as liver by the presence of portal tracts. Fibrous tissue is not appreciably increased, except in longstanding and severe disease when some increased fibrosis may be observed linking portal tracts. Cirrhosis is not seen (McLean 1966; Alleyne et al 1977).

Kwashiorkor affects infants and growing children, particularly after weaning when demand for protein is high. The terms Protein Calorie Malnutrition (PCM) and Protein Energy Malnutrition (PEM), commonly used to describe kwashiorkor and other syndromes of wasting and growth failure, imply a simple nutritional basis. The conventional view is that kwashiorkor is a manifestation of protein deficiency in the presence of adequate caloric intake (in the form of high carbohydrate or high fat diet), while marasmus results from a global deficiency of both protein and calories (Alleyne et al 1977). The biochemical explanation for fatty liver in kwashiorkor is that severe protein deficiency limits lipoprotein synthesis: non-complexed triglycerides are not exported from the liver and continue to accumulate in hepatocytes. Since fat is available in depots, and to some extent in the diet, its influx to the liver continues. On the other hand, where severe deprivation of both proteins as well as fat and calories exists (marasmus), depot fat is rapidly exhausted in providing energy requirements. The absence of fatty liver in marasmus, despite inadequate synthesis of carrier protein, is attributed to marked reduction in availability of lipid to the hepatocyte (Nayak 1979; Coward and Lunn 1981).

However, accumulating evidence now suggests that a purely dietary hypothesis cannot adequately account for these disorders (Behar 1977; Longhurst 1981), nor explain differences between major clinical syndromes (Gopalan 1968). New evidence suggests that orthodox views on the primary role of nutritional deficiency in PEM, and hence in the pathogenesis of the associated hepatic changes, must be reassessed. It is now clear that dietary protein levels that were formerly considered grossly inadequate are capable of sustaining normal growth (Annegers 1973). Food and Agriculture Organization – World Health Organisation (FAO) data comparing the average daily per capita availability of food energy and protein for various countries shows more than adequate availability in all, and little difference in protein energy (P/E) ratios between countries with no malnutrition and those where this problem exists in varying degrees (Behar 1977). While such epidemiological data can be criticised on the grounds that population mean values might obscure areas of real deprivation, detailed long term studies of individual communities have demonstrated that, although various indices of nutrition were favourable through all sections of the community, infant malnutrition remained widespread (Longhurst 1979).

Moreover, the nutritional basis for the distinction between various forms of PEM has been questioned, as no difference has been found in P/E ratios or total food intake in children who ultimately developed marasmus or kwashiorkor (Gopalan 1968).

Animal studies have also failed to provide convincing support for the classical dietary explanation for kwashiorkor. In primates, prolonged low-protein, high-carbohydrate diets, although impairing body growth, did not produce a kwashiorkor-like syndrome. Only after early weaning, and subsequent stressing by prolonged (200–300 days) severe protein and energy restriction, did a condition reminiscent of marasmic-kwashiorkor develop in baboons (Coward and Whitehead 1972). Even at the height of this illness, there was no excess of liver fat, hepatocellular inflammation, or necrosis (Patrick et al 1973). Moreover, although laboratory animals fed restricted diets rapidly regain weight and health when allowed normal diets, hospital mortality rates for kwashiorkor have remained at around 20–30% for many years, despite high protein and calorie feeds. Finally, strenuous and costly efforts to prevent PEM, addressed to improving nutrition (supplements, enrichment, nutrition education) have given disappointing results. Thus, there is a growing realisation that increased food availability is not the solution to infant malnutrition in the developing world, and even if this were possible, it would not eliminate malnutrition in most children who suffer from it (Behar 1977).

The reassessment of the role of diet in the pathogenesis of kwashiorkor and its hepatic complications has led to a renewed interest in the possible role of gut infection, first suggested over 25 years ago (Smythe 1958). More recently, longitudinal studies in children from both malarial (Gambia) and non-malarial regions (Guatemala) have shown that gastro-enteritis is the single most important factor affecting growth. Recurrent episodes of diarrhoea (which affects children with kwashiorkor on average 10–20% of the time) can account for virtually all the growth failure seen in 'malnutrition' (Rowland et al 1977). In many areas there is a significant relationship between the onset of the rainy season, increased water pollution with faecal bacteria, and diarrhoeal disease (Tomkins et al 1978), which seems to be associated with bacterial colonisation of the small intestine. Microbial overgrowth in the upper small bowel has been demonstrated in jejunal aspirates from malnourished infants in studies from West Africa, Central America, and South East Asia (Rowland et al 1977; Gracey 1979). In view of the association of kwashiorkor and marasmus with the weaning and post-weaning period, it seems likely that bacterial overgrowth in the small intestine and diarrhoea at this time is due to the ingestion of bacteriologically contaminated food and water which is unavoidable in endemic areas (Rowland et al 1978).

Experiments with an animal model of jejuno-ileal by-pass have demonstrated that growing rats with bacterial overgrowth in the small intestine develop many of the features characteristic of human kwashiorkor, and suggest that small intestinal bacterial overgrowth could be a *primary* aetiological factor in the development of childhood growth retardation and malnutrition. Rats with a 90% resection of small intestine adapted well, and, after initial weight loss gained weight, thrived, and maintained normal liver function. However, rats with an equivalent small intestinal by-pass (retaining the long excluded segment of bowel as an isoperistaltically emptying loop) showed impaired growth, the rapid onset of hypo-albuminaemia (occasionally with ascites), hepatocellular dysfunction with increased hepatic lipid and substantial mortality (Figure 18.2).

These changes were not the result of enhanced malabsorption due to the excluded loop, as there was no difference in faecal calorie or lipid excretion between resected and by-pass rats, and pair feeding experiments showed the increased weight loss to be due to diminished food intake.

The abnormalities which develop after by-pass in the rat are reminiscent of many of the features of human kwashiorkor and marasmus. The by-passed segment of small bowel is heavily colonised and the excess mortality was corrected, and disturbances in growth and liver function were modified by

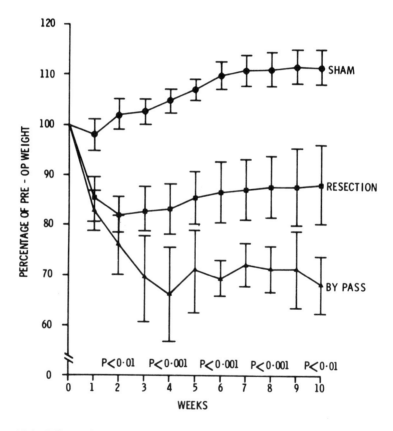

Figure 18.2. Effect of sham operation (●), 90% small bowel resection (■) and equivalent by-pass (▲) on body weight in the rat. After by-pass, rats lost twice as much weight as after resection (*p*<0.001).

antibiotics. Toxins produced by the abnormal intestinal flora could explain diminished appetite, enhanced weight loss, and hepatocellular dysfunction (Maxwell et al 1982). A purely nutritional basis for liver disease in PEM now seems unlikely since chronic gastro-intestinal bacterial overgrowth in association with a nutritional defect appears to reproduce many of the important features of marasmus and kwashiorkor (better than do nutritional models alone).

Starvation in adults does not appear to have important effects on the liver since grossly malnourished German subjects studied after the war, who had substantial weight loss, showed no signs of hepatic disease and had normal liver histology (Sherlock and Walshe 1948). Liver biopsies from patients with anorexia nervosa are also essentially normal.

Clinical and epidemiological studies have also brought into question the relationship between malnutrition and chronic liver disease, since follow-up of children with severe fatty liver of kwashiorkor did not show progression to cirrhosis (Cook and Hutt 1967). The discovery of Australia antigen and rapid developments in detection of hepatitis viruses revealed that they were responsible not only for acute hepatitis, but for much chronic liver disease, particularly in the developing world. Although malnourished populations are at high risk of exposure to hepatitis viruses, there is no evidence that malnutrition 'conditions' the liver to infective agents.

Liver disease after intestinal by-pass surgery for obesity

Just as the critics of the nutritional hypothesis for liver disease appeared to be winning the argument, the occurrence of liver disease after by-pass surgery of the small intestine for obesity revived the controversy and seemed to provide new evidence for the importance of malnutrition in the pathogenesis of fatty liver, hepatocellular necrosis, and cirrhosis.

Jejuno-colic anastomosis, the prototype intestinal by-pass operation for obesity, was abandoned after it became apparent that it had an unacceptably high morbidity and mortality, with almost half the deaths resulting from liver failure (McGill et al 1972). Subsequently jejuno-ileal anastomosis was introduced, and proved to be a much more satisfactory procedure, but liver dysfunction, although infrequent, remained the most serious complication (Maxwell et al 1977).

Prevalence of liver disease after intestinal by-pass

Data from a number of well documented reports from Europe and the USA including at least 50 patients are summarised in Table 18.1. This shows the overall mortality of jejuno-ileal by-pass together with deaths associated with liver failure, and numbers of patients with clinically significant liver involvement. From these reports it appears that liver disturbance occurs in between 3% and 10% of patients after jejuno-ileal bypass. Although the overall mortality is much lower than seen after jejuno-colic anastomosis, deaths associated with liver disease continue to make a substantial contribution — between 25% and 75% — to total deaths.

Table 18.1. Some reports on overall mortality rate, clinically significant liver dysfunction, and deaths associated with liver failure after jejuno-ileal by-pass.

Author	Cases	Overall mortality	Liver dysfunction	Deaths associated with liver failure
DeWind and Payne (1976)	230	19 (8%)	14 (6%)	10 (4%)
Bray et al (1976)	989	47 (4%)	Not stated	11 (1%)
Maxwell et al (1977)	120	5 (4%)	3 (3%)	3 (3%)
Halverson et al (1978)	101	5 (5%)	6 (6%)	3 (3%)
Andersen et al (1980)	2450	123/2450 (5%)	83/1917 (4.3%)	Not stated

Liver changes after intestinal by-pass

When weight loss is achieved by dieting, hepatic histology improves, and there is reduction in steatosis (Drenick et al 1970). This is in striking contrast to weight reduction achieved after jejuno-ileal by-pass, which is followed by worsening steatosis, often accompanied by hepatitic changes and fibrosis. These changes are remarkably similar to those in alcoholic liver disease (Peters et al 1975). The triad of steatosis, hepatocellular necrosis and fibrosis seen in both disorders may persist or progress in apparently healthy patients five or more years after by-pass (Hocking et al 1981).

Fatty change

A striking increase in hepatic fat occurs during the early postoperative catabolic phase of weight loss. Fat accumulation is maximal around six months post-operatively, subsiding to preoperative values about two to three years after surgery (Salmon and Reedyk 1975). The demonstration of a relationship between the extent of weight loss at intervals after by-pass and the degree of fatty change in the liver (Figure 18.3) suggests a relationship between postoperative hepatic steatosis, and the rate of mobilisation of fat from peripheral stores to fulfil calorie requirements. Chemical estimates show a net fat accumulation of at least three times preoperative values 13 months after by-pass. This is largely due to increase in hepatic triglycerides, with little change in cholesterol or phospholipid concentration (Holzbach et al 1974).

Although extensive fatty metamorphosis is the most obvious change in the liver after by-pass, fat accumulation *per se* is generally of little significance. The other morphological changes may be more important determinants of hepatic dysfunction.

Hepatocellular necrosis

Hepatic changes after by-pass are most prominent during the early postoperative period, but can be detected in asymptomatic individuals some years after

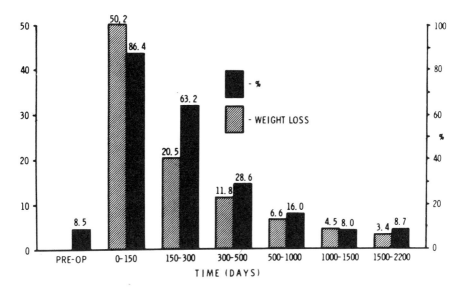

Figure 18.3. Relationship between marked fatty infiltration and weight loss after jejuno-ileal by-pass. Weight lost in each period is expressed as a percentage of total weight lost (shaded columns), and related to percentage of patients with marked hepatic steatosis (solid black columns) in each period. From Salmon and Reedyk (1975), with kind permission of the authors and the editor of *Surgery, Gynecology and Obstetrics.*

surgery, well after weight stabilisation. They are reflected in routine liver function tests by elevation of hepatocellular enzymes, accompanied by small but significant changes in plasma bilirubin, alkaline phosphatase and albumin which are apparent during the early postoperative period, and revert to normal after a new stable weight is achieved (Maxwell et al 1977) (Figure 18.4).

However, unlike fat accumulation, biochemical disturbances after by-pass do not seem to be related to the extent of weight loss, nor are they due to alcohol, halothane or hepatitis B infection. It is of interest that the median time after by-pass for the appearance of clinical liver dysfunction (three months) is precisely the time when the most significant biochemical changes are noted in asymptomatic patients following surgery. Thus the development of jaundice and liver failure after intestinal by-pass seems to represent the tip of an iceberg of widespread asymptomatic liver disturbance, rather than a rare idiosyncratic response.

Hepatic fibrosis/cirrhosis

Although minor degrees of fibrosis (and cirrhosis) may be present in obese individuals before surgery, there is good evidence that these changes may develop *de novo*, or progress, after intestinal by-pass (Maxwell and McGouran 1982). While some cases of cirrhosis occurring after by-pass may be due to alcohol abuse, it is well established that cirrhosis may be a genuine complication of the by-pass procedure itself, with over 9% of patients

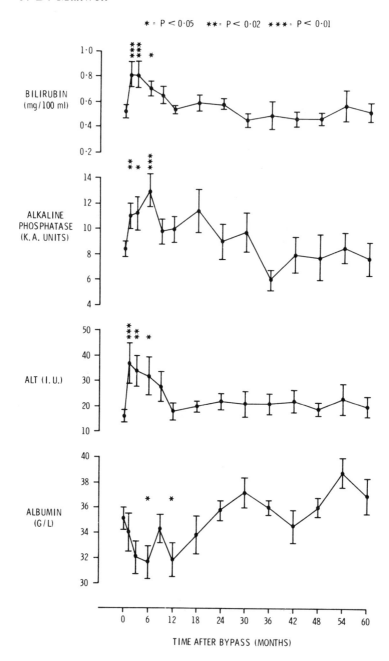

Figure 18.4. Mean (±SEM) plasma concentrations of bilirubin, alkaline phosphatase, alanine aminotransferase (ALT), and albumin in 35 healthy patients followed up to 60 months after jejuno-ileal by-pass. Asterisks denote significant change from preoperative values. From Maxwell et al (1977), with kind permission of the editor of the *British Medical Journal*.

developing this complication on long term follow up (Hocking et al 1981). Interestingly, increased activity of proline hydroxylase (the rate-limiting enzyme in collagen synthesis) has been demonstrated in liver biopsies from patients after by-pass who develop hepatocellular necrosis and fibrosis, but not in biopsies showing only fatty change (Mezey and Imbembo 1978).

Hepatic granulomas

In a small proportion of liver biopsies taken after intestinal by-pass, non-caseating granulomas have been noted, unrelated to tuberculosis, sarcoid or liver failure. Although of no clinical significance, they may provide an insight into the pathogenesis of hepatic disease after intestinal by-pass, as granulomas can result from immune complex deposition (Spector and Heesom 1969).

Nutritional deficiency

Intestinal by-pass operations created a human model which challenged the concept that malnutrition does not cause chronic liver injury in man, and the similarity to the hepatic changes seen in kwashiorkor prompted the suggestion that *protein malnutrition* might account for liver disease after by-pass. This was supported by the observation that in the early catabolic period after by-pass (when fatty change was most marked, and liver function tests most deranged) plasma amino acid profiles were typical of protein-calorie malnutrition (Moxley et al 1974). After weight stabilisation, the concentrations of amino acids returned to normal, and amino acid tolerance tests improved, suggesting improved absorption. However there is no good evidence that protein deficiency, even of extreme degree, can result in hepatocellular necrosis, inflammation or fibrosis in man (Mezey and Imbembo 1978) — the most significant changes following by-pass surgery. Moreover, it is of interest that in contrast to the findings after by-pass, when equivalent weight loss is achieved by dieting, hepatic histology improves, and there is reduction in steatosis (Drenick et al 1970).

Other nutritional factors implicated include deficiency of *essential fatty acids and lipotropes*. It has been speculated that essential fatty acid deficiency (as a result of the short gut and steatorrhoea) might cause disruption of lysosomal membranes and consequent hepatic damage. However there is no evidence from clinical studies to support this suggestion. Although intestinal adaptation is morphologically less pronounced after by-pass than comparable resection, and it has been inferred from this that some (unspecified) nutritional defect might account for by-pass disease (Vanderhoof et al 1981), animals with experimental resection or by-pass show no difference in malabsorption of fat or total calories. As animals which have undergone resection do not develop liver dysfunction (Maxwell and McGouran 1982), selective nutritional deficiency after by-pass seems unlikely. Nor is there any evidence in man to support the suggestion that liver changes after by-pass are related to, or aggravated by, deficiency of *vitamins, minerals* or choline. Experimental evidence in support of the nutritional hypothesis has come from studies in dogs, where progression to liver damage and death was inevitable after 80% by-pass, but could be prevented by daily instillation of 15 g of predigested gelatin, or of 15–30 ml of medium chain triglyceride (MCT) into the proximal end of an exteriorised by-passed loop. However 2 g of sulphathalidine or 5 g of methylcellulose had no such protective effect (McClelland et al 1970). It was concluded that the gelatin and MCT prevented liver damage by providing additional nutrition, but other interpretations are possible. The instilled nutrients might have encouraged the development of a normal flora, or may have exerted a cleansing effect on the by-passed loop.

The alternative hypothesis implicates *intestinal bacteria*. The small bowel does not normally harbour anaerobes or coliforms in significant numbers. However, after jejuno-ileal by-pass, the development of an abnormal colonic type flora is well documented in both experimental animals and clinical studies (Maxwell and McGouran 1982). Significant bacterial overgrowth in the long, excluded segment of jejuno-ileum is accompanied by a similar flora in the small intestine remaining in continuity.

The most persuasive evidence implicating bacteria in hepatic dysfunction after intestinal by-pass comes from a number of experimental animal studies which have demonstrated that liver dysfunction follows experimental jejuno-ileal by-pass, but is not seen after equivalent resection (Maxwell and McGouran 1982) (Figures 18.5 and 18.6).

Further evidence implicating bacteria has come from studies showing that antibiotics can prevent hepatic dysfunction after by-pass in animals (Hollenbeck et al 1975; McGouran and Maxwell 1980) and man (Vanderhoof et al 1981; Drenick et al 1982). Abnormal metabolism by intestinal bacteria of ingested nutrients and *bile acids* could contribute to liver injury after by-pass via the production of endogenous hepatotoxins. Enhanced bacterial deconjugation of bile salts and high plasma levels of potentially hepatoxic secondary bile acids have been demonstrated after jejuno-ileal by-pass (Banwell et al 1974). However it is unlikely that these are responsible for the develop-

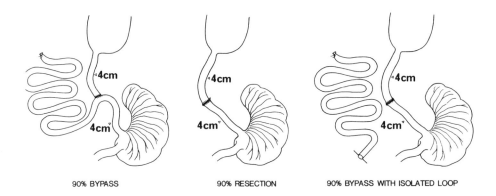

90% BYPASS   90% RESECTION   90% BYPASS WITH ISOLATED LOOP

Figure 18.5. Diagrammatic representation of 90% end-to-side jejuno-ileal by-pass and equivalent resection in the rat. In additional experiments the long by-passed loop was isolated and exteriorised as an ileostomy. Enhanced weight loss and adverse effects on liver function occur, whether or not the excluded segment has direct access to functioning bowel.

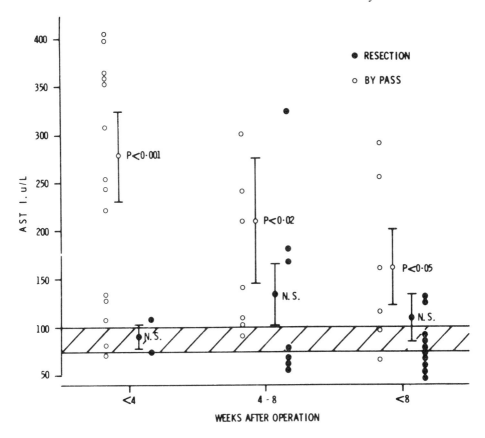

Figure 18.6. Effect of 90% jejuno-ileal bypass (○) and resection (●) in rats on plasma aspartate aminotransferase (AST) for three time periods after surgery. Shaded area denotes mean ±SEM for sham-operated controls. Plasma AST was unaffected by resection, but significantly elevated after by-pass. From McGouran and Maxwell (1980), with kind permission of Academic Press.

ment of liver disease, as this is not seen after equivalent bile salt malabsorption in patients undergoing ileal resection. Furthermore, patients with the bilio-intestinal type of by-pass (where the apex of the excluded jejuno-ileal segment is anastomosed to the gall-bladder, allowing enhanced bacterial deconjugation and subsequent absorption of bile acids from the long excluded segment) do not appear to be at increased risk of liver dysfunction. Intestinal bacterial fermentation of ingested carbohydrate to *alcohol* would provide a satisfactory explanation both for the occurrence of liver disease after by-pass, and its similarity to alcoholic liver disease. Alcohol has been detected after by-pass in venous samples from man and the dog, but levels were very low and insufficient to implicate this as a hepato-toxin (Mezey et al 1975). Additionally it has been suggested that dietary choline could be converted to the lipotrophically inactive form, trimethylamine, by the increased numbers of bacteria present after by-pass. There is no evidence that deficiency of choline or other nutrients, vitamins or minerals ever causes clinically significant liver injury in man.

An ingenious experimental modification of the standard jejuno-ileal operation has also cast doubt on the relevance of intestinal bacterial metabolism (either by producing hepatotoxic products from bile salts or ingested food, or by inactivating dietary lipotropes) in the pathogenesis of liver disease after intestinal by-pass. In these studies, the long excluded segment of jejuno-ileum was separated from the short section of functioning small bowel and exteriorised. (Figure 18.5). Thus there was no longer any connection between the heavily colonised excluded loop, and food or endogenous bile secretions. Nevertheless, adverse effects on the liver were identical to those seen after standard jejuno-ileal by-pass (Edmiston et al 1979; McGouran and Maxwell 1980).

Thus a *direct hepatotoxic effect of bacteria* seems the most likely explanation for liver dysfunction after intestinal by-pass, but this conclusion is tentative and reached only after exclusion of possible indirect bacterial mechanisms discussed above. There is no evidence to implicate bacterial colonisation of the liver after by-pass. Although portal pyaemia is not infrequent, liver disease due to direct bacterial involvement is rare, and has not been reported after intestinal by-pass. Circulating immune complexes have been implicated in skin and joint disease after by-pass surgery and it is possible that immunological sequelae of intestinal bacterial overgrowth may also be involved in disturbances of liver structure and function. Granulomas, which are occasionally found in the liver after by-pass, can be produced by immune complexes (Spector and Heesom 1969). However bacterial endotoxins absorbed via the portal vein to the liver also seem likely candidates, and certainly are capable of causing hepatocellular damage and cholestasis and of inhibiting liver phagocytes (Nolan 1978).

Thus current evidence suggests that liver injury after intestinal by-pass is due to some enterohepatic factor related to bacterial overgrowth in the long, excluded segment. Nevertheless, associated nutritional deficiency may play a permissive role, as indicated by the need for an extensive by-pass before liver disturbance occurs (Burney et al 1977), and from studies showing that protein deficiency enhances the effects of certain hepatotoxins (Lieber 1974; Carey et al 1966).

Parenteral nutrition and liver disease

Cholestasis has developed in infants given long term parenteral nutrition for neonatal intestinal obstruction, and a mixed cholestatic-hepatitic picture can develop in adults on total parenteral nutrition (TPN) for two weeks or longer.

Components of the TPN solutions (fat; amino acids) have been incriminated, and experimental studies have also shown that both nitrogen containing and hyperosmolar solutions may have an anti-choleretic effect (Cano and Gerolami 1983).

Intrahepatic cholestasis during TPN may also be related to gut flora changes, with overgrowth of bacteria favouring endotoxin and lithocholic acid production. Reports indicating that metronidazole treatment can prevent cholestasis during TPN support this suggestion (Capron et al 1983). For further discussion of TPN see Chapter 16.

REFERENCES

Alleyne G A O, Hay R W, Picou D, Stanfield J P & Whitehead R S (1977) *Protein Energy Malnutrition* London: Arnold.

Anderson T, Juhl E & Quaade F (1980) Jejuno-ileal bypass for obesity—what can we learn from a literature study. *American Journal of Clinical Nutrition* 33: 440–445.

Annegers J F (1973) The protein–calorie ratio of West African diets and their relationship to protein-calorie malnutrition. *Ecology of Food and Nutrition* 2: 225–235.

Baddeley R M (1976) Results of jejuno-ileostomy for gross refractory obesity. *British Journal of Surgery* 63: 801–806.

Banwell J G, Lockwood D H, Sherr H P, Nair P P & White J J (1974) Bile acid metabolism and hepatic disease following small bowel bypass for obesity. *American Journal of Clinical Nutrition* 27: 1369–1379.

Behar M (1977) Protein-calorie deficits in developing countries. *Annals of the New York Academy of Science,* 300: 176–187.

Bray G A, Barry R E, Benfield J R et al (1976) Intestinal bypass as a treatment for obesity. *Annals of Internal Medicine* 85: 97–109.

Brown R G, O'Leary J P R & Woodward E R (1974) Hepatic effects of the jejuno-ileal bypass for morbid obesity. *American Journal of Surgery* 127: 53–58.

Brunt P W, Kew M C, Scheuer P J & Sherlock S (1974) Studies in alcoholic liver disease in Britain. *Gut* 15: 52–58.

Burney D P, Burnham S J, Hough A J & Scott H W (1977) Experimental short gut: hepatic alterations after jejuno-ileal resection, by-pass and vibramycin therapy. *American Surgeon* 43: 778–786.

Cano N & Gerolami A (1983) Intrahepatic cholestasis during total parenteral nutrition. *Lancet* 1: 985.

Capron J-P, Gineston J-L, Herve M-A & Braillon A (1983) Metronidazole prevention of cholestasis associated with total parenteral nutrition. *Lancet* 1: 446–447.

Carey J B, Wilson I D, Zaki F G & Hanson R F (1966) The metabolism of bile acids with special reference to liver injury. *Medicine* (Baltimore) 45: 461–470.

Cook G C & Hutt M S R (1967) The liver after kwashiorkor. *British Medical Journal* 3: 454–457.

Coward W A & Lunn P G (1981) The biochemistry and physiology of kwashiorkor and marasmus. *British Medical Bulletin* 37: 19–24.

Coward D G & Whitehead R G (1972) Experimental protein-energy malnutrition in baby baboons. *British Journal of Nutrition* 30: 171–179.

DeWind L T & Payne J H (1976) Intestinal bypass surgery for morbid obesity—long term results. *JAMA* 236: 2298–2301.

Drenick E J, Simmons F & Murphy J F (1970) Effect on hepatic morphology of treatment of obesity by fasting, reducing diets, and small bowel bypass. *New England Journal of Medicine* 282: 829–834.

Drenick E J, Fisler J & Johnson D (1982) Hepatic steatosis after intestinal by-pass. Prevention and reversal by metronidazole, irrespective of protein-calorie malnutrition. *Gastroenterology* 82: 535–548.

Edmiston C E, Hulsey T K, Scott H W, Hoyumpa A M & Wilson F A (1979) Microbial colonisation and hepatic abnormalities in jejuno-ileal by-pass with resection, mucous fistula and ileo-colostomy. *Journal of Infectious Diseases* 140: 358–369.

Galambos J T & Wills C E (1978) Relationship between 505 paired liver tests and biopsies in 242 obese patients. *Gastroenterology* 74: 1191–1195.

Gopalan C (1968) Kwashiorkor and marasmus: Evolution and protein deficiencies. In McCance R A & Widdowson E M (eds) *Calorie Deficiencies*, pp 49–58. London: Churchill.

Gracey M (1979) The contaminated small bowel syndrome. *American Journal of Clinical Nutrition* 32: 234–243.

Halverson J D, Wise L, Wazna M F & Ballinger W F (1978) Jejuno-ileal by-pass for morbid obesity. *American Journal of Medicine* 64: 461–475.

Himsworth H P (1950) *Lectures on the Liver and its Disease*, 2nd edn, p 91. Oxford: Blackwell.

Himsworth H P & Glynn L E (1944) Massive hepatic necrosis and diffuse hepatic fibrosis (acute yellow atrophy and portal cirrhosis): their production by means of diet. *Clinical Science* 5: 93–123.

Hocking M P, Duerson M C, Alexander R W & Woodward E R (1981) Hepatic histopathology after jejuno-ileal by-pass for morbid obesity. *American Journal of Surgery* **141**: 159–163.

Hollenbeck J I, O'Leary J P, Maher J W & Woodward E R (1975) The pathogenesis of liver failure after bypass for obesity. *Review of Surgery* **32**: 149–152.

Holzbach R T, Wieland R G, Lieber C S et al (1974) Hepatic lipid in morbid obesity. Assessment at and subsequent to jejuno-ileal by-pass. *New England Journal of Medicine* **290**: 296–299.

Juhl E & Quaade F (1970) Obesity in patients with cirrhosis of the liver. *Scandinavian Journal of Gastroenterology* **5** (Suppl. 7): 207–212.

Klatskin G, Krehl W A & Conn H O (1954) Effect of alcohol on choline requirement. *Journal of Experimental Medicine* **100**: 605–614.

Lelbach W K (1975) Cirrhosis in the alcoholic and its relation to the volume of alcohol abuse. *Annals of the New York Academy of Sciences* **252**: 85–105.

Lieber C S (1974) Effects of ethanol upon lipid metabolism. *Lipids* **9**: 103–107.

Lieber C S, Spritz N & De Carli L M (1969) Fatty liver produced by dietary deficiencies: its pathogenesis and potentiation by ethanol. *Journal of Lipid Research* **10**: 283–287.

Lieber C S, Seitz H K, Garro A J & Worner T M (1979) Alcohol related diseases and carcinogenesis. *Cancer Research* **39**: 2863–2886.

Longhurst R W (1979) Malnutrition and the community — the social origins of deprivation. *Proceedings of the Nutrition Society* **38**: 11–16.

Maxwell J D (1980) Liver disease. In Maxwell J D, Gazet J-C & Pilkington T R E (eds) *Surgical Management of Obesity* pp 235–255. London: Academic Press.

Maxwell J D & McGouran R C (1982) Jejuno-ileal by-pass. Clinical and experimental aspects. *Scandinavian Journal of Gastroenterology* **17** (Suppl. 74): 129–147.

Maxwell J D, Sanderson I, Butler W H, Gazet J-C & Pilkington T R E (1977) Hepatic structure and function after modified jejuno-ileal by-pass surgery for obesity. *British Medical Journal* **2**: 726–729.

Maxwell J D, Ang L, Cleeve H J W & McGouran R C (1982) Intestinal by-pass in the rat: a model for growth failure, liver disease and jejunal bacterial overgrowth in marasmus and kwashiorkor. *Journal of Pediatric Gastroenterology and Nutrition* **1**: 417–425.

McGill D B, Humpherys S R, Baggenstoss A H & Dickson E R (1972) Cirrhosis and death after jejuno-ileal shunt. *Gastroenterology* **63**: 872–875.

McGouran R C & Maxwell J D (1980) Animal models of intestinal by-pass. In Maxwell J D, Gazet J-C & Pilkington T R E (eds) *Surgical Management of Obesity*, pp 159–169. London: Academic Press.

McLean A E M (1966) Enzyme activity in the liver and serum of malnourished children. *Clinical Science* **30**: 129–137.

McLelland R N, Deshazo C U, Heimbach D M, Eigenbrodt E H & Dowdy A B (1970) Prevention of hepatic injury after jejuno-ileal by-pass by supplemental jejunostomy feedings. *Surgical Forum* **21**: 368–370.

Mezey E & Imbembo A L (1978) Hepatic collagen proline hydroxylase activity in heaptic disease following jejuno-ileal by-pass for morbid obesity. *Surgery* **83**: 345–353.

Mezey E, Imbembo A L, Potter J J, Rent K C, Lombardo R & Holt P R (1975) Endogenous ethanol production and hepatic disease following jejuno-ileal by-pass for morbid obesity. *American Journal of Clinical Nutrition* **28**: 1277–1283.

Morgan M (1982) Alcohol and nutrition. *British Medical Bulletin* **38**: 21–29.

Moxley R T, Pozefsky T & Lockwood D H (1974) Protein nutrition and liver disease after jejuno-ileal by-pass for morbid obesity. *New England Journal of Medicine* **290**: 921–926.

Nayak N C (1979) Nutritional liver disease. In MacSween R N M, Anthony P P & Scheuer P J (eds) *Pathology of the Liver*, pp 221–231. Edinburgh: Churchill-Livingstone.

Nolan J P (1978) Bacteria and the liver. *New England Journal of Medicine* **299**: 1069–1071.

Patek A J (1979) Alcohol, malnutrition and alcholic cirrhosis. *American Journal of Clinical Nutrition* **32**: 1304–1312.

Patek A J, Toth I G, Saunders M G, Castro G A M & Engel J J (1975) Alcohol and dietary factors in cirrhosis: an epidemiological study of 304 alcoholic patients. *Archives of Internal Medicine* **135**: 1053–1057.

Patrick R S, Mackay A M, Coward D G & Whitehead R G (1973) Experimental protein-energy malnutrition in baby baboons. 2. Liver pathology. *British Journal of Nutrition* **30**: 171–179.

Peters R L, Gay T & Reynolds T B (1975) Post jejuno-ileal by-pass hepatic disease: its similarity to alcohol hepatic disease. *American Journal of Clinical Pathology* **63**: 318–331.

Rowland M G M, Cole T J & Whitehead R G (1977) A quantitative study into the role of infection in determining nutritional status in Gambian village children. *British Journal of Nutrition* **37**: 441–450.

Rowland M G M, Barrell R A E & Whitehead R G (1978) Bacterial contamination in traditional Gambian weaning foods. *Lancet* **1**: 136–138.

Rubin E & Lieber C S (1968) Alcohol induced hepatic injury in non-alcoholic volunteers. *New England Journal of Medicine* **278**: 869–876.

Rubin E & Lieber C S (1974) Fatty liver, alcoholic hepatitis and cirrhosis produced by alcohol in primates. *New England Journal of Medicine* **290**: 128–135.

Salmon P A & Reedyk L (1975) Fatty metamorphosis in patients with jejuno-ileal by-pass. *Surgery, Gynecology and Obstetrics* **141**: 75–84.

Sherlock S & Walshe V (1948) Effect of undernutrition in man on hepatic structure and function. *Nature* London **161**: 604.

Sidransky H & Farber E (1960) Liver choline oxidase activity in man and several species of animals. *Archives of Biochemistry* **87**: 129–133.

Smythe P M (1958) Changes in intestinal bacterial flora and role of infection in kwashiorkor. *Lancet* **2**: 724–727.

Spector W G & Heesom N J (1969) The production of granulomata by antigen–antibody complexes. *Journal of Pathology* **98**: 31–39.

Tomkins A M, Drasar B S, Bradley A K & Williamson W A (1978) Water supply and nutritional status in rural northern Nigeria. *Transactions of the Royal Society of Tropical Medicine and Hygiene* **72**: 239–243.

Trowell H C, Davies J N P & Dean R F A (1954) *Kwashiorkor*, pp 128–144. London: Edward Arnold.

Vanderhoof J A, Tuma D J, Antonson D L & Sorrell M F (1981) Effect of antibiotics in the prevention of jejuno-ileal dysfunction. *Digestion* **23**: 9–15.

Chapter 19
Liver Disorders Associated with Dietary Constituents

J. D. Maxwell

In this chapter I shall first discuss liver damage caused by normal dietary constituents, and then hepatic disease associated with dangerous foods and dietary contaminants. In genetically normal individuals, abnormally high intake of specific dietary components may produce adverse liver changes, and in certain rare inborn metabolic disorders components of the diet cause liver disease even when taken in normal quantities. Moreover complex dietary factors may also have subtle influences on liver function.

EFFECTS OF SPECIFIC DIETARY CONSTITUENTS

Vitamins

Early arctic explorers found to their cost that eating polar bear liver caused lethargy, headaches, vomiting and later skin desquamation. This disease is now known to be caused by the enormous amounts of vitamin A stored in polar bear liver.

Chronic hypervitaminosis A is usually caused by protracted intake of large doses, often by health food enthusiasts, of at least 90 000 IU/day for over a year (RDA 5000 IU/day). Large dose capsules are available without prescription.

Toxicity is thought to occur when excessive amounts of vitamin A circulate that are not bound to retinol binding protein, and may be precipitated by protein deficiency (Weber et al 1982). Clinically the condition is characterised by loss of hair, dry skin, itch, cheilosis, gingivitis, headache, anorexia, fatigue, musculo-skeletal pains, hepatomegaly and abnormal liver function. Histological changes in the liver include perisinusoidal fat deposition in Ito cells located between sinusoids and hepatocytes. Excessive deposition leads to transformation of these cells into fibroblasts, with subsequent collagen formation, cirrhosis and portal hypertension (Russell et al 1974). Alcoholics are unusually susceptible to toxicity of vitamin A (Leo and Lieber 1983).

Minerals

Iron

In distinction to the relatively innocuous reticulo-endothelial iron deposition, parenchymal iron overload of sufficient intensity and duration is considered to

288

be responsible for the clinical manifestations of *haemochromatosis*. It is usually the result of increased iron absorption which may be caused by a number of factors including inborn error of metabolism (idopathic haemochromatosis), enhanced absorption by increased erythropoiesis (iron loading anaemias), absence of feedback regulation of iron absorption (congenital atransferri-naemia) and high dietary iron intake. Only this last category is relevant to the present discussion.

Dietary iron overload. Approximately 70% of adult male South African blacks have excessive tissue iron deposits at autopsy (Charlton et al 1973) with maximum siderosis in the 40–60 year age group. Available evidence indicates that iron overload in these individuals results from extremely high dietary iron intake, mostly derived from home brewed alcoholic beers prepared in iron containers. Because of the high acidity of these brews significant quantities of inorganic iron are dissolved, resulting in a daily oral intake of 50–100 mg of iron, which is absorbed as efficiently as simple ferric salts. The estimated daily positive iron balance is 1–3 mg, and about 20% have hepatic iron concentrations in excess of 5000 µg/g wet weight. Haemosiderin deposits are found in hepatocytes as well as Kupffer cells (Bantu siderosis) and RE cells in spleen and marrow. Although portal fibrosis of various degrees is seen in most severely siderotic individuals, only a small proportion develop micronodular cirrhosis. This has suggested that other toxic factors, including alcohol, malnutrition or unidentified contaminants of the homemade beers, may be necessary for the development of cirrhosis.

Dietary iron overload is rarely seen outside the black population of South Africa. Its development depends not only on the absolute amounts of iron in food, but also on the availability of dietary iron for absorption. When cooked with cereals, iron salts are poorly absorbed, as shown by a survey from Ethiopia where the staple dietary cereal (teff) provides several hundred milligrams of iron per day, yet body iron stores were not increased.

Iron overload in cirrhosis is often seen, although not of the magnitude found in idiopathic haemochromatosis. The cause is multifactorial, related both to factors initiating liver disease such as alcohol, as well as to results of liver disease such as porto-caval shunts, and impaired transferrin synthesis. Alcohol stimulates iron absorption in normal subjects, probably indirectly through stimulation of hydrochloric acid secretion, which in turn increases the solubility of ferric iron and its availability for absorption. Some wines also have a high iron content. Furthermore the development of siderosis appears to accelerate after onset of porto-caval shunting (either surgical or spontaneous). Some increased iron absorption in cirrhosis may also be due to chronic pancreatitis, since normal pancreatic secretions inhibit iron absorption by non-specific binding of ionic iron to proteins, or formation of insoluble iron complexes with bicarbonate.

Additional factors include folate deficiency, common in alcoholism and cirrhosis, which interferes with iron utilisation by the marrow; and increased haemolysis of hypersplenism in cirrhotics. This could increase delivery of iron to tissue stores, and enhance iron absorption in response to increased plasma iron turnover.

However, hepatic siderosis is found only in the final stages of cirrhosis, when destructive tissue changes are almost complete, and (in contrast to idiopathic haemochromatosis where excessive iron deposition precedes cirrhosis) seems to play little or no part in the development of tissue damage (Hershko 1977).

Copper

Hepatic parenchymal overload with copper may also be responsible for serious liver disease, and has interesting parallels with iron in that this may result from an inborn error of metabolism (Wilson's disease) or follow various chronic (usually cholestatic) forms of liver disease. More recently, evidence has accumulated to suggest that enhanced dietary intake of copper is responsible for a rare form of liver disease, Indian childhood cirrhosis (ICC), a fatal disease of children between the ages of 1 and 3 years which occurs throughout India, predominantly among rural, middle income Hindu families. Affected children develop progressive abdominal distension, and a hard liver edge is palpable. Jaundice often heralds the terminal stage, with death within weeks or months from bleeding, anaemia, bacterial infection or liver failure.

Liver biopsy is required for diagnosis, since clinical features may be non-specific, and liver function tests (including serum copper and ceruloplasmin concentrations) are unreliable. Biopsy shows damaged hepatocytes, with ballooning vacuolation or necrosis. Hyaline inclusions identical to those seen in alcoholic liver disease, Wilson's disease or late PBC (primary biliary cirrhosis) may be found. There is variable inflammatory infiltrate, and aggressive intralobular pericellular fibrosis, with small groups of cells surrounded by collagen forming 'micro-micronodular cirrhosis'. Almost every hepatocyte contains dark brown, orcein-staining granules of copper-associated protein, an appearance seen in no other hepatic disorder in this age group. Very high hepatic copper concentrations (>1300 μg/g dry weight compared with <55 μg/g in normal infants) are found (Tanner et al 1979) and the pattern of copper distribution differs from that in Wilson's disease and prolonged cholestasis, suggesting a different mechanism of accumulation (Popper et al 1979).

There is a family history in 30% of cases, but as the disease is almost entirely confined to Indians living in the sub-continent, this indicates that environmental factors (rather than genetic) must be at least partially responsible. Brass and copper household utensils have been incriminated as a possible source of gross hepatic copper accumulation in ICC. Milk takes up copper from such utensils avidly, and animal milk stored in such containers could supply a copper intake from 6% to 20% greater than that of the breast fed infant. Children with ICC are breast fed for a shorter time, and have animal milk introduced at an earlier stage than controls (Figure 19.1). Thus early introduction of copper contaminated animal milk is considered to be of aetiological importance, and explains many of the epidemiological features of ICC. However it is not yet known whether dietary copper loading alone is responsible for ICC, or whether a second hepatic insult is necessary to initiate disease in a copper loaded liver (Tanner et al 1983).

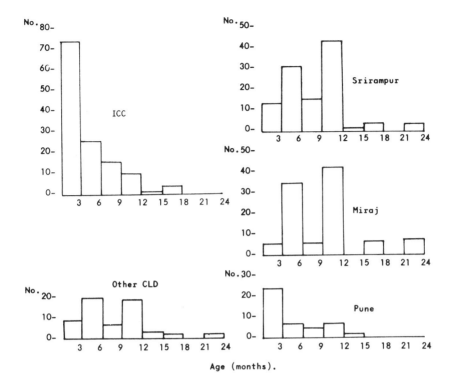

Figure 19.1. Age of introduction of animal milk feeds in children with ICC, children with other hepatic disorders (CLD), and healthy children in two rural areas (Sirampur and Miraj) and urban Pune. From Tanner et al (1983), with kind permission of the authors and the editor of *Lancet*.

Carbohydrate

Galactosaemia may result from two inherited disorders of galactose metabolism, both transmitted by autosomal recessive inheritance. The genetic disturbance is due to deficiency of either galactokinase or galactose-1-phosphate uridyl transferase, the enzymes catalysing the first and second reactions in galactose metabolism in glucose.

The clinical manifestations of galactokinase deficiency are mild and mainly manifest by cataract, but toxic effects of transferase deficiency are much more serious. The condition presents after introduction of milk, with failure to thrive, vomiting, diarrhoea and development of impaired liver function with jaundice. Death may result in the first few weeks, but survivors develop cataracts, mental deficiency and finally cirrhosis and portal hypertension.

The reason for hepatotoxicity is obscure, but galactosaemia should be considered in all young children with cirrhosis. Initial liver manifestations are of diffuse, fatty change followed by characteristic acinar formation, with pseudoglandular or ductular structures around canaliculi, and eventually macronodular cirrhosis. There may be numerous giant cells.

Diagnosis is suggested by detection of galactose in blood or urine, and is established by demonstration of the enzyme deficiency in peripheral blood cells. Dietary treatment (withdrawal of milk and milk products) is life-saving as it prevents liver damage and cataracts but the effect on intellectual development is variable. The requirement for a galactose free diet also necessitates a lactose free diet as the disaccharidase is hydrolysed in the gut to galactose and glucose (Segal 1983).

Three defects of fructose metabolism are known, all inherited as autosomal recessive traits. *Essential fructosuria* (due to fructokinase deficiency) is a benign asymptomatic metabolic anomaly. Hereditary *fructose-1,6-diphosphatase deficiency* is characterised by episodic spells of hyperventilation, apnoea, hypoglycaemia, ketosis and lactic acidosis due to impairment of gluconeogenesis. It often follows a lethal course in newborns. Later episodes may be triggered by fasting or infections, but tolerance to fasting grows with age. Hereditary *fructose intolerance*, due to deficient fructose-1-phosphate aldolase, is characterised by severe hypoglycaemia and vomiting after intake of fructose. Prolonged fructose ingestion in infants leads to failure to thrive, vomiting, hepatomegaly, renal tubular dysfunction with amino-aciduria, cirrhosis, and finally death from hepatic failure.

If a strict fructose-free (and hence sucrose-free) diet is used, the prognosis is good. Protein foods are allowed and some vegetables are acceptable, but others (such as carrots, peas and leeks) should be avoided as they contain sucrose. It is essential to have detailed dietary advice, as a sudden intake of fructose can cause a severe metabolic upset (Gitzelman et al 1983).

Amino acids

Tyrosinosis is another rare metabolic disorder with autosomal recessive inheritance. It is accompanied by elevated levels of tyrosine and its metabolites, and although the origin of the disorder is still under debate, deficiency of fumaryl aceto-acetate hydrolyase has been proposed.

The acute form presents in the first few months of life with failure to thrive, vomiting, diarrhoea and a cabbage-like odour. Hepatomegaly is frequent, and if untreated, death from liver failure ensues in six to eight months. Similar but milder features are seen in the chronic form, with cirrhosis, renal tubular disorders and vitamin D resistant rickets dominating the clinical picture by one year of age. Hypoglycaemia may be a problem, and hepatocellular carcinoma is a late complication in over one-third of cases. It is very rare except in Quebec where the incidence is greater than that of phenylketonuria, and where it occurs on a hereditary rather than a sporadic basis.

Dietary restriction of tyrosine and phenylalanine (and often methionine) has been advocated, and may result in improvement of some of the manifestations in children with the chronic type. However, infants with the acute form usually die, despite dietary restriction. Liver transplantation has been successfully performed to treat the metabolic abnormality, and in an attempt to prevent hepatoma (Goldsmith 1983).

COMPLEX DIETARY EFFECTS AND LIVER DISEASE

Hepatic porphyrias (Figure 19.2)

Diet is an important influence on the clinical expression of the hereditary hepatic porphyrias (*acute intermittent porphyria; variegate porphyria; hereditary coproporphyria*). A low caloric intake, usually instituted in an effort to lose weight, is a common contributing cause to acute attacks and increased excretion of porphyrin precursors. Even brief periods of starvation during weight reduction, after surgery, or with intercurrent illness, should be avoided in these patients.

In acute intermittent porphyria, 60–80% reduction in optimal calorie intake was associated with a significant rise in urinary excretion of both porphyrin precursors, aminolevulinic acid (ALA) and porphobilinogen (PBG). Isocaloric substitution of fat for carbohydrate and/or protein also increased porphyrin precursor excretion. These changes were reversible on return to an optimal diet. Moreover excretion of PBG decreased if added carbohydrate was given to a patient already on an adequate diet, or if carbohydrate intake increased from 150 to 300 g daily (substituting carbohydrate for fat).

In experimental animals starvation enhances, and glucose or protein can repress, the inducing effect of porphyrogenic drugs on ALA synthetase (the initial and rate limiting enzyme in haem synthesis) and PBG excretion. There is no clear explanation for this 'glucose effect', but repression of ALA synthetase may be mediated by glucose itself (Kappas et al 1983).

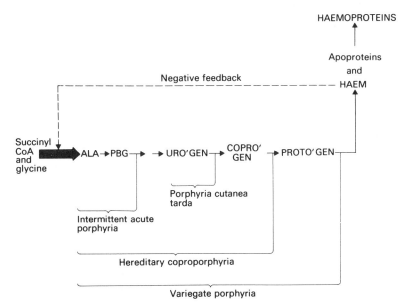

Figure 19.2. Pathway of porphyrin and haem synthesis showing characteristic precursor excretion in various porphyrias, and negative feedback control of the initial and rate limiting enzyme, ALA synthetase.

Hepatotoxins

Diet may also have important indirect influences in promoting (or inhibiting) hepatotoxins, through its effect on the hepatic microsomal enzyme cytochrome-P450-dependent biotransformation system, involved in the metabolic conversion of many structurally diverse compounds. In man, alcohol induces the activity of hepatic microsomal enzyme systems so that there is potential enhancement of susceptibility to agents which are activated by microsomal enzymes to hepatotoxic metabolites (for example industrial solvents, plant alkaloid toxins, and drugs such as paracetamol and isoniazid). Induction by alcohol of microsomal systems which activate pro-carcinogens also raises the possibility that this might contribute to the enhanced incidence of cancer, including possibly primary liver cancer, in alcoholics (Lieber et al 1979). Numerous other dietary factors induce microsomal enzymes in experimental animals (vegetables, polycyclic hydrocarbons in charcoal broiled meat, dietary flavones, etc.) but their clinical relevance is unknown.

Conversely, a low protein diet inhibits the activity of microsomal biotransformation systems, and this is a likely explanation for the increased susceptibility of protein deficient animals and individuals to certain hepatotoxins (alcohol, aflatoxins, bile acids), but their relative protection from toxins which require metabolic activation (see above).

Biliary tract cancer

Finally, ethnic differences in dietary habits may contribute to geographical differences in prevalence of liver disease. For example, in addition to various known risk factors identified for biliary tract cancer, epidemiological studies from Japan have also shown a possible association with consumption of dried noodles and pork, while expenditure on fat and protein-rich Western type foods were negatively associated for this cancer (Tominaga et al 1979).

LIVER DISEASE ASSOCIATED WITH DANGEROUS FOODS OR INGESTED HEPATOTOXINS

Alcohol

Alcohol is undoubtedly the most important diet-related cause of liver disease worldwide. Evidence that it is directly hepatotoxic, independent of any nutritional effect, was presented in Chapter 18.

Mycotoxins

So-called 'mushroom poisoning' results from the ingestion of toxic fungi which resemble the edible field mushroom. Liver disease is associated with *Amanita phalloides* (Death cap) and *Amanita verna* (Fool's mushroom) (Editorial, *Lancet* 1980).

Aflatoxins are a group of chemicals produced by the common moulds *Aspergillus flavus* and *Aspergillus parasiticus*. These fungi readily grow on nuts, pulses and cereals when stored in warm humid conditions. Aflatoxins were first isolated in 1961 after an outbreak of acute liver disease, which killed 100 000 turkeys in England, was traced to contaminated poultry feed. They are amongst the most potent experimental hepatotoxins known, but there are marked species differences in response. Acute toxicity is associated with jaundice and liver necrosis, while chronic toxicity in animals has been shown to produce cirrhosis and primary liver cancer. There is some evidence that animals which metabolise the toxin rapidly are susceptible to acute toxicity, while slow metabolisers are more susceptible to chronic liver damage. Both protein restriction and pre-existing liver damage potentiate the effects of aflatoxins, which may be clinically relevant (Editorial, *Nutrition Reviews* 1971).

Epidemiological evidence has suggested that man may be susceptible to both acute and chronic hepatotoxicity from aflatoxins.

An outbreak of *acute hepatitis* ascribed to aflatoxicosis, characterised by jaundice, rapidly developing ascites and portal hypertension with high mortality has been reported from India (Krishnamachari et al 1975). The disease spared children, and was confined to the poorest section of the community, who had subsisted mainly on maize heavily contaminated with *A. flavus* as a result of excessive rains and poor storage. The estimated daily aflatoxin load of affected individuals was 2–6 mg for a month. Liver histopathology showed extensive bile duct proliferation with periductal fibrosis and multinucleated giant cells, which seem to be characteristic of aflatoxin hepatotoxicity in man.

The development of *hepatic fibrosis* and *cirrhosis* in children with kwashiorkor, who were fed spoilt peanut flour as a supplement for periods of up to 30 days has been described, and some evidence has linked *Reye's Syndrome* in children, an acute and often fatal condition with encephalopathy and fatty degeneration of viscera, including the liver, to aflatoxin ingestion (Editorial, *Nutrition Reviews* 1971; Editorial, *Food and Cosmetics Toxicology* 1976).

Aflatoxin B1 is the most potent hepatocarcinogen in animals, and the search for an association between aflatoxin and *primary liver cell cancer* (PLC) in man has concentrated on areas of the world with highest recorded rates for this cancer. Epidemiological studies have shown a positive relationship between estimated current exposure of the population to aflatoxin and the occurrence of PLC (Murray-Lyon 1983), and case control studies have shown a strong positive association between ingestion of increasing levels of aflatoxin (and alcohol) and the relative risk of developing PLC (Jayme et al 1982). However the validity of these studies must be questioned since they are susceptible to confounding factors (e.g. variation in methods of food preparation) and are critically dependent on the accuracy of data on incidence of PLC. Moreover, none of these studies considered exposure to other potential causes of PLC, such as exposure to hepatitis B virus, nitrosamines, pyrrolizidine alkaloids, malnutrition and parasitic disease in producing liver cancer (Editorial, *Food and Cosmetics Toxicology* 1976).

In the USA, a careful comparison of PLC mortality in rural white males from areas of high (south-east: 13–197 mg/kg body weight) and low aflatoxin exposure (north-west: 0.2–0.3 mg/kg body weight) showed that the former had 10% excess of PLC deaths. However this difference was far less than would have been anticipated from experiments with rats, or prior epidemiological studies in Africa and Asia (Stoloff 1983). PLC undoubtedly has a multifactorial aetiology, but these findings suggest that any hepatocarcinogenic role in man is questionable, particularly since chronic hepatitis B virus infection has now been strongly implicated in the pathogenesis of PLC in Africa and Asia (Oon and Friedman 1982). Perhaps, rather than acting as a primary carcinogen in man, aflatoxins may suppress cell-mediated immunity and encourage chronic infection with hepatitis B virus (Lutwick 1979).

Plant toxins

Pyrrolizidine alkaloids are widely distributed through the plant kingdom, and many occur in common weeds throughout the world. Over 240 species of plants are known to contain such alkaloids, and clinical poisoning usually arises from ingestion of members of the *Crotalaria, Heliotropium* and *Senecio* genera. Only some are hepatotoxic, and these all have the basic pyrrolizidine nucleus with a double bond in position 1–2, and are esterified in one or more positions (McLean and Mattocks 1979).

Poisoning in humans arises in one of two ways. Sometimes plants (which by bad luck or judgement may include species containing toxic pyrrolizidine alkaloids) are used for medicinal purposes, or to prepare herbal infusions (bush tea) as an inexpensive alternative to commercial tea. This practice was endemic in the West Indies where it gave rise to veno-occlusive disease

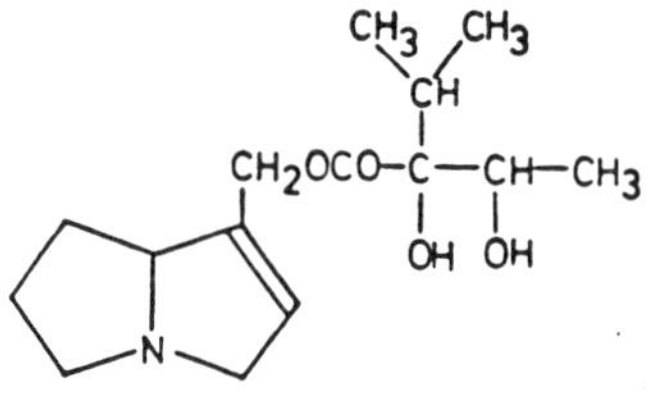

Supinine

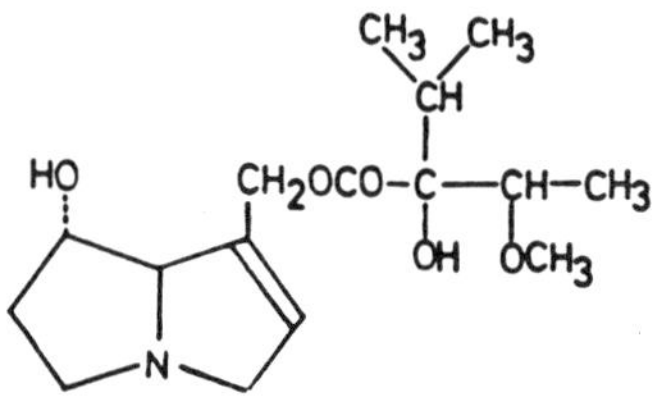

Heliotrine

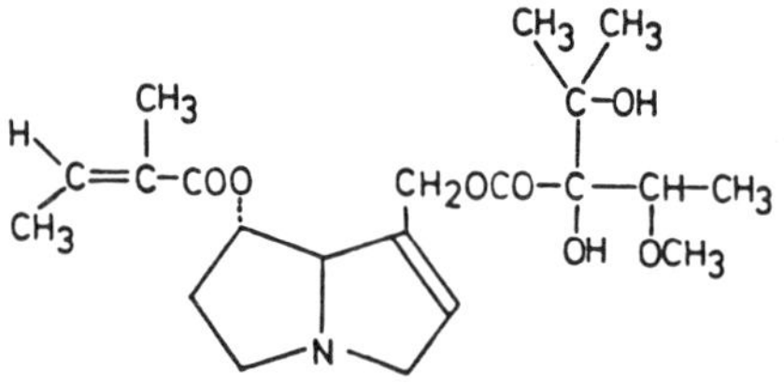

Lasiocarpine

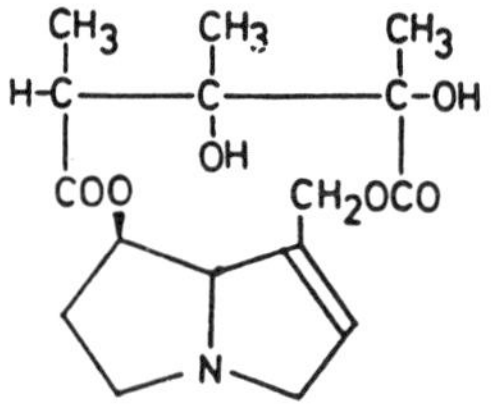

Monocrotaline

Figure 19.3. Chemical structure of some hepatotoxic pyrrolizidine alkaloids. From McLean and Mattocks (1979), with kind permission of the authors and the publisher, Marcel Dekker.

(VOD) of the liver, and was thought to account for approximately one-third of cirrhoses found at autopsy in Jamaica. Sporadic cases have been described from India, USA and the UK (McLean and Mattocks 1979).

At other times, cereal crops have become contaminated with alkaloid-containing weeds. Epidemics of liver disease arising in this way have been reported from South Africa, USSR, India and Afghanistan (Tandon et al 1978). Fatal poisoning of domestic animals is a major economic problem in arid regions.

Clinical poisoning results in abdominal pain, vomiting and fever, followed by rapid development of hepatosplenomegaly, tense ascites and venous collateral vessels over the abdomen (Figure 19.4). Liver function tests indicate hepatic necrosis, but jaundice is mild or absent in early stages. Initial histological changes are of centrilobular haemorrhagic necrosis, with damage to vascular endothelium. At a later stage cirrhosis with reversed lobulation develops (so called because each cirrhotic nodule has a portal triad at its centre). Severe hepatic congestion is due to multiple occlusion of terminal branches of the hepatic venous tree. This is characteristic of VOD which can be distinguished histologically from other types of Budd–Chiari syndrome by the existence of dilated sinusoids in the hepatic parenchyma which act as by-pass channels. Megalocytosis has been found in animals, but not in humans.

The extraordinary specificity of these alkaloids in damaging centrilobular hepatocytes and adjacent vascular endothelium is thought to be due to metabolic activation of the toxins to pyrrole derivatives by the hepatic microsomal hydroxylating system. These pyrrolic metabolites are reactive compounds, capable of alkylating cell constituents, and their cytotoxic effects are due to irreversible chemical interaction with intracellular organelles, while adjacent vascular endothelium is damaged by spillover (McLean and Mattocks 1979).

Although liver cell tumours have been described following administration of alkaloids to laboratory animals, it is questionable whether these toxins are relevant to human PLC.

Cycads are a primitive botanical family intermediate between ferns and flowering plants, which have a palm-like appearance. They are used in Africa and the East Indies as forage crops, and at times of food shortage, as a source of starch by man. The plant contains a glycoside, cycasin, which is metabolically activated in the gut by bacterial β-glucosidase to a toxic aglycone. The plant's toxicity as a food stuff depends on the precise method of preparation, but acutely fatal liver damage has been described. There is no evidence that cycasin contributes to PLC or other cancers (McLean and Mattocks 1979).

The fruit of a West African plant (*Blighia sapida*) brought to the West Indies by Captain Bligh after he had survived the mutiny on the Bounty, is known as ackee. Ripe ackee is a prized delicacy, but ingestion of unripe fruit causes Jamaican vomiting sickness (JVS). The illness is characterised by an acute onset with severe vomiting, followed usually by convulsions, coma and death. JVS is accompanied by severe hypoglycaemia, and before the cause was recognised, had a high mortality. At autopsy the most prominent finding was of depletion of liver glycogen, and a peculiar diffuse fatty infiltration with small lipid droplets in liver and other organs (McLean and Mattocks 1979).

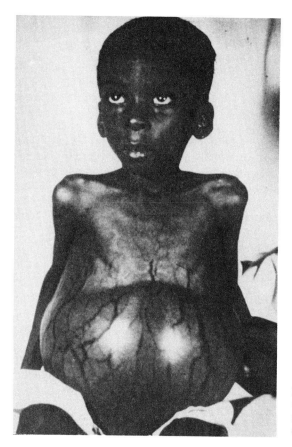

Figure 19.4. Jamaican child with hepatic veno-occlusive disease. Photograph by courtesy of Dr E K McLean.

The toxin isolated from unripe ackee, named *hypoglycin*, is an unusual amino acid whose mode of action has been extensively studied. (Figure 19.5).

Hypoglycin is metabolised to its toxic form, methylene cyclopropylacetic acid, which strongly inhibits transport of long chain fatty acids into mitochondria, thus suppressing their β oxidation. This causes depression of gluconeogenesis and, eventually, hypoglycaemia, after glucose has been mobilised from all available stores, leading to complete depletion of liver glycogen, and later fatty change.

Urinary excretion of the toxic metabolite of hypoglycin, as well as the presence of abnormal urinary metabolites (dicarboxylic acids and short chain fatty acids) has been demonstrated after ackee poisoning, but is not found in Reye's syndrome which has clinical and histological similarities to JVS (Tanaka et al 1976).

Tannins are a very diverse group of chemical compounds, largely of vegetable origin. In addition to their commercial use in dyeing, printing, and in the preparation of leather, they occur in tea and coffee, and are also extensively used as food and drink additives. This widespread dietary

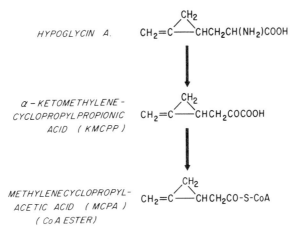

Figure 19.5. Structure and metabolism of hypoglycin A. From Tanaka et al (1976), with kind permission of the authors and the editor of *New England Journal of Medicine.*

exposure, and their chemical ability to catalyse the formation of diethylnitrosamine, has attracted attention to their possible toxicity.

Liver necrosis has been reported following treatment of burns with tannic acid and fatal liver failure has occurred after use of barium enemas containing tannic acid. However, animal studies suggest that oral administration is less harmful than parenteral adminstration (McLean and Mattocks 1979) and there are no reports suggesting toxicity after oral administration in humans. Dietary exposure to tannins is unlikely to result in significant hepatotoxicity in man, since the daily intake of food grade tannic acid, estimated from levels in food and drinks, is considerably less than the acceptable daily intake calculated from toxicological data from animals fed the food grade material (Editorial, *Food and Cosmetics Toxicology* 1969).

Chemicals

Acute and chronic liver disease as a result of exposure to hepatotoxic drugs is well recognised, but chemical contamination of foodstuffs resulting in liver injury has been reported only rarely. Three examples will be given.

Epping jaundice

In February 1965 an unusual outbreak of jaundice occurred in the Epping district of Essex. In all, 84 individuals were known to have been affected, and the clinical features included acute onset of upper abdominal and lower chest pain, fever with an influenza-like illness, rigors and increasing jaundice with pruritus. Hepatomegaly was noted, and the illness lasted some weeks before recovery. Liver function tests showed a mixed cholestatic-hepatitic picture. In cases who underwent liver biopsy, damage to both parenchyma and biliary tree was seen with inflammatory infiltrate and cholestasis, and in some patients cholangitis.

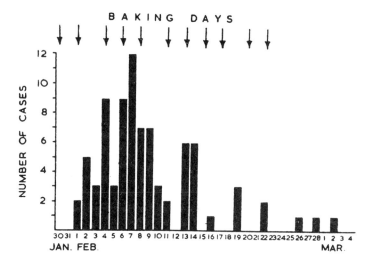

Figure 19.6. Incidence of cases of Epping jaundice on the days of onset of symptoms. Baking days shown by arrows. From Kopelman et al (1966), with kind permission of the authors and the editor of *British Medical Journal*.

Careful enquiry revealed that all those affected had eaten wholemeal bread made at a local bakery (Figure 19.6), and that the flour from which the bread was baked had been contaminated in transit by spillage of a chemical hardener for epoxy resin — 4,4'-diaminodiphenylmethane — an aromatic amine. Animal experiments produced changes similar to those seen in human liver biopsy specimens (Kopelman et al 1966).

Hexachlorobenzene and acquired porphyria

Between 1955 and 1959 an outbreak of cutaneous hepatic porphyria occurred in three provinces of south-eastern Turkey, involving an estimated 3000 cases. Children and adolescents were predominantly affected and the clinical features were similar to porphyria cutanea tarda, with photosensitivity, marked porphyrinuria (see Figure 19.2) and hepatomegaly, but without the excretion of porphyrin precursors, abdominal pain or neurological dysfunction characteristic of acute porphyria. Epidemiological studies strongly suggested the possibility that the disease was related to ingestion of seed wheat treated with a newly introduced fungicide containing hexachlorobenzene. When fed to rats, hexachlorobenzene caused hepatomegaly and high liver concentrations of uro-, copro-, and proto-porphyrins (Ockner and Schmid 1961).

Spanish toxic oil syndrome

Between May 1981 and the end of 1982, an outbreak of a unique disease syndrome occurred in Spain, with over 20000 cases and many deaths. The condition, thought to result from consumption of adulterated rapeseed oil bought from itinerant salesmen, had a multiplicity of symptoms including nausea, vomiting, abdominal pain, fever, myalgia, headaches, skin eruptions and respiratory distress. Hepatomegaly and raised liver enzymes were characteristic findings. The causative chemical has not yet been identified and there is no experimental model. However there is a clinical parallel with human graft versus host disease (GVHD). It has been suggested that heterocyclic compounds, structurally similar to drugs known to produce allergic/auto immune side-effects similar to GVHD, may have been formed from isothiocyanates present in unrefined rapeseed oil (Kammuller et al 1984).

Acknowledgements

I am indebted to Professor A E McLean, Dr E K McLean, Dr M Morgan, Professor W B Robertson and Dr M S Tanner for their advice, and to Marion Amos for expert secretarial assistance.

REFERENCES

Charlton R W, Bothwell T H & Seftel H C (1973) Dietary iron overload. *Clinics in Haematology* **2**: 383–403.

Editorial (1969) Tannic acid again. *Food and Cosmetics Toxicology* **7**: 364–365.

Editorial (1971) Aflatoxin, monkeys and humans. *Nutrition Reviews* **29**: 230–232.

Editorial (1976) Possible effects of aflatoxin consumption by man. *Food and Cosmetics Toxicology* **14**: 151–152.

Editorial (1980) Mushroom poisoning. *Lancet* **2**: 351–352.

Gitzelmann R, Steinman B & Van Den Berghe G (1983) Essential fructosuria, hereditary fructose intolerance and fructose-1,6-diphosphatase deficiency. In Stanbury J B, Wyngaarden J B, Fredrickson D S, Goldstein J L & Brown M S (eds) *The Metabolic Basis of Inherited Disease,* pp 118–140. 5th edition. New York: McGraw-Hill.

Goldsmith L A (1983) Tyrosinemia and related disorders. In Stanbury J B, Wyngaarden J B, Fredrickson D S, Goldstein J L & Brown M S (eds) *The Metabolic Basis of Inherited Disease*, 5th edn., pp 287–299. New York: McGraw-Hill.

Hershko C (1977) Storage iron regulation. *Progress in Hematology* **10**: 105–148.

Jayme S B, Almero E M, Castro M C A, Jardeleza M T R & Salamat L A (1982) Case control dietary study of primary liver cancer risk from aflatoxin exposure. *International Journal of Epidemiology* **11**: 112–119.

Kammuller M E, Penninks A H & Seinen W (1984) Spanish toxid oil syndrome is a chemically induced GVHD-like epidemic. *Lancet* **1**: 1174–117.5

Kappas A, Sassa S & Anderson K E (1983) The porphyrias. In Stanbury J E, Wyngaarden J B, Fredrickson D S, Goldstein J L & Brown M S (eds) *The Metabolic Basis of Inherited Disease*, 5th edn., pp 1301–1384. New York: McGraw-Hill.

Kopelman H, Robertson M H, Sanders P G & Ash I (1966) The Epping jaundice. *British Medical Journal* **1**: 514–516.

Krishmachari K A V R, Bhat R V, Nagarajan V & Tilak T B G (1975). Hepatitis due to aflatoxicosis: an outbreak in western India. *Lancet* **1**: 1061–1063.

Leo M A & Lieber C S (1983) Interaction of alcohol with vitamin A: alcoholism. *Clinical and Experimental Research* **7**: 15–21.

Lieber C S, Seitz H K, Garro A J & Worner T M (1979) Alcohol related diseases and carcinogenesis. *Cancer Research* **39**: 2863–2886.

Lutwick L I (1979) Relation between aflatoxin, hepatitis B virus, and hepatocellular carcinoma. *Lancet* **1**: 755–757.

McLean E K & Mattocks A R (1979) Environmental liver injury: plant toxins. In Farber E & Fisher M (eds) *Toxic Injury of the Liver*, Part B, pp 517–539. New York and Basel: Marcel Dekker.

Murray-Lyon I M (1983) Primary and secondary cancer of the liver. In Gazet J-C (ed) *Carcinoma of the Liver, Biliary Tract and Pancreas*, pp 1–81. London: Edward Arnold.

Ockner R K & Schmid R (1961) Acquired porphyria in man and rat due to hexachlorobenzene intoxication. *Nature* **189**: 499.

Oon C-J & Friedman M A (1982) Primary hepatocellular carcinoma. *Cancer Chemotherapy and Pharmacology* **8**: 231–235.

Popper H, Goldfischer S, Sternlieb I, Nayak N C & Madhavan T V (1979) Cytoplasmic copper and its toxic effects: studies in Indian childhood cirrhosis. *Lancet* **1**: 1205–1208.

Russell R M, Boyer J L, Bagheri S A & Hruban Z (1974) Hepatic injury from chronic hypervitaminosis A resulting in portal hypertension and ascites. *New England Journal of Medicine* **291**: 435–440.

Segal S (1983) Disorders of galactose metabolism. In Stanbury J B, Fredrickson D S, Goldstein J L & Brown M S (eds) *The Metabolic Basis of Inherited Disease* 5th edn., pp 167–191. New York: McGraw-Hill.

Stoloff L (1983) Aflatoxin as a cause of primary liver cell cancer in the United States: A probability study. *Nutrition and Cancer* **5**: 165–186.

Tanaka K, Kean E A & Johnson B (1976) Jamaican vomiting sickness: biochemical investigation of two cases. *New England Journal of Medicine* **295**: 461–467.

Tandon H D, Tandon B N & Mattocks A R (1978) An epidemic of veno-occlusive disease of the liver in Afghanistan. *American Journal of Gastroenterology* **70**: 607–613.

Tanner M S, Portmann B, Mowat A P, Williams R, Pandit A N, Mills C F & Bremner I (1979) Increased hepatic copper concentration in Indian childhood cirrhosis. *Lancet* **1**: 1203–1205.

Tanner M S, Kantarjian A H, Bhave S A & Pandit A N (1983) Early introduction of copper-contaminated animal milk feeds as a possible cause of Indian childhood cirrhosis. *Lancet* **2**: 992–995.

Tominaga A, Kuroishi T, Ogawa H & Shimizu H (1979) Epidemiologic aspects of biliary tract cancer in Japan. *National Cancer Institute Monograph* **53**: 25–34.

Weber F L, Mitchell G E, Powell D E, Reiser B J & Banwell J G (1982) Reversible hepatotoxicity associated with hepatic vitamin A accumulation in a protein deficient patient. *Gastroenterology* **82**: 118–123.

Index